VASCULAR TUMORS AND MALFORMATIONS
OF THE OCULAR FUNDUS

Monographs in Ophthalmology

VOLUME 14

The titles published in this series are listed at the end of this volume.

VASCULAR TUMORS AND MALFORMATIONS OF THE OCULAR FUNDUS

J. J. DE LAEY AND M. HANSSENS

Department of Ophthalmology, University Hospital,
Ghent, Belgium

With collaboration of

P. Brabant, L. Decq, R. De Gersem, A. Hoste, P. Huyghe,
V. Lenaerts, M. Leys, L. Pollet, H. Priem,
A. Van Cleemput, R. Van Hijfte, and
E. Vrielynck

KLUWER ACADEMIC PUBLISHERS
DORDRECHT / BOSTON / LONDON

Library of Congress Cataloging-in-Publication Data

```
De Laey, J. J.
     Vascular tumours and malformations of the ocular fundus / by J.J.
De Laey and M. Hanssens ; with the collaboration of P. Brabant ...
[et al.].
        p.   cm. -- (Monographs in ophthalmology ; 14)
     "Report for the Belgian Ophthalmological Society"--Pref.
     ISBN 0-7923-0750-X (alk. paper)
     1. Fundus oculi--Blood-vessels--Tumors.  2. Fundus oculi-
-Abnormalities.   I. Hanssens, M.   II. Belgian Ophthalmological
Society.  III. Title.  IV. Series.
     [DNLM: 1. Eye Neoplasms.  2. Fundus Oculi--abnormalities.
3. Neoplasms, Vascular Tissue.  4. Retinal Diseases.  5. Retinal
Vessels.   W1 MO586D v. 7 / WW 270 D341v]
RE545.D4   1990
616.99'284--dc20
DNLM/DLC
for Library of Congress                                  90-4664
                                                            CIP
```

ISBN-13: 978-94-010-6753-9   e-ISBN-13: 978-94-009-0589-4
DOI: 10.1007/ 978-94-009-0589-4

Published by Kluwer Academic Publishers,
P.O. Box 17, 3300 AA Dordrecht, The Netherlands.

Kluwer Academic Publishers incorporates
the publishing programmes of
D. Reidel, Martinus Nijhoff, Dr W. Junk and MTP Press.

Sold and distributed in the U.S.A. and Canada
by Kluwer Academic Publishers,
101 Philip Drive, Norwell, MA 02061, U.S.A.

In all other countries, sold and distributed
by Kluwer Academic Publishers Group,
P.O. Box 322, 3300 AH Dordrecht, The Netherlands.

Table of Contents

Preface

This report for the Belgian Ophthalmological Society concerns a number of fundus diseases, which most ophthalmologists only rarely encounter. Still it is of importance that they should be able to recognize them, not only because most of these eye diseases are treatable when they are diagnosed early enough, but also because they are sometimes associated with major visceral and neurological problems. The ophthalmologist may be the first practitioner to suspect a von Hippel-Lindau's disease or a neurofibromatosis. He should realize at that moment that his role is not only to treat the eyes but also to advise his patient, refer him to other specialists and consider the genetical implications of his diagnosis.

Clinicopathologic correlations are of great importance and we felt that it was necessary to emphasize the histopathological aspect of these diseases.

A report has to overview the literature on a specific topic. The literature on vascular tumors of the fundus is extremely vast and even if we tried to be as complete as possible, we must confess that we did not cite every author who published on such cases.

A third aspect, which was considered as important, was to provide sufficient clinical and histopathologic examples of the various disease, which are reviewed. We are indebted to a large number of friends who kindly authorized the publication of their material. In particular we wish thank Prof. A. Brini (Strasbourg), Dr. D. de Wolff-Rouendaal (Leiden), Prof. P. Dhermy (Paris), Dr P. C. Donders (Groningen). Dr A. Hamburg (Utrecht), Prof. A. Kint (Ghent), Prof. W. R. Lee (Glasgow), Dr A. Leys (Leuven), Prof. W. Manschot (Rotterdam), Prof. E. P. Messmer (Essen). Dr B. Mosny (Hamburg), Prof. A. Raspiller (Nancy), Dr B. Snyers (Louvain) and Dr C. Verougstraete (Brussels). We also thank all the ophthalmologists who referred their patients and who will recognize some of the illustrations.

We acknowledge the help of Mr R. Verdonck, photographer of the Department of Ophthalmology, who prepared most of the illustrations and the secretarial assistance of Mrs S. De Meyer who typed the manuscript.

Finally we are grateful to the Board of Directors of the Belgian Ophthalmological Society, who gave us the possibility to write this report.

J. J. De Laey and M. Hanssens

1   Choroidal hemangioma

The first clinical description of a choroidal hemangioma was published in 1860 by Schirmer [62]. In 1868 Leber [38] described a case of choroidal hemangioma as a cavernous spindle cell sarcoma. However, it is mainly since the publications by Panas & Remy [52], by Miller [46] and by Nordenson [49] that this tumor has been clinically recognized. Although Reese [56] in 1963 could only trace 128 cases of choroidal hemangiomas in the literature, these tumors are probably much more common. They are even considered as the second most frequent tumor of the choroid after malignant melanoma [35]. However, they are often not recognized. Sometimes they are found on routine examination, sometimes because they are part of Sturge-Weber syndrome or when they cause visual symptoms.

I. Pathogenesis

Although the pathogenesis of choroidal hemangiomas is still obscure [55, 76], most authors consider them to be of congenital origin [6, 7, 13, 16, 24, 41, 56, 76], although they usually remain undetected up to the third decade of life [23]. The lesions were described as angiomatous malformations [12], as a teleangiectatic type of an angioma venosum racemosum [4], as vascular hamartomas [15, 67], as benign developmental tumors or hamartomas [55] or as congenital hamartomas [1, 76].
It is possible that the lesion may develop after birth from a pre-existing vascular hamartoma. Local hemodynamic factors could then contribute to its development. A possible relationship between tumor and short posterior ciliary arteries was postulated. These arteries would then be seen as feeder vessels [15, 33]. Other mechanisms were also proposed, such as the potential role of chorioretinal scars in altering local hemodynamics [55], persistent arteriovenous shunts [76] or even alteration of the parasympathetic part of the cerebrospinal nerves [34].

II. Clinical forms

Choroidal hemangiomas may be isolated or be part of Sturge-Weber syndrome. They may also be found in association with retinitis pigmentosa

[5], cloverleaf syndrome [73], von Hippel's angiomatosis [69] or tuberous sclerosis [42]. Some of these associations are probably fortuitous, others however indicate that choroidal hemangiomas have to be seen as part of the phakomatosis.

1. Solitary choroidal hemangioma

Approximately 50% of choroidal hemangiomas occur as a localized tumor [13, 56] usually situated in the posterior pole of the fundus. About 70% of solitary hemangiomas are situated temporal to the disc, almost always close to the short posterior ciliary arteries [76]. Right and left eyes are equally affected and there is no sex predilection [13, 76]. Some authors believe that all choroidal hemangiomas are related to Sturge-Weber syndrome and consider a solitary hemangioma as a monosymptomatic form of the syndrome [6, 13, 19]. For others [7, 35, 76] the solitary hemangioma is to be considered as a separate entity. There are so many differences between solitary and diffuse hemangiomas as well clinically as histopathologically

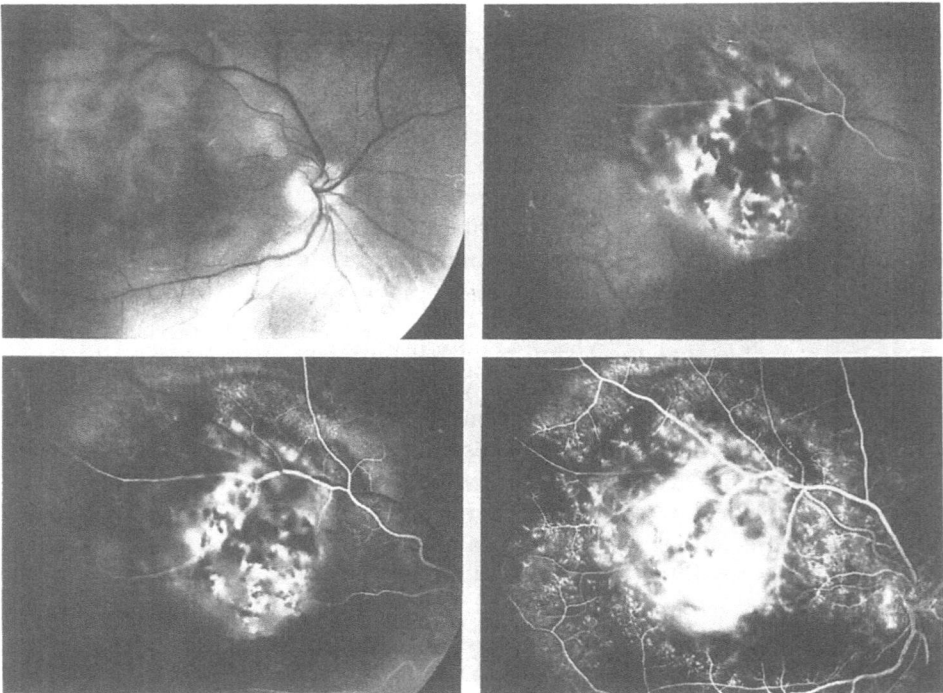

Figure 1-1.   Choroidal angioma with exudative retinal detachment involving the macula. The vascular structures of the tumor are well seen on the early phases of the fluoroangiography. Intense diffusion and pigmentary changes.

that the solitary choroidal hemangioma cannot be regarded as a forme fruste of Sturge-Weber syndrome.

2. *Sturge-Weber syndrome*

The complete Sturge-Weber syndrome consists of an ipsilateral naevus flammeus or facial hemangioma, episcleral and choroidal hemangioma, congenital glaucoma, angiomas of the meninges and brain and cerebral calcification. When the facial hemangioma, which is always present, affects the upper eyelid, intra-ocular involvement is certain [68]. According to Duke-Elder [16] 100 of the approximately 250 cases of Sturge-Weber, which were described up to then, proved to have on histopathology a choroidal hemangioma. Exceptionally bilateral involvement is possible [40].

Sturge-Weber syndrome is more common in males than in females and affects preferably the left side.

III. Symptoms

1. *Solitary choroidal hemangioma*

A circumscribed choroidal hemangioma is rarely detected early in life. Its rate of growth is probably maximal during the normal growth period [23]. It

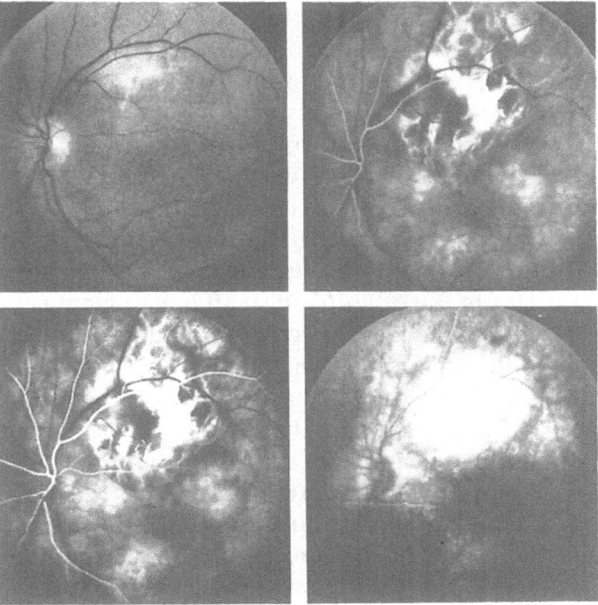

Figure 1–2.   Circumscribed choroidal angioma.

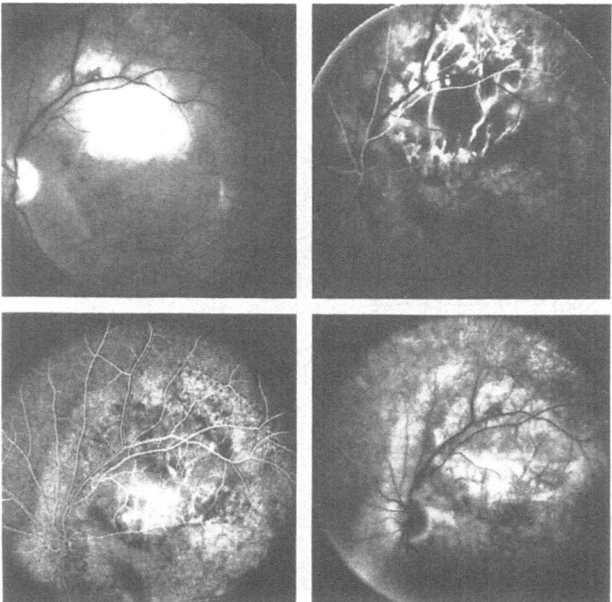

Figure 1–3.   Same eye as fig. 1–2 two years later. Note that the exudative detachment affects the whole macula. Fluorescein angiography underlines the increased pigmentary changes.

will usually cause symptoms after the third decade. The median age at diagnosis for solitary choroidal hemangioma was 38.7 years [76].

The symptoms are related to a serous detachment of the retina overlying the tumor (Figs 1–1, 1–2, 1–3). This detachment spreads towards the fovea and first causes metamorphopsia or visual blurring. It is therefore not surprising that a number of choroidal hemangiomas are referred with the clinical diagnosis of central serous chorioretinopathy. A subfoveal heman-gioma may cause progressive visual loss due to the cystoid degeneration of the overlying retina [2] or may be the cause of a progressive hypermetropia of up to 10 D [61]. On the other hand small hemangiomas may remain silent and are sometimes detected on routine examination. Choroidal hemangiomas are best seen with indirect ophthalmoscopy. Solitary hemangiomas are usually dome-shaped tumors in the vicinity of the optic disc or in the macular region. Their sizes vary between 3 to 12 mm in diameter and between 1 to 6 mm in elevation. The color of the tumor is orange to salmon red. The fibrous tissue, which is often present between the tumor and the retina, may give it a grayish-white appearance. Yellowish mottling associated with pigmentary changes due to proliferation or hyperplasia of the retinal pigment epithelium are not unfrequently seen. This yellowish pigment may possibly represent lipofuscin accumulated in pigment epithelial cells. Its presence is indicative of a severe and recent damage of the pigment

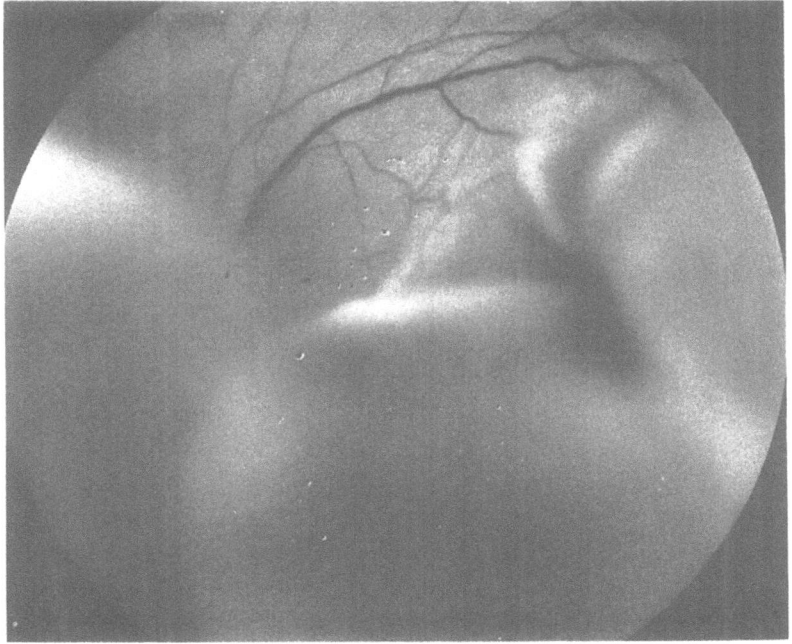

Figure 1–4. Bullous retinal detachment in a case of Sturge-Weber syndrome

epithelium [22]. The presence of lipofuscin is certainly not specific for choroidal hemangiomas; it may also be found in metastatic tumors, in localized serous detachments of the RPE, in naevi and especially in malignant melanomas. The vascular tumor provokes a progressive exsudative retinal detachment which at first may be limited to the region of the tumor, but may also progress to a bullous detachment (Fig. 1–4). The exudation may increase during pregnancy and regress after delivery [54]. The presence of large depigmented zones starting from the inferior limit of the tumor and progressing towards the inferior retinal periphery indicates previous episodes of serous detachment or longstanding subclinical serous detachment (Fig. 1–5). The aspect of these tracks is very similar to what is observed in very chronic cases of central serous choroidopathy. Visual loss may also result from cystoid macular edema or preretinal membrane formation.

2. *Sturge-Weber syndrome*

In Sturge-Weber syndrome the choroidal hemangioma is usually diagnosed at a much younger age than in cases of solitary choroidal hemangioma. In the series of Witschel and Font [76] the median age at diagnosis of choroidal

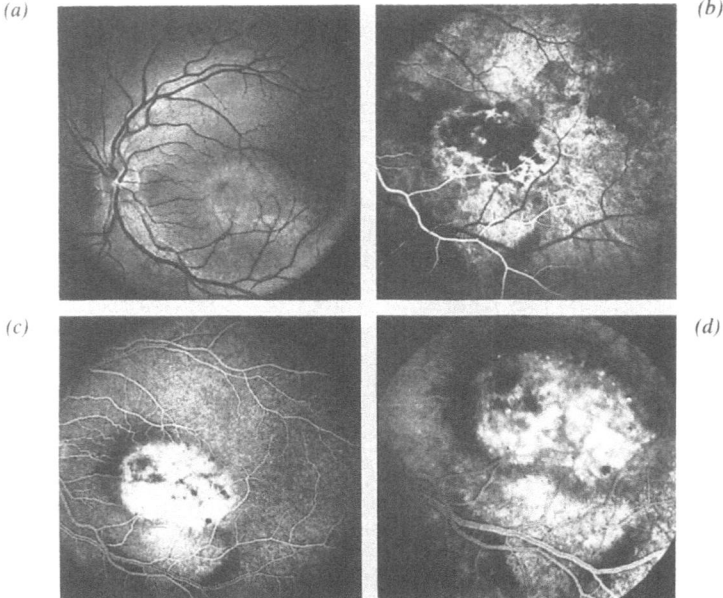

Figure 1–5.   Submacular choroidal hemangioma with pigmentary tracks starting from the inferior limit of the tumor. This is especially well seen in d.

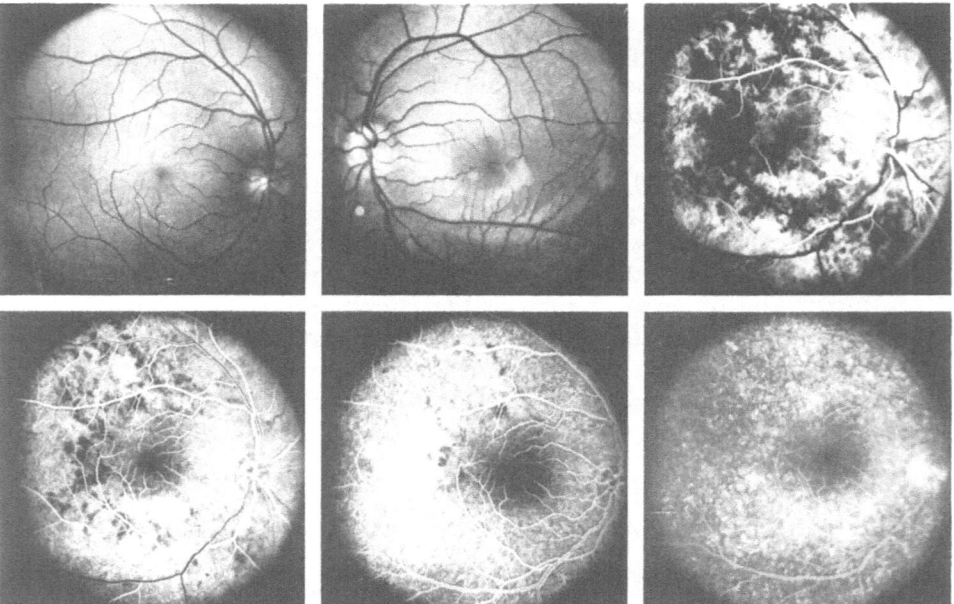

Figure 1–6.   Right and left eye of a patient with Sturge-Weber syndrome affecting the right side. Fluorescein angiography of the right eye reveals delayed choroidal filling and widespread pigmentary changes.

hemangioma associated with Sturge-Weber syndrome was 7.6 years. The associated features of the syndrome and mainly the facial hemangioma and the congenital glaucoma prompt an ophthalmological examination.

In Sturge-Weber syndrome the hemangioma presents as a more diffuse thickening, affecting a large proportion of the choroid. This gives a deep-red 'tomato-ketchup' appearance at the affected fundus [68]. This aspect can especially be appreciated when comparing the two fundi of the patient with indirect ophthalmoscopy. The difference in color is then striking.

As in solitary hemangiomas cystic degeneration and exudative detachment of the overlying retina are possible complications of the diffuse hemangioma.

IV. Complications

1. Retinal complications

The retinal complications such as exudative detachment and cystic degeneration of the retina have already been described.

2. Glaucoma

Marked glaucoma is an almost inevitable complication of untreated choroidal hemangioma [13, 16, 44, 56] and is especially frequent in Sturge-Weber syndrome. In Witschel and Font's series [76] glaucoma occurred in 13 of their 17 Sturge-Weber cases and was either of the congenital or adult type. The incidence of the congenital type with buphthalmos and features of immature anterior chamber angle varies between 23% [76] and 70% [6]. The histological characteristics may be the same of those of congenital glaucoma without angioma. Barkan's membrane is present in some sections [74].

The adult type of glaucoma may develop at any age and is associated in 30% [6] to 70% of the cases [76] with secondary angle closure.

Other mechanisms are however also possible. The breakdown of the blood-aqueous barrier may result in plasmoid aqueous which blocks the angle. The congenital vascular anomalies in choroidal angiomas may result in increased aqueous production with secondary changes in the filtration angle [6]. Engorged episcleral vessels or episcleral vascular hamartomas are frequently mentioned [53, 74, 76] and are considered as highly characteristic of Sturge-Weber syndrome (Fig. 1–7). In 50% of the cases they are associated with elevated episcleral venous pressure and may thus play an important role in the pathogenesis of secondary glaucoma in these eyes. Eyes with solitary hemangioma are not unfrequently complicated by neovascular glaucoma. This was the case in 18 out of 45 patients [76].

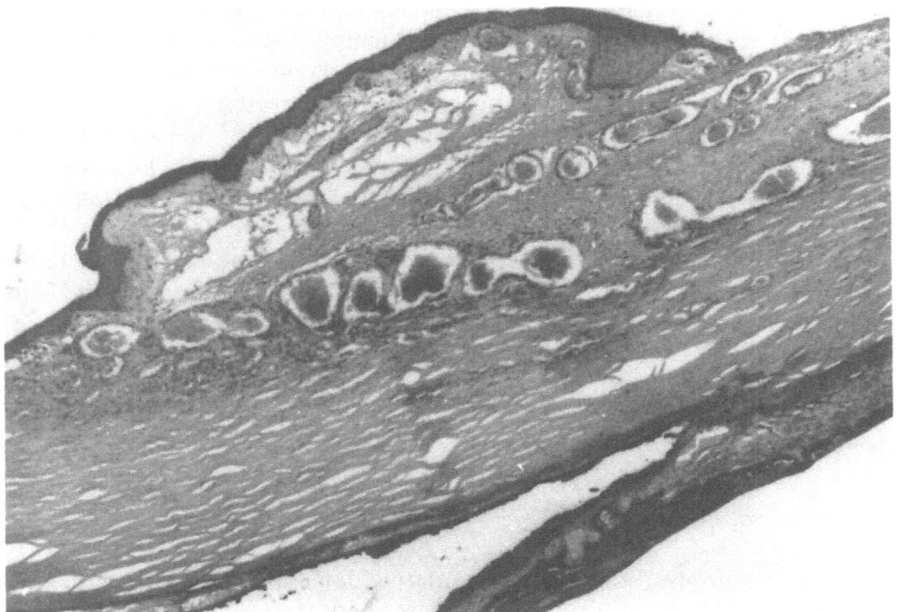

Figure 1–7.   Episcleral vascular hamartoma in Sturge-Weber syndrome. Engorged and dilated thin walled vessels in the episcleral and subconjunctival perilimbal tissue. 12.586 PAS (Courtesy of Dr. B. Mosny, Hamburg)

V. Diagnosis

1. Ophthalmoscopy

The clinical characteristics of choroidal hemangioma have been described in a previous section. Especially in such cases the diagnosis of choroidal hemangioma will be more readily made with indirect ophthalmoscopy than with direct ophthalmoscopy or even with slit lamp fundus biomicroscopy. The diagnosis is indeed based on the color and shape of the lesion and can best be appreciated using a large field of observation. This allows the comparison with surrounding fundus areas.

2. Diaphanoscopy

In contrast with malignant melanomas of the choroid, hemangiomas are easily transilluminated. However, RPE proliferations may interfere with the light transmission [18]. Together with ophthalmoscopy, diaphanoscopy is probably the most important diagnostic method in cases of choroidal hemangiomas.

3. Fluorescein angiography

Since McLean and Maumenee [44] described the intense staining of choroidal hemangioma after the intravenous injection of fluorescein, fluorescein angioscopy and later angiography have become essential tools in the differential diagnosis of suspected fundus lesions. Fluoroangiographic differentiation between choroidal hemangiomas and other choroidal tumors is not always possible [50]. According to Wessing [75] the irregular appearance of choroidal vessels in the early sequences is suggestive. This has been confirmed by Gass [22, 23], who also insists on the irregular and dense fluorescence and the accumulation of the dye in cystoid spaces during the late sequences (Fig. 1–8). This last feature is an indication of degeneration and edema of the outer retina. The pattern of fluorescence may be variable and fluorescein angiography is not always very helpful [14, 50, 64]. It provides however an objective document with clear delineation of the extent of the pathological process. It thus permits a better follow-up of suspected lesions. Not uncommonly choroidal hemangiomas are surrounded by a darker rim. The reason for this hypofluorescent border is still unclear, although it may correspond to the layer of compressed melanocytes seen on histology [76]. The pigmentary changes which are induced by chronic exudation are also better seen in fluorescein angiography (Fig. 1–5). Their aspect in comet tail is sometimes an important argument in the differentiation with malignant melanomas. Indeed, comet tails are indicative of a slowly progressive exudative process, which may cause recurrent detachments. This is less likely to occur in malignant, rapidly growing tumors, such as malignant melanomas or choroidal metastasis.

In diffuse angiomas pathological choroidal vessels are not always recognized. The abnormal filling pattern of the choroid, associated with pigmentary changes indicate the extent of the lesion (Fig. 1–6).

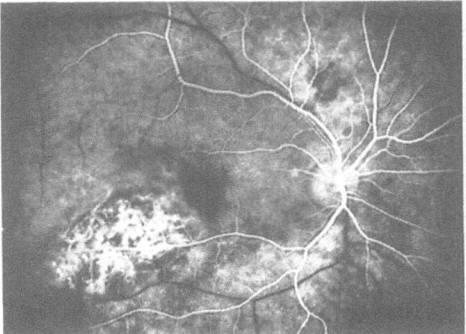 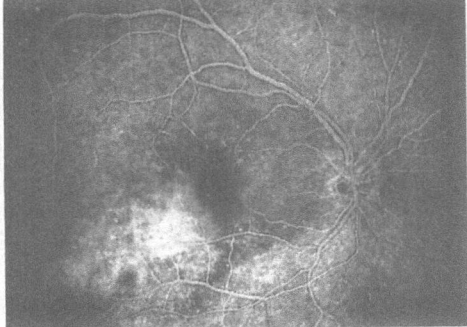

Figure 1–8.   Fluorescein angiographic appearance of a circumscribed angioma.

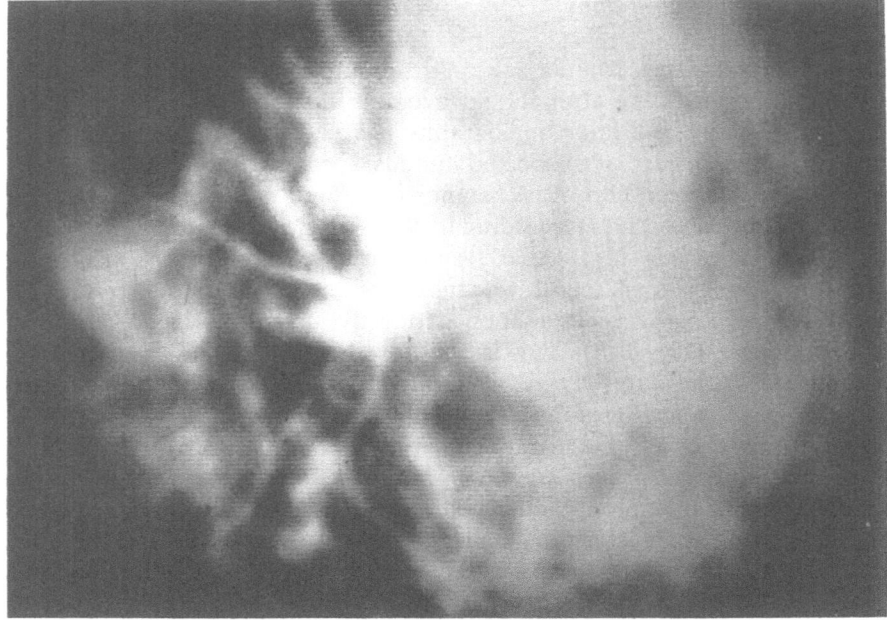

Figure 1–9.   Infrared video-angiography of a choroidal hemangioma.

4. Infrared angiography

M. Bonnet [8] has suggested the diagnostic value of infrared absorption angiography using indocyanin green as a dye. In our experience [47] infrared fluorescence video-angiography may provide supplementary arguments in doubtful cases. The experience is still limited but this technique may more readily indicate choroidal vascular structures (Fig. 1–9) and in contrast with malignant melanomas of the choroid late diffusion may be less pronounced in cases with choroidal hemangiomas.

5. Radiophosphorus uptake test

The ^{32}P uptake test is difficult to perform because of the posterior position of choroidal hemangiomas. The technique may still be justified in doubtful cases. The ^{32}P uptake is much lower than in melanomas of comparable size [29, 36]. However, false positive tests may occasionally occur [64].

6. Ultrasonography

Ultrasonography is one of the most important tests in differentiating choroidal hemangiomas from other tumors (Fig. 1–10). The accuracy of

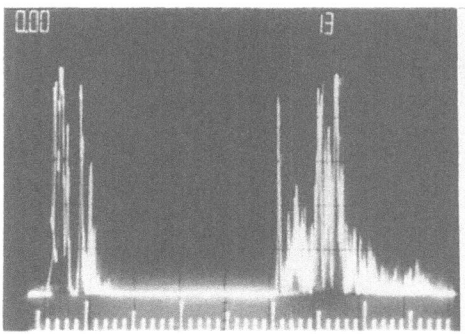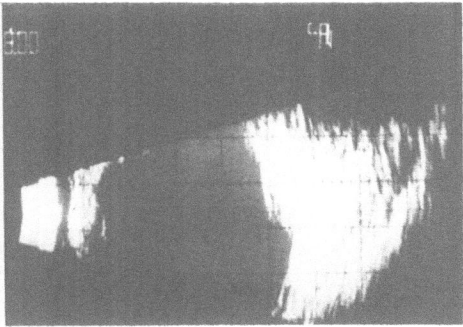

Figure 1–10.   A- and B-scan echography of a choroidal angioma.

ultrasonic differentiation of intraocular tumors goes up to 95% [51]. Ultra-sonography may detect solid tumors of the choroid if their prominence from the sclera exceeds 1 mm. Tissue differentiation becomes possible in tumors of over 1.5 mm [26]. In A-scan echography a choroidal hemangioma is characterized by a high internal reflectivity between 50 and 100%. This is related to the histological structure with prominent large internal tissue surface. A malignant melanoma usually has a reflectivity of less than 50%. Only large melanomas may become more heterogenous and present a higher reflectivity. In these cases the prominence differentiates them from the usually flatter hemangiomas. Hemangiomas do not present an elevation of more than 5 to 6 mm [11]. Spontaneous vascular movements, which are present in 70 to 80% of melanoma cases are rarely seen in hemangiomas [26]. With B-scan the lesion presents a rounded tumor pattern with a distinct anterior border and internal acoustic solidity [64]. Choroidal excavation and acoustic hollowness, which are characteristic findings in malignant mela-nomas, are rarely seen in choroidal hemangiomas.

7. Radiography

A plain radiography of the skull may be helpful and indicates possible ossification of the choroid [37]. A partial ossification of the choroid is not an unusual finding in choroidal hemangiomas [13, 76].

VI. Histopathology

In the older literature extensive histological descriptions were given by Wagenmann [71], Meller [45], Reis [57], Salus [59], Mülock-Houwer [48], von Hippel [70], Jaensch [31] and Brons [9]. More recent summarizing articles were published by Rosen [58], Danis [13] and Witschel and Font

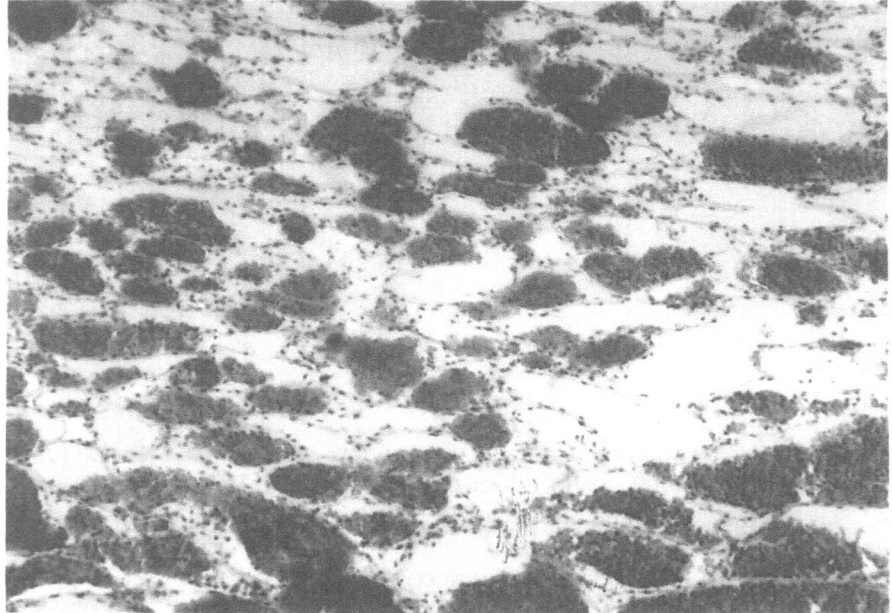

Figure 1–11.   Choroidal hemangioma: large thin-walled, blood filled vascular spaces lined by flat endothelium and separated by thin septa (cavernous type). 9011 H.E (Courtesy of Dr A Hamburg, Utrecht).

[76]. These last authors added 71 personal cases to the 130 cases reported which have been verified histologically [16, 33].

Many authors consider that all choroidal hemangiomas pass imperceptedly into the normal choroid [13, 44, 63]. Others however consider that solitary hemangiomas have sharp limits [6, 76], even although they are not encapsulated [6, 63]. In 75% of the cases there are well demarcated peripheral margins separating the tumor from the uninvolved choroid. This margin is made by compressed melanocytes and choroidal lamellae [76]. The diffuse hemangiomas, on the other hand, have unclear limits. Diffuse angiomatosis may affect more than half of the whole choroid, while the rest exhibits large engorged vessels [33, 76].

From a histologic point of view, the choroidal hemangiomas may be divided in cavernous, capillary or mixed types.

The *cavernous type* (Fig. 1–11) is composed of large, thin-walled, blood-filled, vascular spaces, lined by flat endothelium [6, 13, 16, 56, 63, 76]. These spaces are generally separated by thin, intervascular septa [6, 13, 16, 41, 63, 72, 76]. The spaces are of sensibly, uniform caliber, although they are larger than any normal ocular vessel [13]. They can also be more irregular and of varying size [63]. Telangiectasis may be seen dispersed between these spaces [3, 10].

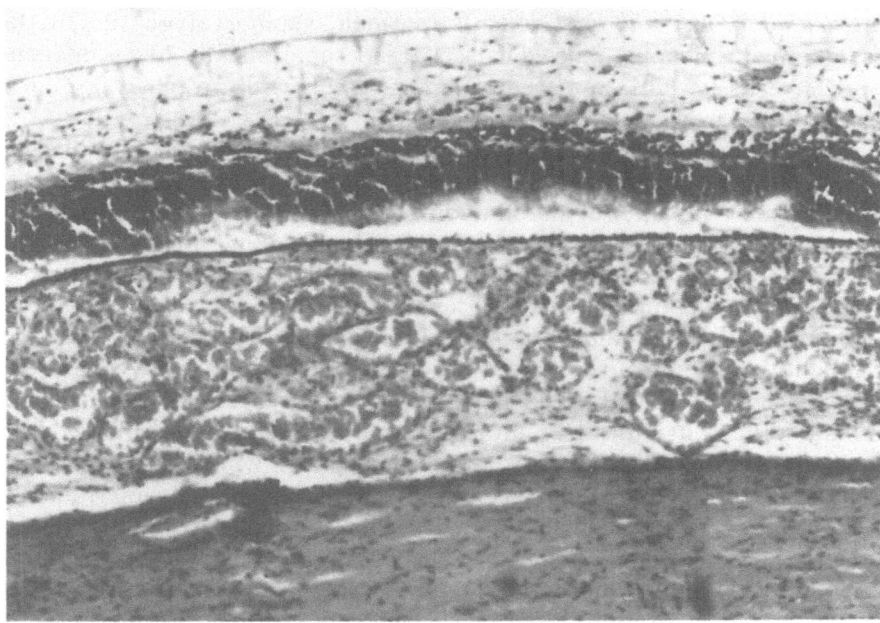

Figure 1–12.   Diffuse choroidal hemangioma in Sturge-Weber syndrome 1424.60 H.E.S.

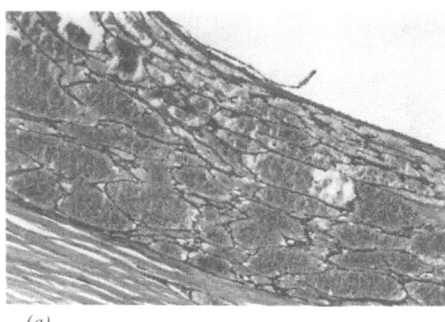

(a)

Figure 1–13.   Diffuse hemangioma in Sturge-Weber a. central part b. peripheral part 12.586 PAS (Courtesy of Dr B. Mosny, Hamburg).

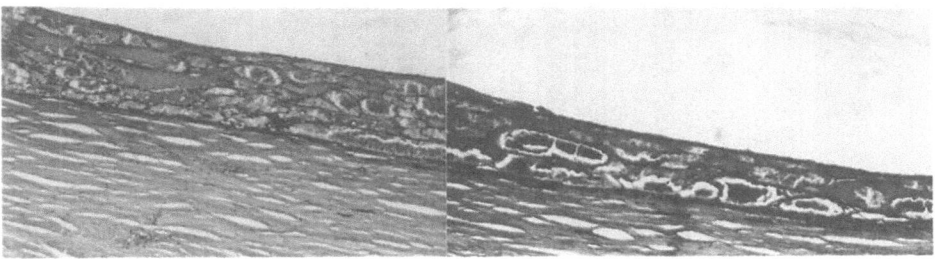

(b)

The *Capillary hemangioma* consists of small, capillary type vessels, lined by flat, inconspicuous endothelial cells and separated by loose edematous connective tissue [76]. Sometimes, larger vessels with proper walls can also be found [63].

Mixed hemangiomas present features both of cavernous and capillary type [76]. In Sturge-Weber syndrome (Figs. 1–12, 1–13) the angiomas are always of the mixed type [19, 76] and in addition large numbers of extremely tilted, thin-walled vessels are found in the episcleral and subconjunctival, perilimbal tissue.

Solitary hemangiomas are usually cavernous [16, 19, 41, 56]. However, capillary and mixed solitary angiomas have also been described [43, 49]. Transitions between the different forms may be found in one and the same tumor [63].

Some authors however did not find any difference between isolated or associated hemangiomas [13]. In less typical cases the tumor may consist of an extensive and diffuse choroidal telangiectasis which appears in some areas as a convolution of vessels and in other parts of the same tumor as a capillary or cavernous hemangioma. Thus, the same tumor may take various forms [16].

There are neither smooth muscles in the vessel walls nor abnormalities of the basement membrane in any of the three types of angiomas [76]. Never was any sign of histologic malignancy observed [13]. The complete absence of proliferation of elements of the vessel wall strongly suggests that these

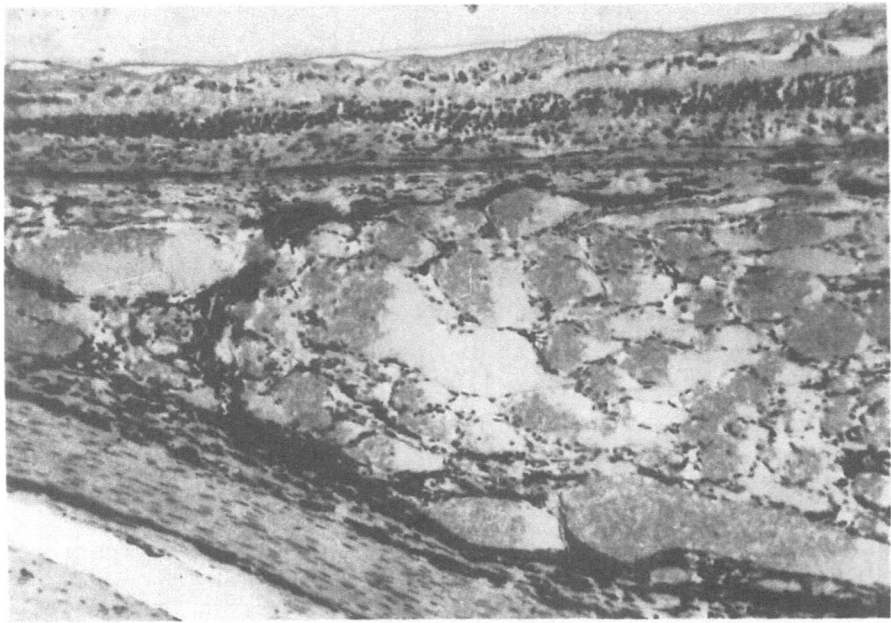

Figure 1–14.   Cavernous hemangioma of the choroid: compressed melanocytes at the margin of the tumor 10.584 H.E.S. (Courtesy of Prof. P. Dhermy, Paris).

tumors are non-proliferative lesions [76]. The frequent occurrence of ganglion cells was reported by some [20] but could not be confirmed by others
[7].

The *secundary changes*, induced by choroidal hemangiomas, are essentially similar in diffuse and in circumscribed tumors [76]. However they
appear early [56] and are generally more severe in Sturge-Weber syndrome
[56, 76].

In over two thirds of the cases of solitary hemangiomas the *choroidal
melanocytes* are pushed towards the sclera, the choriocapillaris and the
peripheral margins of the tumor [76] (Fig. 1–14). Proliferation of melanocytes was observed by some [33] but this finding could not be confirmed by
others [76].

The *choriocapillaris* may show different stages of obliteration and
sclerosis or be destroyed and present areas of chorioretinal scarring [76].

Bruch's membrane is frequently hyperthrophied [16, 72], may present
hyaline bodies [72] (Fig. 1–15), but may also well be intact [6, 7, 10, 13, 45],
interrupted or even absent [6, 7]. *The retinal pigment epithelium* may be
intact [7] or mildly atrophic [76]. Desquamated, swollen or pigment-laden
cells may be seen in the subretinal space [6]. Sometimes, the RPE even
disappeared [13]. Most commonly however, proliferation of RPE cells is
observed [6, 7, 13, 56, 76] (Fig. 1–16). This occurs in over two third of

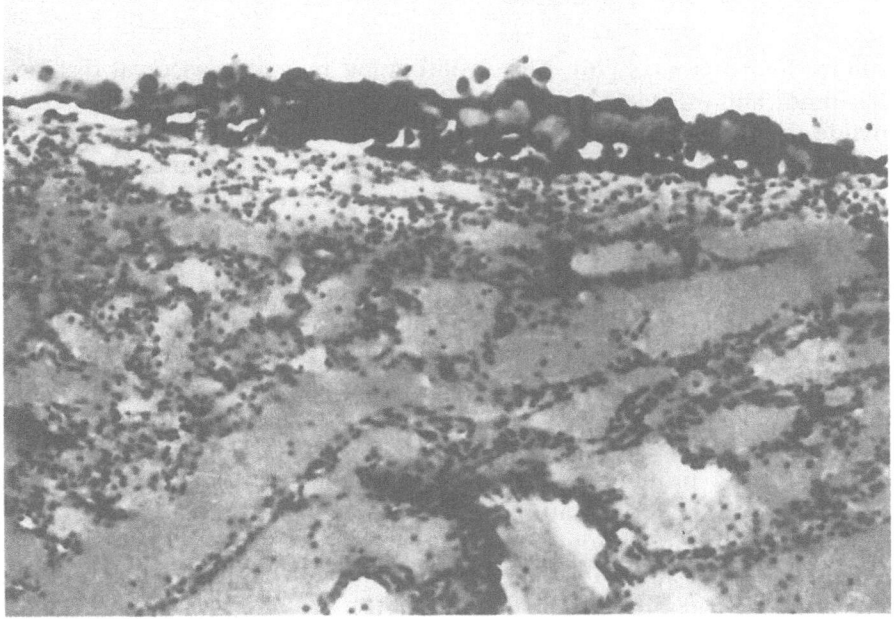

Figure 1–15. Large drusen over a choroidal hemangioma in a case of Sturge-Weber
syndrome. 3285.72 H.E.

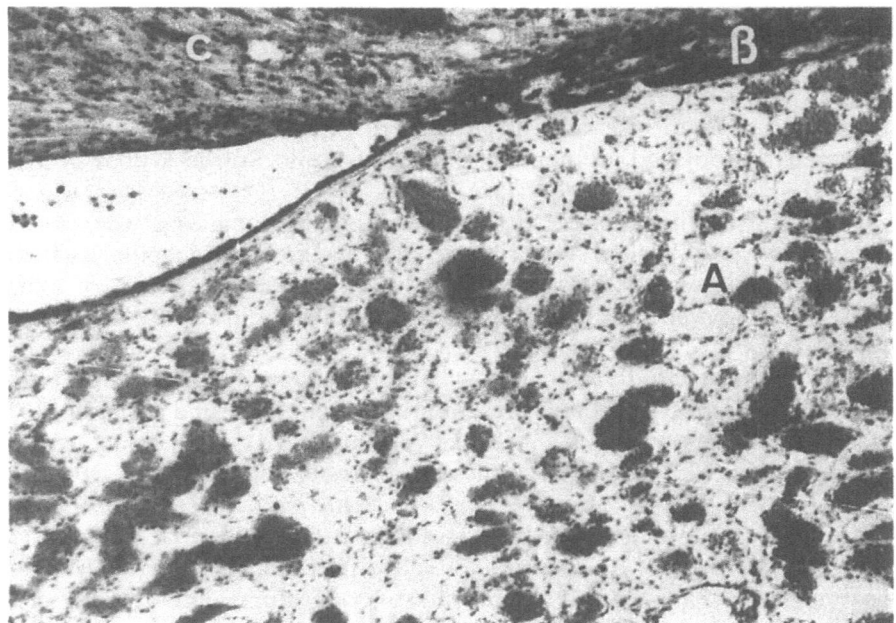

Figure 1–16.   Choroidal hemangioma (A). Proliferation of retinal pigment epithelium (B) Disorganized and gliotic retina (C). 9011 H.E. (Courtesy of Dr A. Hamburg, Utrecht).

solitary hemangiomas [76]. This proliferation may also occur at distance of the tumor and especially in the macular area [13, 31, 33, 57]. RPE cells may invade the retina [13], sometimes mimicking retinitis pigmentosa [76]. Even in small angiomas can early and marked degenerative changes occur of the overlying *retina* [76]. These changes include atrophy or edema [56], chorio-retinal adhesions [63, 76], atrophy or loss of photoreceptors [13, 76], gliosis [13, 76] and cystoid degeneration [6, 13, 44, 56, 63, 72, 76] (Fig. 1–17). A localized or total retinal detachment is seen in 50% [76] to 90% [56] of the cases and is related to subretinal exudation [13, 44, 56, 76] or hemorrhage [56]. These changes are related to the duration of the evolution [13] and are probably the consequence of the breakdown of the blood-retinal barrier at the level of the RPE [67]. They may provoke secondary inflammatory reactions and glaucoma [13].

Endarteritis proliferans of the posterior ciliary arteries has also been reported in the older literature [3, 24, 52]. An *epichoroidal membrane* is a common finding in choroidal hemangiomas [6, 7, 9, 13, 15, 16, 48, 56, 57, 63, 69, 72, 76] (Figs. 1–18, 1–19). It can be observed in 2/3 of circumscribed and in half of the diffuse hemangiomas [76].

Such an epichoroidal membrane may be localized over the surface of the tumor or even at distance and then most often at the macula [48, 57, 69]. It

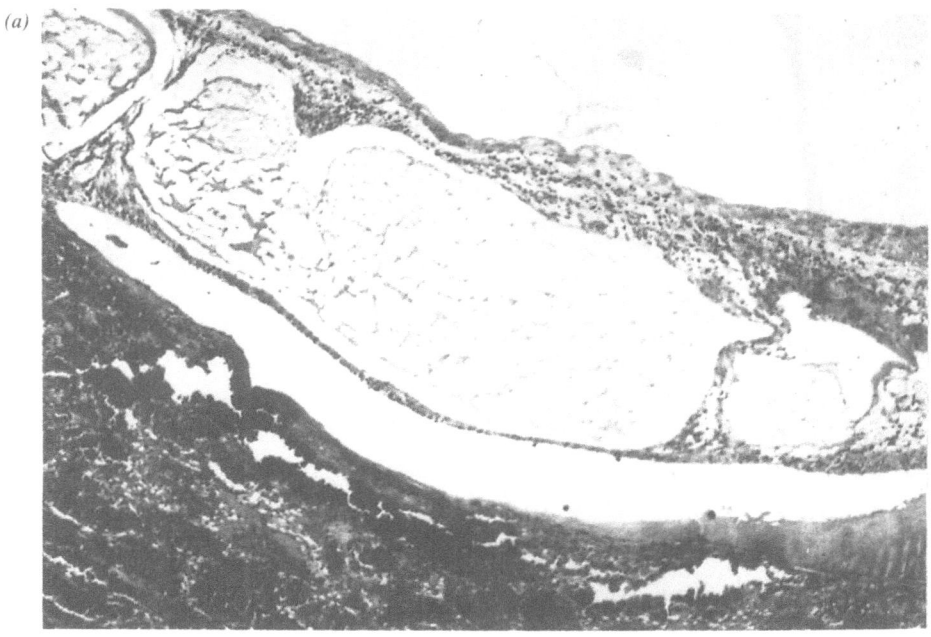

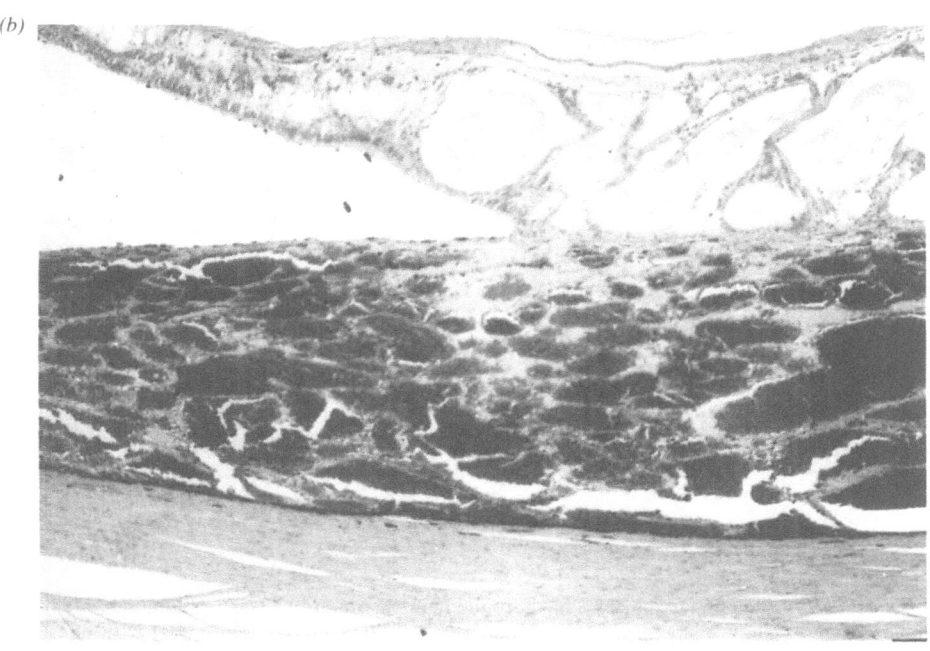

Figure 1–17. Hemangioma of the choroid with extensive cystoid, degeneration of the overlying retina. 657.54 H.E.

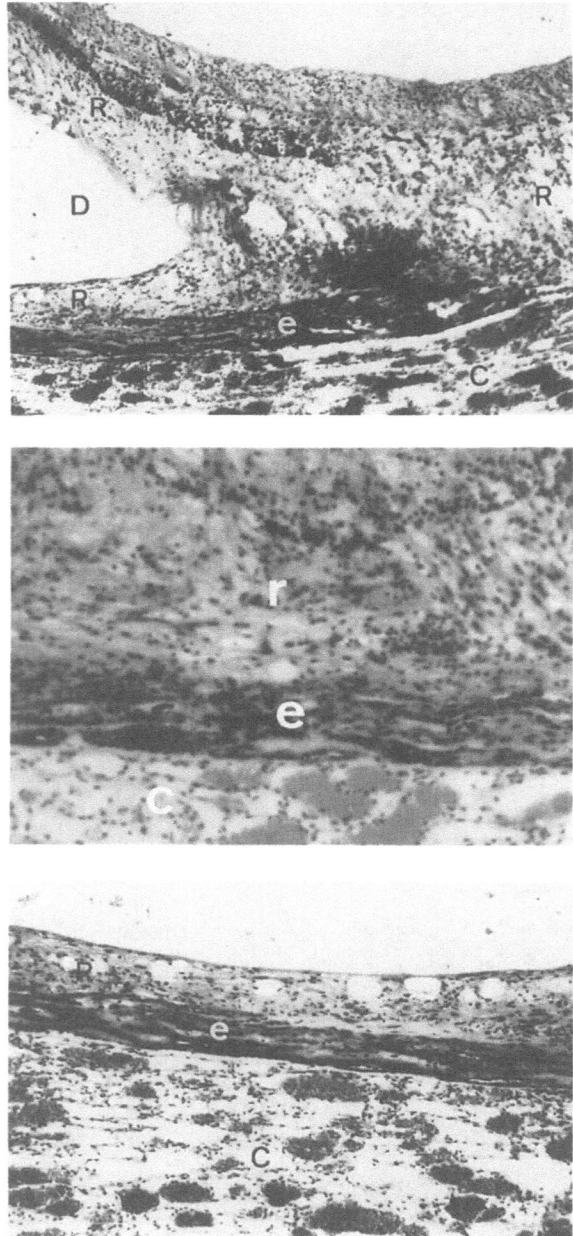

Figure 1-18.   Secondary changes in choroidal hemangioma (C). Epichoroidal membrane with proliferated retinal pigment epithelium (E). Severely disorganized retina (R) with gliosis and cystoid degeneration (D). 9011 H.E. (Courtsey of Dr A. Hamburg, Utrecht).

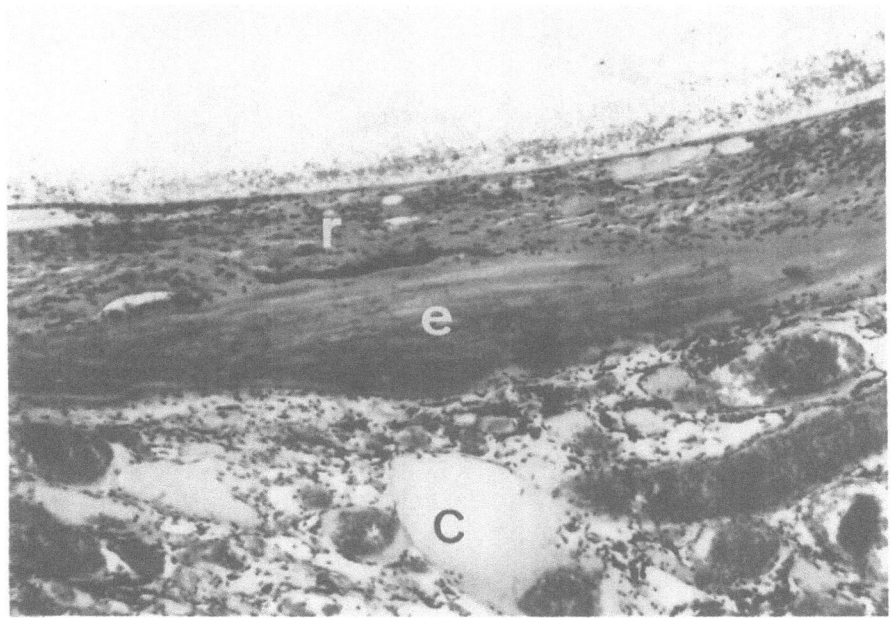

Figure 1–19. Fibrous epichoroidal membrane (E) over a choroidal hemangioma (C). Severe retinal degeneration (R). B839 case of Prof. Casanovas, Barcelona.

is situated at the inner side of the tumor between retina and choroid [7, 6, 13, 15, 16, 48, 57, 63, 69], with sometimes thin lamellae of fibrillar tissue between choroid and RPE [25, 31]. The membrane is composed of pauci-nuclear, fibrillar tissue [48, 57, 69], resembling the cuticular elements of Bruch's membrane [56] or fibrous tissue [6, 13, 16, 56, 63, 72, 76].

This membrane is believed to be ectodermal in origin [39, 45, 57, 60] with possible later involvement of mesenchymal tissue [7]. It may thus represent a fibrous transformation of proliferated pigment epithelium [7, 10, 16, 56, 76]. According to some, the epichoroidal membrane is not of mesodermal origin [59].

According to Mülock-Houwer [48] and Salus [59] the slow transsudation of fluid through the walls of the dilated vascular spaces of the tumor provokes retinal degeneration and detachment, this in turn could irritate the RPE and the choroid and cause the formation of the epichoroidal plaque and chorioretinal fusion [13]. *Calcification* [7, 56] and *ossification* [6, 7, 13, 16, 56, 63] are far from being exceptional and have been reported in 20% of circumscribed and in 64% of diffuse hemangiomas [76]. The importance seems to correlate with the duration of the disease [76] and is sometimes so extensive that the lesion may be mistaken for a primary osteoma [56].

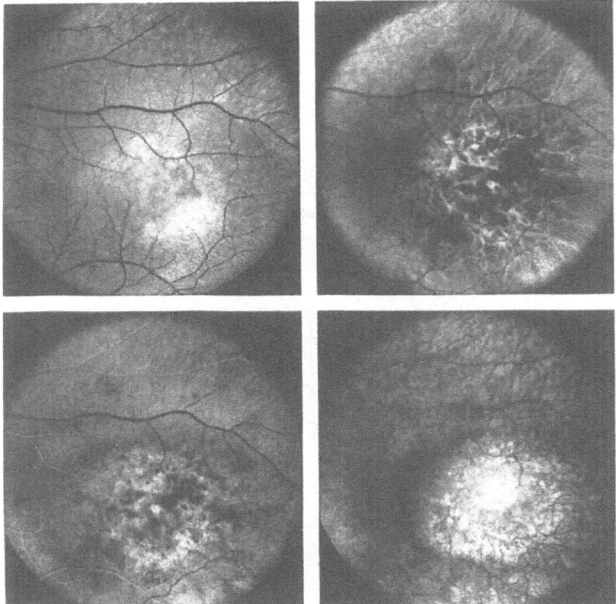

Figure 1–20.   Choroidal hemangioma before Argon laser photocoagulation.

Most authors localize the ossification in the epichoroidal membrane [6, 7, 13, 16, 56, 63, 76] although ossification was also seen at the external side of Bruch's membrane, in the choroid or even at distance of the tumor [13].

Plaques of proliferated or transformed RPE seem always intimately related to the bony trabeculae, suggesting that the ossification occurs primarily in areas of previous RPE proliferation and not within the choroidal angioma [76]. Vessels from the choroid may penetrate into the areas of ossification through breaks in Bruch's membrane [76]. In some cases a calcific impregnation of ganglion cells, retinal capillaries and inner limiting membrane has also been reported [21].

VII. Treatment

Since the tumor grows very slowly, treatment is only to be considered if the patient becomes symptomatic. When the diagnosis of choroidal hemangioma is made at the occasion of a routine examination, patients should be followed at least annually.

1. Photocoagulation

Photocoagulation is the treatment of choice [2, 22, 23, 43]. The purpose of the treatment is mainly to achieve a resolution of subretinal fluid. No

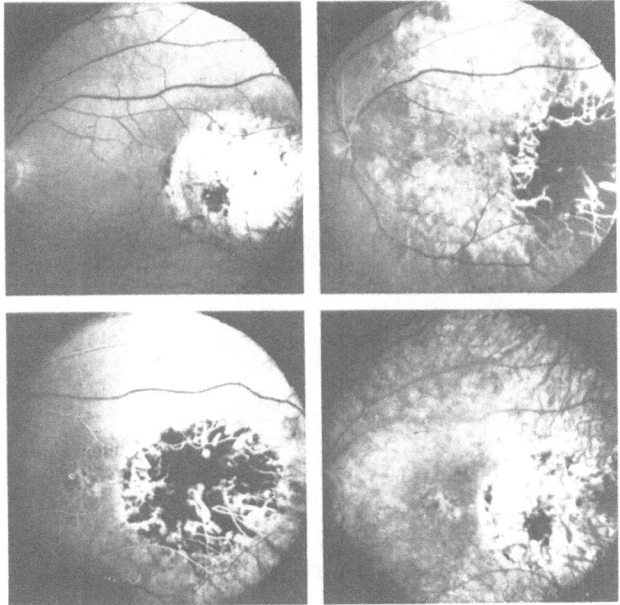

Figure 1–21.   Same eye as Fig. 1–20, 3 years after photocoagulation.

attempt should be made to destroy the tumor as this results in a higher amount of complications related to intense treatment [2, 60]. The treatment can be done with the Xenon lamp or with the laser (Argon or Dye) (Figs. 1–20, 1–21). As the treatment is often partial, recurrences of retinal detachment are possible. These recurrences and the associated, degenerative changes in the overlying retina ultimately result in a poor long term visual prognosis.

2. Retinal detachment surgery in diffuse hemangiomas

Since retinal detachment is more severe in diffuse hemangiomas, treatment here is usually more difficult. In eyes with an extensive retinal detachment, drainage of subretinal fluid followed by photocoagulation may be appropriate. Alternatively cryotherapy [30] or diathermy may be used.

3. Radiotherapy

Radiotherapy has initially been used with variable results. Improvement of radiotherapeutic techniques and especially the introduction of the linear accelerator have renewed the interest of radiotherapy in the treatment of complicated choroidal hemangiomas [27, 28]. A total dosis of 2,000 to 3,000 rads is delivered in fractionned doses. This results not only in a resorption of subretinal fluid but also in a possible normalization of intraocular pressure.

References

1. Andersen S R (1975): Varix of the iris. *Arch Ophthalmol*, 93: 32–33.
2. Augsburger J J, Shields J A, and Moffat K P (1981): Circumscribed choroidal hemangiomas. Long-term visual prognosis. *Retina*, 1: 56–61.
3. Bergmeister R (1911): Ein Fall von Angiom der Chorioidea. *Von Graefe's Arch Ophthalmol*, 79: 285–292.
4. Bergstrand H, Olivecrona H, and Tonnis W (1936): Gefässmissbildungen und Gefässgeschwülste des Gehirns. Thieme Verlag, Leipzig.
5. Berkow J W (1966): Retinitis pigmentosa associated with Sturge-Weber syndrome. *Arch Ophthalmol*, 75: 72–76.
6. Berliner M L and Breinin G M (1951): Angioma of the choroid. A clinicopathologic report of two cases of partial and complete encephalotrigeminal angiomatosis. *Arch Ophthalmol*, 96: 39–48.
7. Boke W (1957): Ein Beitrag zur Klinik, Morphologie und Pathogenese des Aderhautangioms. *Ophthalmologica*, 139: 373–379.
8. Bonnet M, Habozit P, and Magnard M G (1976): Valeur de l'angiographie en infrarouge au vert d'indocyanine dans le diagnostic clinique des angiomes de la choroïde (observation anatomoclinique). *Bull Soc Ophthalmol Fr*, 76: 713–716.
9. Brons C (1936): Kavernöses Angiom der Chorioidea. *Klin Mbl Augenkl*, 97: 43–51.
10. Campos R (1947): Su di un angioma della coroide con ossificazione della vitrea. *Boll Oculist*, 26: 145–170.
11. Coleman D J, Lizzi F L, and Jack R J (1977): *Ultrasonography of the eye and orbit*. Lea and Febiger Co, Philadelphia.
12. Cushing H and Bailey P (1928): Tumors arising from the blood vessels of the brain. Thomas, Springfield Ill.
13. Danis P (1952): L'angiome de la choroïde. *Arch Ophtalmol*, 12: 487–509.
14. De Laey J J (1978): Fluoroangiographic study of the choroid in man. *Doc Ophthalmol*, 45: 140–167.
15. Dhermy P, Raynaud G and Coscas G (1971): Angiome de la choroïde et pseudo-rétinite pigmentaire. *Arch Ophtalmol*, 31: 845–858.
16. Duke-Elder A and Perkins E S (1966): in System of Ophthalmology, Diseases of the uveal tract, Henry Kimpton, London, vol. IX, 808–813.
17. Ferry A P (1964): Lesions mistaken for malignant melanoma of the posterior uvea. A clinicopathologic analysis of 100 cases with ophthalmoscopically visible lesions. *Arch Ophthalmol*, 72: 463–469.
18. Francois J (1978): Diagnostic de l'hémangiome de la choroïde. *J Fr Ophtalmol*, 1: 313–316.
19. Francois J, Rabaey M, Evens L, and Eliaerts H (1959): Hémangiome de la choroïde. *Bull Soc Belge Ophtalmol*, 123: 550–564.
20. Fuchs A (1951): El diagnostico clinico del hemangioma de la coroides y su relacion con il sistema nervoso. *Rev Oto-Neuro-Oftalm*, 26: 99–108.
21. Garrow A and Loewenstein A (1943): A case of monocular hydrophthalmia with special reference to its possible relation to the Sturge-Weber syndrome. *Br J Ophthalmol*, 27: 335–354.
22. Gass J D M (1974): Differential diagnosis of intra-ocular tumors: a stereoscopic presentation. The C V Mosby C°, St. Louis, 123.
23. Gass J D M (1987): Stereoscopic atlas of macular diseases: diagnosis and treatment. Third edition. The C V Mosby C°, St. Louis, 172–177.
24. Ginsberg S (1978): Angiom. Handb. der speziellen pathologische Anatomie und Histologie, *XI/1*, 539–541. Henke & Lubarsch, J. Springer, Berlin.
25. Giulini (1890): Uber das kavernöse Angiom der Aderhaut. *Von Graefe's Arch Ophthalmol*, 36: 247.

26. Goes F and Benozzi J (1980): Ultrasonographic aid in the diagnosis of choroidal hemangioma. *Bull Soc Belge Ophtalmol*, 191: 97–111.
27. Greber H, Alberti W, and Scherer E (1985): Strahlentherapie der Aderhauthämangiomen. *Fortschr. Ophthalmol*, 450–452.
28. Greber H, Wessing A, Alberti W, and Scherer E (1984): Die erfolgreiche Behandlung eines Aderhautshämangioms mit Sekundärveränderungen bei Sturge-Weber-Syndrom. *Klin Mbl Augenheilk*, 185: 276–278.
29. Hoskins J C and Kearncy J J (1977): A case of negative P$_{32}$-test in a histologically proven choroidal hemangioma. *Arch Ophthalmol*, 95: 438–439.
30. Humphrey W T (1979): Choroidal hemangioma: response to cryotherapy. *Ann Ophthalmol*, 11: 100–104.
31. Jaensch P S (1932): Schwierigkeiten und Irrtümer bei der Diagnose des Aderhautsarkoms. *Klin Mbl Augenheilk*, 88: 622–643.
32. Jahnke W (1931): Histologisches Befund bei Glaukom und gleichseitiger Naevus flammeus faciei *Ztschr Augenheilk*, 74: 165–176.
33. Jones T S and Cleasby G (1959): Hemangioma of the choroid: a clinico-pathologic analysis. *Am J Ophthalmol*, 48: 612–628.
34. Kautzky R (1949): Dtsche Ztschr. Nervenheilk., 161: 506.
35. Kreibig W (1941): Zur klinischen Diagnose des Aderhautangioms *Klin Mbl Augenheilk*, 107: 597–621.
36. Lanning R and Shields J A (1979): Comparison of radio-active phosphorus (P$_{32}$) uptake test in comparable sized choroidal melanomas and hemangiomas *Am J Ophthalmol*, 87: 769–772.
37. Larmande A (1948): Les angiomes calcifiés et ossifiés de la choroïde *Bull Soc Ophtalmol Fr*, 48: 96–99.
38. Leber T (1868): Fall von kavernösem Sarkom der Aderhaut. *Von Graefe's Arch Klin Ophthalmol*, 14: 221–227.
39. Lent E and Lyon M (1926): Hemangioma of the choroid. *Am J Ophthalmol*, 9: 804–811.
40. Lindsay P S, Shields J A, Goldberg R E, Augsburger J J, and Frank P E (1981): Bilateral choroidal hemangiomas and facial nevus flammeus. *Retina*, 1: 88–95.
41. Lister A and Morgan G (1963): Choroidal hemangio-endothelioma. *Br J Ophthalmol*, 47: 215–221.
42. Loewenstein A and Steel J (1941): Retinal tuberous sclerosis (Bourneville's disease). *Am J Ophthalmol*, 24: 731–741.
43. Mackensen D and Meyer-Schwickerath G (1980): Diagnostik und Therapie des Aderhauthämangioms. *Klin Mbl Augenheilk*, 177: 16–23.
44. Mc Lean A L and Maumenee E (1959): Hemangioma of the choroid. *Trans Am Ophthalmol Soc*, 57: 171–194.
45. Meller J (1907): Ein Fall von Angiome der Chorioidea. *Ztschr Augenheilk*, 17: 50–54.
46. Milles W J (1884): Naevus of right temporal and orbital region, naevus of the choroid and detachment of the retina in the right eye. *Trans Ophthalmol Soc U.K.*, 4: 168–171.
47. Molnar I., Brabant P, and De Laey J J (1987): Video-angiographie infrarouge et tumeurs de la choroïde *Ophtalmologie*, 1: 539–542.
48. Mülock-Houwer A W (1925): Beitrag zur pathologischen Anatomie und zur klinischen Diagnose des kavernösen Angioms der Chorioidea. *Klin Mbl Augenheilk*, 75: 657–670.
49. Nordenson E (1885): Ein Fall von kavernösem Aderhautsarkom mit Knochenschale bei einem 11-jährigen Mädchen. *Von Graefe's Arch Ophthalmol*, 81: 59–72.
50. Norton E W & Gutman F (1967): Fluorescein angiography and hemangiomas of the choroid. *Arch Ophthalmol*, 78: 121–125.
51. Ossoinig K C & Blodi F C (1974): Pre-operative differential diagnosis of tumors with echography. III. Diagnosis of intra-ocular tumors. in Blodi F C, editor. Current concepts in Ophthalmology, The C V Mosby C°, St. Louis, vol. 4, p. 296.
52. Panas F & Remy A (1879): Contribution à l'anatomie pathologique de l'oeil. Martinet, Paris, p. 88.

53. Phelps C D (1978): The pathogenesis of glaucoma in Sturge-Weber syndrome. *Ophthalmology*, 85: 276–286.
54. Pitta C, Bergen R & Littwin St. (1979): Spontaneous regression of a choroidal hemangioma following pregnancy. *Ann Ophthalmol*, 11: 772–774.
55. Pitta CG, Shingleton BJ, Harris PJ and Regan CD (1979): Solitary Choroidal hemangioma. *Am J Ophthalmol*, 88: 698–701.
56. Reese A B (1963): Tumors of the eye. 2nd ed., Harper and Row, New York pp. 392–402.
57. Reis W (1911): Zur Kenntnis des Angioma chorioidea. *Ztschr Augenheilk*, 26: 308–317.
58. Rosen E (1950): Hemangioma of the choroid. *Ophthalmologica*, 120: 122–149.
59. Salus R (1913): Angiom der Aderhaut. *Ztschr Augenheilk*, 30: 317–326.
60. Sanborn G E, Augsburger J J, and Shields J A (1982): Treatment of circumscribed choroidal hemangiomas. *Ophthalmology*, 89: 1374–1380.
61. Schepens C L and Schwartz A (1958): Intra-ocular tumours. Bilateral hemangioma of the choroid *Arch Ophthalmol*, 60: 72–83.
62. Schirmer R (1860): Ein Fall von Telangiektasie. *Von Graefe's Arch Ophthalmol*, 7: 119–121.
63. Schwab F (1966): Die Tumoren der Netzhaut und der Aderhaut mit Ausnahme des Retinoblastoms und des bösartigen Melanoms der Aderhaut *Ophthalmologica*, 151: 231–259.
64. Shields J A (1983): Intra-ocular tumors. The C V Mosby C°, St. Louis.
65. Shields J A and Zimmerman L E (1973): Lesions simulating malignant melanoma of the posterior uvea. *Arch Ophthalmol*, 89: 466–471.
66. Smith J L, David N J, Hart L M, Levenson D S and Tillett C W (1968): Hemangioma of the choroid. Fluorescein photography and photocoagulation. *Arch Ophthalmol*, 69: 85–88.
67. Spencer W H (1986): Ophthalmic Pathology: an Atlas and Textbook. 3rd ed., vol. 3, W B Saunders C°, Philadelphia, London, Toronto, pp. 1425–1427.
68. Susac J O, Smith J L and Scelfo R J (1974): The 'tomato-catsup' fundus in Sturge-Weber syndrome. *Arch Ophthalmol*, 82: 69–70.
69. Von Hippel E (1911): Die anatomische Grundlage der von mir beschriebenen 'sehr seltenen Erkrankung der Netzhaut'. *Von Graefe's Arch. Ophthalmol*, 79: 350–377.
70. Von Hippel E (1931): Ueber das Angiom der Aderhaut. *Von Graefe's Arch Ophthalmol*, 127: 46–56.
71. Wagenmann A (1900): Ueber ein kavernöses Angiom der Aderhaut bei ausgedehnter Teleangiektasie der Haut. *Von Graefe's Arch Ophthalmol*, 51: 532–549.
72. Watillon M, Gilson M, Comhaire-Poutchinian Y & De Corte M.Th (1970): Hémangiome de la choroïde: fluorétinographie et anatomopathologie. *Bull Soc Belge Ophtalmol*, 156: 590–597.
73. Watters E C, Hiles D A, Johnson B L (1973): Cloverleaf skull syndrome. *Am J Ophthalmol*, 76: 716–720.
74. Weiss D J (1973): Dual origin of glaucoma in encephalo-trigeminal hemangiomatosis. *Trans Ophthalmol Soc U.K.*, 93: 477–493.
75. Wessing A (1968): Fluoreszenzangiographie der Retina. Lehrbuch und Atlas. Georg Thieme, Stuttgart, 143–166.
76. Witschel H & Font R L (1976): Hemangioma of the choroid. A clinicopathologic study of 71 cases and a review of the literature. *Survey Ophthalmol*, 20: 415–431.

2   Retinal angiomatosis — von Hippel-Lindau's Disease

The first reports on retinal angiomatosis are attributed to Magnus (1874), Jackson (1878), and Panas and Remy (1879) [58, 43, 65]. Fuchs (1882) published the description and drawings of the classical red peripheral tumor with the typically dilated artery and veins, but considered the lesion to be an arterio-venous aneurysm [23]. Collins (1894) gave the first pathological description of thin-walled vessels and cystic spaces, but called it a capillary naevus [15], while Czermak (1905) described it as a capillary angioma [16]. von Hippel (1911) identified the tumor as a hemangioblastoma and gave it the name of angiomatosis retinae [86]. In later years the entity was described by some authors as angiogliosis or angiogliomatosis [10, 27, 39]. In his classical paper Lindau (1926–1927) described the lesion as a primary hemangioma, noted the association of angiomatosis retinae with cerebellar cysts and proved the histological similarity of both cerebellar and retinal tumors [54, 55]. Van Der Hoeve (1932) finally classified the lesion among the congenital phakomatoses [85]. The disease has since been the subject of many publications under the denomination of angiomatosis retinae or von Hippel-Lindau's disease.

Retinal angiomatosis may be defined as a hereditary and congenital angiomatous hamartoma of the retina [26]. It may manifest itself as an isolated manifestation and is then called 'von Hippel's disease' or in association with cerebellar and/or visceral involvement or von Hippel-Lindau's disease.

I. Pathogenesis

In the earlier literature the tumor was considered as a primary retinal gliosis with angiomatous differentiation [34, 60] or as a primary angioma with secondary reactive gliosis [15, 16, 24, 75]. It was thought that the development of the retinal angioma could be followed by dilatation of afferent and efferent vessels on the basis of a disturbed circulation, whereby arterio-venous anastomoses [12, 18, 24, 45, 46, 59, 71] as well as arteritis or phlebitis of the vessel wall might play a preponderant role. Van Der Hoeve classified the disease among the congenital phakomatoses and since several authors also stressed the hamartomatous nature of the tumor [5, 31, 92].

According to some the disease process is from the very beginning an abnormality of the entire vascular unit of artery, vein and capillary, giving rise to hypertrophy and hyperplasia of the components [31, 92].

Some have suggested that the tumor may arise from a congenital rest of undifferentiated cells, from an 'anlage' of capillary endothelium, from a previously normal retinal vessel [45] or from small circumscribed angiomas [67]. Peripheral tumors have been reported to occur de novo in previously normal areas [90].

Some early lesions consist of only one or a group of small vessels, without any tumefaction, forming a direct connection or arteriovenous communication between artery and vein. Later on, transformation into a tumor nodule occurs [90].

It has also been stressed that early nodules lay essentially in the capillary area with communications to both the arterial and venous systems [45].

As to the correct denomination of the tumor, some consider them as 'hemangioblastoma' or 'hemangio-endothelioma' [92] while others find the term 'capillary hemangioma' more correct [64].

II. Incidence

The reported incidence of retinal angiomatosis is one on 22.500 patients seen by an ophthalmologist [92]. This figure is probably too low as a number of cases remain asymptomatic up to an advanced age [29]. Elliot [20] in 1957 found less than 170 cases in the literature, whereas Go et al. [29] compared in 1981 their cases with 384 other reported cases.

Retinal angiomatosis has no race nor sex predilection; women are as commonly affected as men.

The ocular lesions usually become symptomatic in the third decade. In Go and Lamiell's family the mean age of clinical onset of the disease was 26.2 years. Systematic family investigation however allows an earlier diagnosis even in children or in babies.

The youngest patient with retinal angiomatosis was one day old [56]. On the other hand patients of over 80 years of age may still be asymptomatic [29]. Usually, the younger the patient develops clinical symptoms, the more evolutive the lesions are [11]. In 50% of the cases both eyes are affected [92], although the lesions in one eye may be much further progressed than the lesions in the fellow eye. Multiple tumors in the same eye are frequently seen. Depending on the follow-up period, the incidence of multiple retinal tumors in the same eye may be up to 71% [91].

III. Heredity

In cases of retinal angiomatosis (von Hippel's disease) a hereditary pattern may be found in 20 to 30 % of the cases. von Hippel-Lindau's disease is inherited in an autosomal dominant way with variable expression [3, 29, 37, 41, 45, 57, 70, 72, 82, 89]. Some of the largest families were reported by Ridley et al. [70] (94 family members examined, 24 affected), Salazar and Jamiell [72] (a large Hawaian family of which 111 members were examined and 17 found to be affected) and Go et al. [29] (220 members of the same family with 41 of them with vHL disease).

Chromosomal abnormalities were found in 2 patients with vHL disease by Kobayashi and Shimada [50] and in two other vHL patients by Kawasaki et al. [48]. These anomalies consisted of chromosomal breakage, aneuploidy, polyploidy and trisomy D. However, other studies could not reveal chromosomal anomalies or a specific HLA-type [29] responsable for vHL disease.

IV. Ocular findings

1. Retinal angiomatosis

The evolution of a retinal angioma has been divided into 4 stages [19, 84]:
– Stage 1: arterial and venous dilatation. Formation of one or multiple small angiomas
– Stage 2: appearance of retinal hemorrhages and/or of lipoid exudates
– Stage 3: massive exudation and retinal elevation
– Stage 4: functional loss of the eye by secondary glaucoma, uveitis or phtisis
Since the systematic examination of family members of vHL patients and since the introduction of fluorescein angiography more attention is given to the incipient lesions [2, 45, 59, 72, 90). It seems thus justified to modify the previous clasification:
– Stage 1: incipient lesion
– Stage 2: young angioma
– Stage 3: mature angioma
– Stage 4: complicated angioma

Stage 1. Incipient lesion
Retinal angiomas may arise de novo in apparently normal retina [45, 46, 70, 90]. The first lesion consists of a knot or conglomerate of capillaries which become manifest as a red spot barely to be seen. There are no feeder vessels and no signs of altered vessel wall permeability such as hemorrhages or lipoid exudates. These clusters do not leak fluorescein [59]. Such early lesions are usually located at the equator or in the pre-equatorial retina [45]. These lesions are asymptomatic. At autopsy early angiomas may be found which were not detected on ophthalmoscopy [31, 46].

De Jong et al. [17] noted that in von Hippel's disease retinal arteries and venules may run a strict parallel course for more than one disc diameter. Because of the crowding of the vessels at the optic disc they insist that these

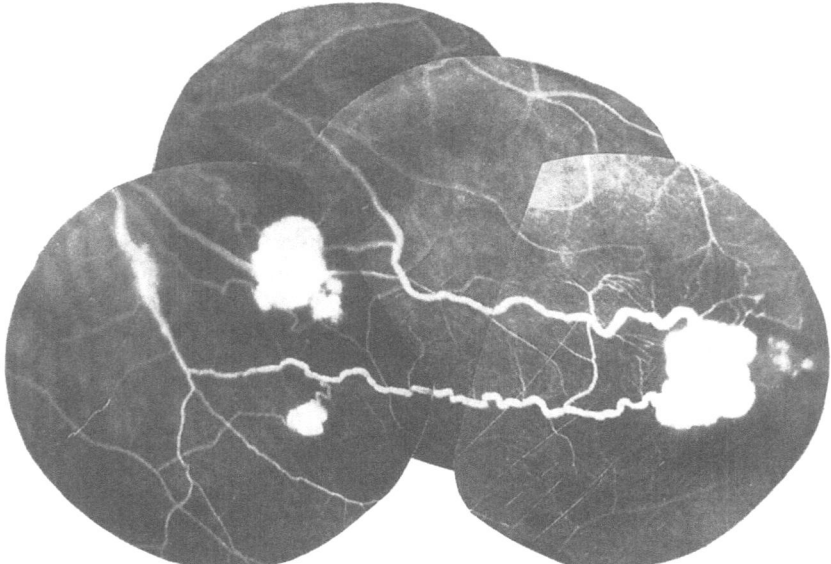

Figure 2–1.   Multiple small retinal angiomas in different stages of evolution in the same fundus. Note the capillary dilatation around the larger tumor.

'twin vessels' should be observed more than two disc diameters away from the disc. They examined 23 members of three subships with vHL disease and found twin vessels in the 8 patients with angiomas, in 16 eyes of 12 family members without angiomas and in only one of 23 controls.

Stage 2. Young angioma
The pretumoral stage nearly always progress to a typical angioma. This progression may take a few weeks up to several years. First a slight elevation of the nodule becomes apparent. The feeder vessels appear somewhat enlarged. In that stage fluorescein leakage is usually observed as well as capillary changes in the vicinity of the angioma (Fig. 2–1).

Stage 3. Mature angioma
The tumor enlarges in size and has a diameter from 1 up to 6 disc diameters. The lesion is usually situated in the midperiphery of the fundus. A progressive dilatation of the feeder vessels results from increased blood flow through the angioma [59]. The angioma usually appears as a red mass, but because of glial proliferations at the surface it may also be completely white (Fig. 2–2). The afferent (arterial) and efferent (venous) feeders may be differentiated easily with fluorescein angiography. These vessels may be

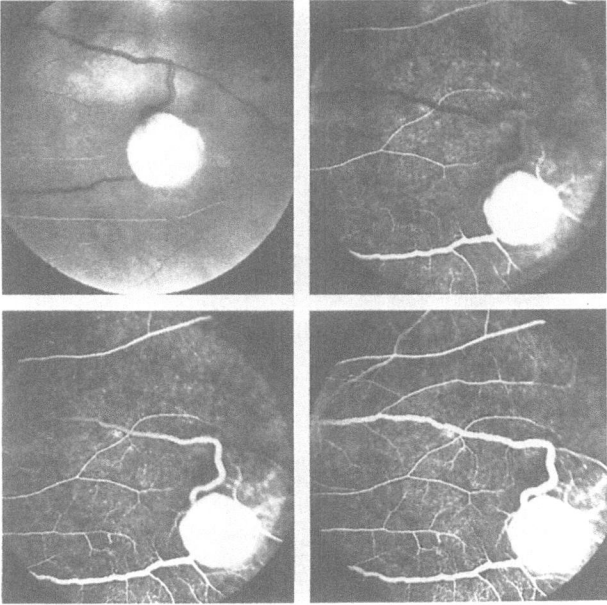

Figure 2–2.   Retinal angioma with its feeder vessels. The angioma appears completely white on the redfree picture.

dilated up to the optic disc and the detection of such abnormal vessels on routine ophthalmoscopy must lead to a systematic examination of the whole fundus in search of angiomatous lesions (Fig. 2–3).

The capillary bed around the lesion is often dilated (Fig. 2–4). Fluorescein angiography may demonstrate a slowing down of the retinal circulation

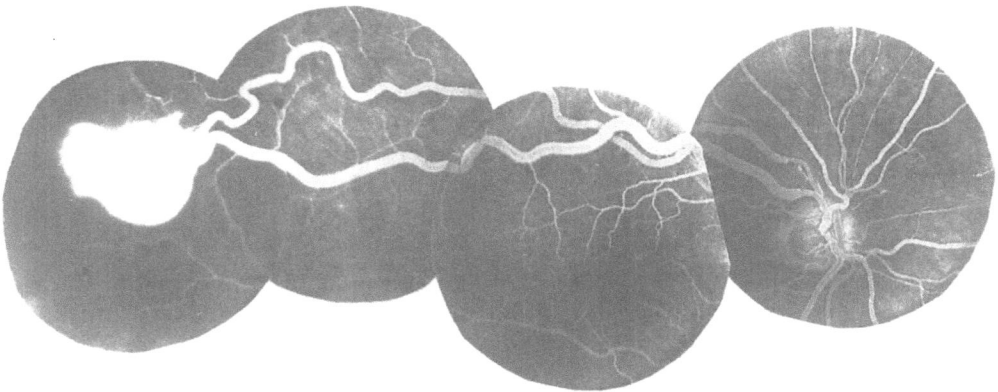

Figure 2–3.   Large retinal angioma with dilated feeders up to the optic disc.

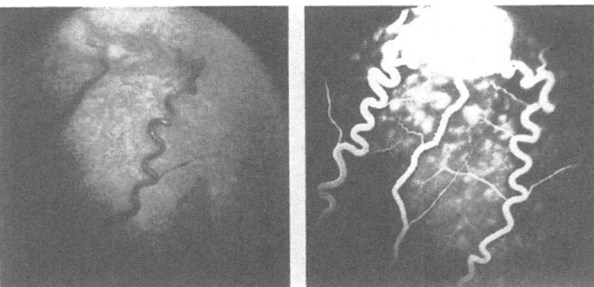

Figure 2–4.   Diffuse leakage from a retinal angioma and from the retinal capillaries surrounding it.

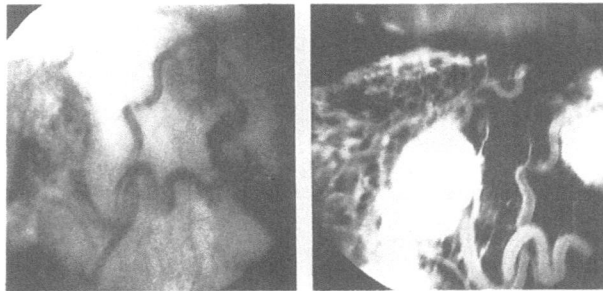

Figure 2–5.   Large retinal angioma associated with retinal neovascularization.

peripheral to the tumor and capillary dropout. This may explain the association of an angiomatous tumor with surface retinal newvessels (Fig. 2–5). The tumor leaks fluorescein profusely, indicating endothelial incompetence, which is also manifested by the presence of lipoid exudates (Figs 2–16a, 2–17a).

Lipoid exudates are a frequent manifestation of the angioma. They are often found in the immediate vicinity of the lesion or in the macular region. The massive deposit of lipoid exudates in the macular region, called by Wise and Wangvivat [94] 'the exagerated macular response' is not specific for von Hippel's disease but may also occur in association with other vascular lesions, whether congenital, such as retinal telangiectasia or Coats' disease or acquired.

The ophthalmoscopic appearance in this stage is more the consequence of exudates than of hemorrhages. Hemorrhages occur seldom spontaneously in retinal angiomas, usually they are the consequences of traction phenomenons or are induced by the treatment.

Progressive exudation from the angioma results first in a localized, later possibly in a massive retinal detachment.

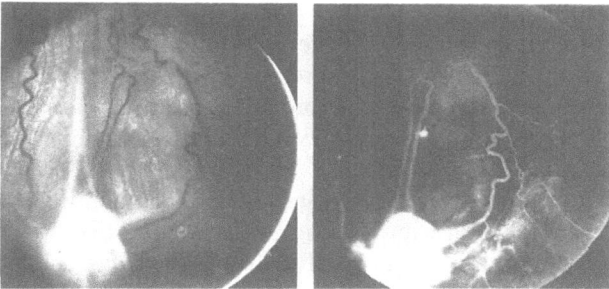

Figure 2-6.   Retinal angioma with fibroglial tissue formation along its feeders.

Fibroglial tissue proliferation is a common feature of evoluated retinal angiomatosis. It usually starts at the level of the tumor and may mask it. The glial proliferation may accompany the secondary neovascularization. It may also progress along the feeder vessels up to the posterior pole (Fig. 2-6). From stage 3 on, the disease becomes symptomatic. As a result of the exudation the patient gradually loses vision. The first sign may be metamorphopsia due to a serous detachment in the macular region. If the treatment is applied consequently, reabsorption of the exudates may be accompanied by restoration of central vision.

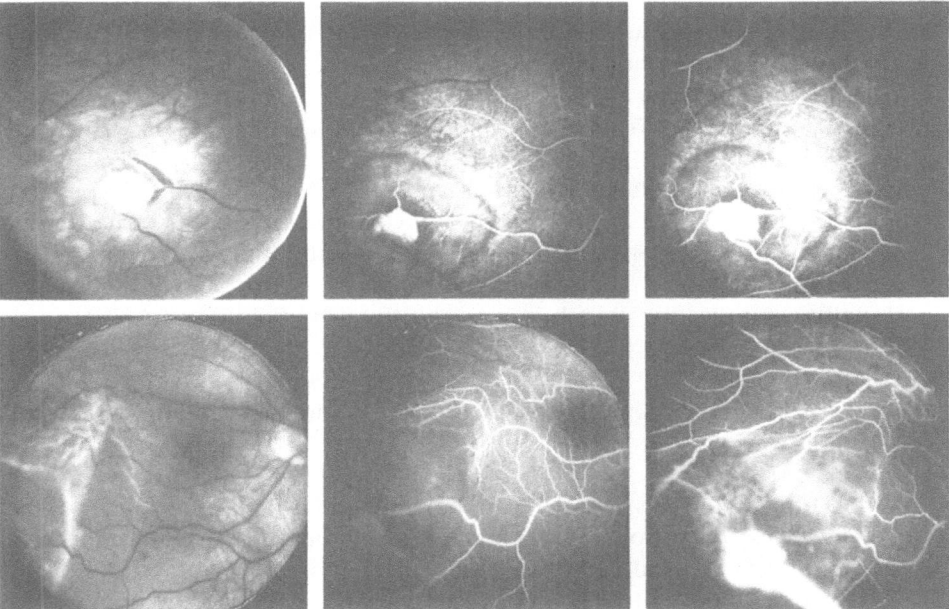

Figure 2-7.   Retinal tear in association with a retinal angioma. Top aspect in October 1980. The patient refused any treatment and was seen again in April 1984 with a rhegmatogenous retinal detachment (bottom).

Stage 4. Terminal angioma
This stage is characterized by the major complications of retinal angiomatosis. Retinal detachment is usually a result of massive exudation but may also be the consequence of traction phenomenons caused by the fibroglial tissue. Such a traction may provoke a retinal tear (Fig. 2–7) or a tractional retinal detachment.

Further complications after total retinal detachment are neovascular glaucoma, uveitis, total cataract and phtisis of the eye.

If multiple angiomas are present or in bilateral cases, the evolution of the different lesions is not necessarily symmetrical. In the same eye, angiomas in various stages of their development may be found. One eye may already be lost, whereas the other eye, although presenting typical lesions, still maintains normal vision.

2. Optic disc angiomas

Because of the specific aspects of optic disc hemangiomas, they will be discussed separately in a following chapter.

3. Optic nerve hemangiomas

Uehara and Ichinomiya [83] described a patient who lost one eye by retinal angiomatosis and who developed nine years later proptosis of the fellow eye. Histopathology of the intra-orbital tumor revealed it to be a hemangioblastoma of the optic nerve.

4. Ocular symptoms from intracranial manifestations of vHL diseases

In vHL diseases hemangiomas of the posterior fossa and of the spinal cord may be found as well as other visceral involvement. In cases of neurological involvement the visual disturbances are usually the result of increased intracranial pressure. Massive dilatation of the third ventricle may exceptionally compress the chiasm, giving rise to visual field defects [52].

V. Associated neurological and visceral involvement or von Hippel-Lindau's disease

Von Hippel-Lindau's disease can be defined as an autosomal dominant precancerous condition characterized by angiomatous tumors and cysts of the retina, the central nervous system and the viscera [29, 88].

It is estimated that 20% of the patients with a retinal angioma will have the familial type and thus present other features of vHL disease [70]. There is a marked clinical variability and seldom does one patient present the complete syndrome [37]. The syndrome may be present in various gradations and a number of subclinical lesions will possibly only be detected after a prolonged follow-up period, through scrutinous examination or even at autopsy.

The diagnosis of vHL disease can be made if an individual presents with retinal or cerebellar hemangioblastoma associated with one or more visceral manifestations of the disease or if a patient presents a single lesion of the syndrome, provided another family member is known to have a cerebellar hemangioblastoma [17].

They are more than 25 distinct lesions in vHL disease [3, 7, 37, 41, 42, 46, 57, 70, 82, 88, 92]: angiomas or hemangioblastomas of the retina, the cerebellum, the medulla oblongata, the spinal cord, liver, kidney, spleen, lung, adrenal cortex, ovaries, bones, epididymis, cysts of cerebellum, pancreas, liver, kidneys, spleen, lungs, omentum, epididymis, ovaries, adrenal cortex, pheochromocytoma, sympathetic paraganglioma, cerebellar ependymoma, syringomyelia, renal cell carcinoma, polycythemia. From these various lesions however 6 produce frequently disease: retinal angiomatosis (53%), cerebellar (36%), medullary (4%) or spinal (4%) hemangioblastoma, pheochromocytoma (10%) and renal cell carcinoma [41].

Horton et al. [41] found in their series pancreatic and renal cysts in over half of the affected individuals; hepatic cysts or renal and epididymal adenomas were also not unfrequently found. However these lesions did usually not cause clinical symptoms, they were mostly detected incidently or at autopsy.

Life threatening conditions are mainly cerebellar hemangioblastoma which causes the highest morbidity and mortality in these patients and renal cell carcinoma. Retinal angiomas are usually the first lesion to become clinically manifest, followed by pheochromocytoma and cerebellar hemangioblastoma. In the pedigree examined by Ridley et al. [70] the median age at diagnosis was 19 years for retinal angiomas (range 4–42 yr), 22 years for pheochromocytoma (range 11–58 yr) and 30 years for cerebellar hemangioblastoma (range 22–58 yr). Renal cell carcinoma becomes symptomatic usually at a later age (mean age 41 years). In Horton's et al. Series [41] it was metastatic in one half of the cases and was lethal in nearly one third.

The association with pheochromocytoma deserves special attention. Pheochromocytoma was first associated with vHL disease by Glushien et al [28]. Since this publication the association was confirmed by others [35, 56, 70]. According to Ridley et al. [70] pheochromocytoma is even the second most frequent manifestation of vHL disease after retinal angiomas. In their family an affected patient had a 42% chance of developing a pheochromocytoma and a 21% chance of developing a cerebellar lesion.

Pheochromocytoma appears frequently in some vHL families but is seldom or absent in other families. This strongly suggests that there seems to be a predisposition in some vHL families to the development of pheochromocytoma [41].

Pheochromocytomas are sporadic in 92% of the cases and familial in 8% [35]. Only 10% of sporadic cases present multiple tumors compared to 55% of the familial cases. Often these tumors may be in obscure places, complicating their detection and treatment. Familial pheochromocytoma is an autosomal dominant disease and may be associated with neurofibromatosis, von Hippel-Lindau's disease or incontinentia pigmenti [21].

Polycythemia is especially frequent in patients with hemangioblastoma of the central nervous system. This could be related to the erythropoietic activity of the tumor [7, 42].

VI. Association of vHL disease with other diseases

1. Association with other phakomatoses

There are a number of similarities between the six diseases which have been combined by Van Der Hoeve under the general term of phakomatoses. These six diseases are Sturge-Weber syndrome (meningo-cutaneous angiomatosis), von Recklinghausen's neuro-fibromatosis, Bourneville disease (tuberous sclerosis), von Hippel-Lindau's disease, Louis Bar syndrome (ataxia teleangiectasia) and Wyburn-Mason syndrome. Associations of two phakomatoses in the same individual or in the same family are however rare. The concurrent presence of vHL disease and von Recklinghausen disease have been demonstrated in a few families [14, 22, 80, 81]. In the family described first by Tischler [81] and later by Thomas et al. [80] 11 members presented only signs of neurofibromatosis at first examination. Three of these patients subsequently developed retinal angiomas, two members presented signs of vHL disease. One patient had at first examination neurofibromatosis (cutaneous neurofibromata and 'café-au-lait' spots). She died after a surgical exploration which revealed a cerebellar hemangioblastoma. Post mortem examination also showed a left renal cell carcinoma, bilateral pheochromocytomas and multiple cysts of the pancreas.

It is worth noting that as well von Recklinghausen as vHL disease may be associated with pheochromocytoma. There is still as yet little evidence to suggest that a single gene may be the cause of these various diseases [81].

2. Association with retinitis pigmentosa

Kollarits et al. [51] observed von Hippel tumors in 2 brothers and one sister with retinitis pigmentosa. General investigations including CT-scan of brain, kidneys, liver and pancreas were unremarkable. The question arises if these were truly retinal angiomas or rather acquired retinal angiomatosis, which is a possible complication of retinitis pigmentosa and will be discussed in chapter 10 of this volume.

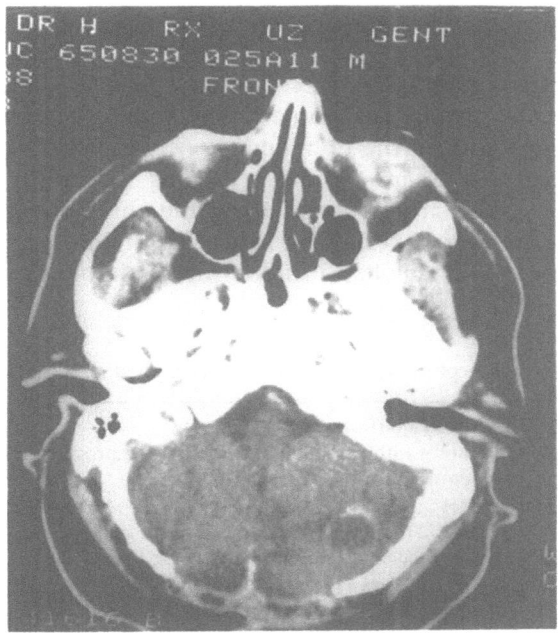

Figure 2–8. Ct-scan of a cerebellar hemangioblastoma in a patient with von Hippel-Lindau's disease.

VII. Diagnosis

1. Retinal angiomatosis

The typical angiomatous lesion of von Hippel's disease does not pose a diagnostic problem. However, it is important to recognize early lesions, especially as they are the most easy to treat. Therefore, a systematic fundus examination including fundus biomicroscopy and fluorescein angiography is essential.

As new lesions may appear, patients should be examined at least each six months. Fluorescein angiography is especially helpful in detecting small angiomas, although incipient lesions do not necessarily leak fluorescein. Fluorescein angiography may also be helpful in differentiating the arterial from the venous feeder and this may be of some importance in the treatment of such lesions. Fluorescein angiography and echography may also be of value in differentiating large or atypical angiomatous tumors. This is specifically the case in hemangiomas of the disc which will be discussed in the next chapter.

2. Von Hippel-Lindau's disease

vHL Disease is a potential lethal condition. Once the diagnosis is made not only the patient, but also his whole family should be screened. This is the specific responsability of the ophthalmologist who will often be the first to make the diagnosis. A prospective screening of family members of vHL disease will reveal in a number of them life threatening lesions [37]. The screening should be performed by a team including a geneticist, a neurologist, an internist, a radiologist and an ophthalmologist (Table 1) [37, 42, 70].

Table 1. Screening protocol in case of vHL disease (modified after Ridley et al. [70])

1. Annual examination by an internist:
   - full physical examination with special attention to blood pressure, both lying and standing
   - 24 hours urine collection for urinary catecholamines
   - plasma catecholamines
   - abdominal echography
   - abdominal CT-scans if biochemical abnormalities are found
   - intravenous pyelogram in cases of doubt on echography
2. Annual neurologic examination with specific attention to cerebellar signs:
   - baseline CT-scan
   - repeated CT-scan if there are suspicious neurological findings
3. Cerebral and renal angiography in case of doubt.

VIII. Differential diagnosis

The early lesion of von Hippel's disease is sometimes difficult to differentiate from an astrocytoma. Although a hemangioblastoma is usually red in color and has feeder vessels and an astrocytoma appears white without feeding vessels, there are some forms which are difficult to differentiate, especially as some astrocytomas may show a marked vascularity [77].

Large or evoluated tumors have to be differentiated from a number of vascular conditions and tumors such as Coats' disease, cavernous or racemose hemangiomas, macro-aneurysmata, acquired angiomas, retinoblastoma and retinoma, Eales disease, sickle cell retinopathy, dominant exudative vitreoretinopathy or choroidal tumors.

IX. Pathology

We will limit our review to publications of the 1975–1985 period. From a pathologic point of view the angiomas can be divided in peripheral and papillary or optic disc lesions. The optic disc lesions will be discussed in the next chapter.

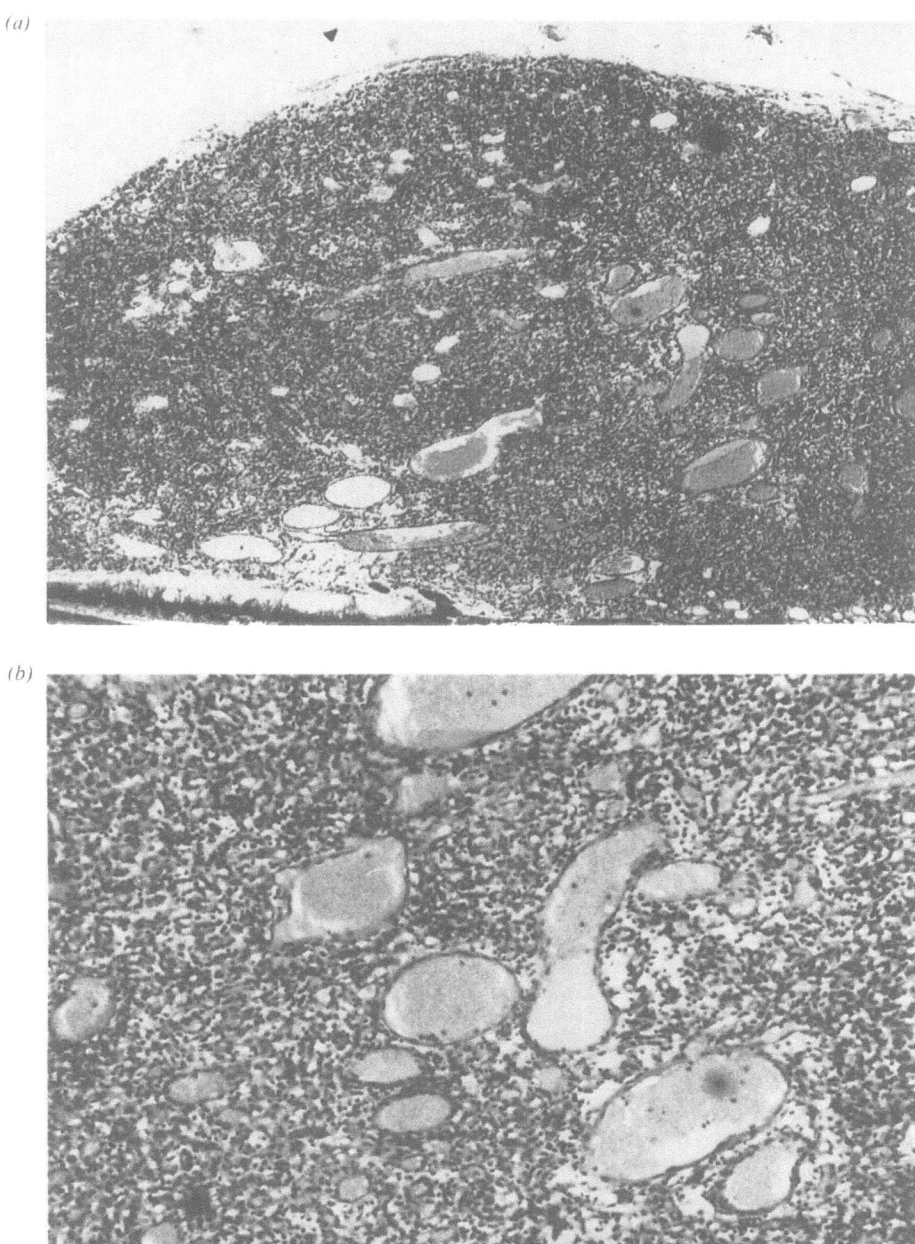

Figure 2–9. Peripheral retinal hemangioma in von Hippel's disease. Appearance of well differentiated capillary hemangioma, together with solid masses of angioblastic cells and large cavernous vessels. (a. general view, b. higher magnification) 6796 HE (Courtesy of Dr Hamburg, Utrecht).

(a)

(b)

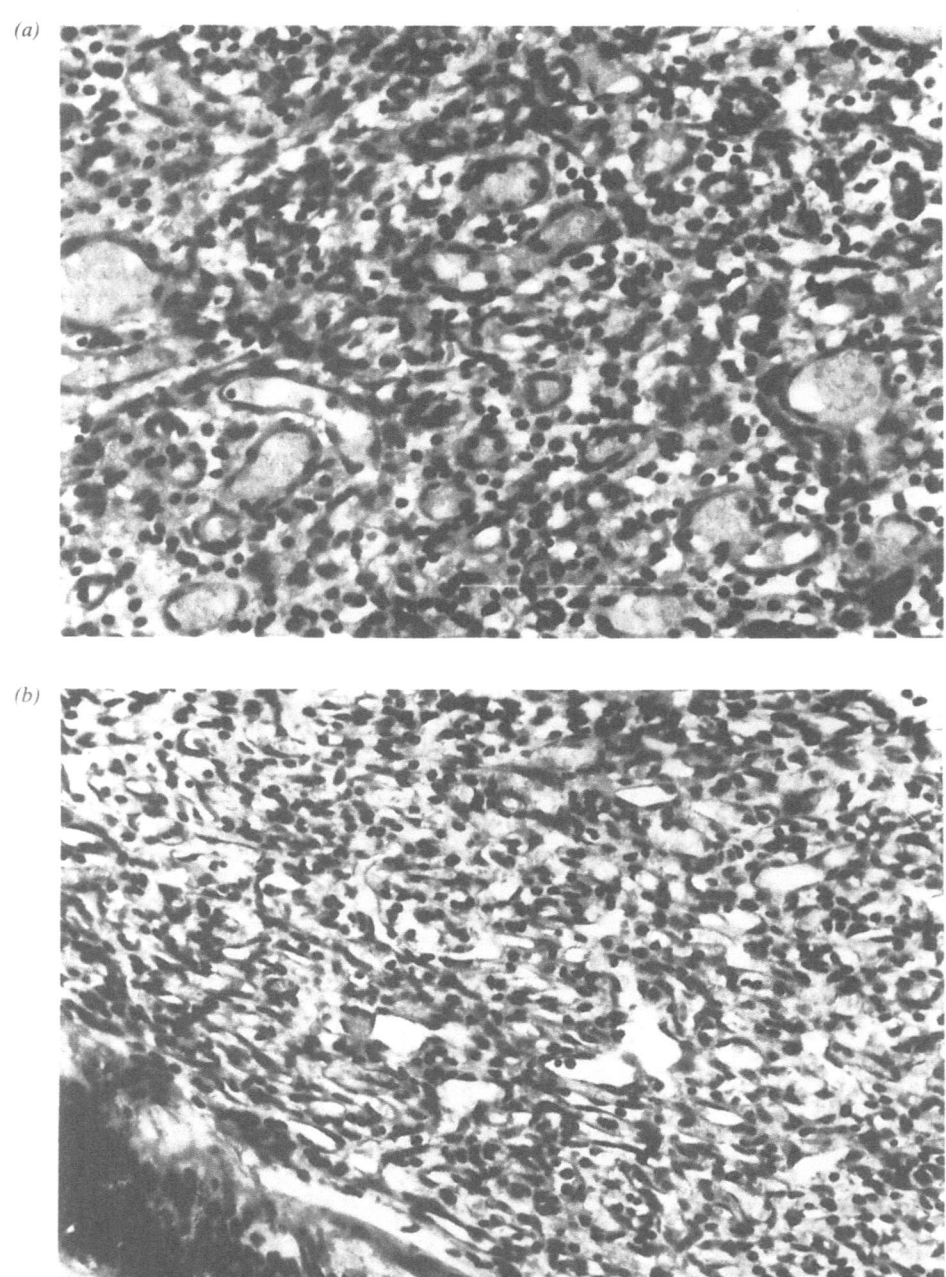

Figure 2–10.   Peripheral retinal hemangioma in von Hippel's disease. Capillaries and small blood vessels forming an anastomosing network. 6796 HE (Courtesy of Dr Hamburg, Utrecht).

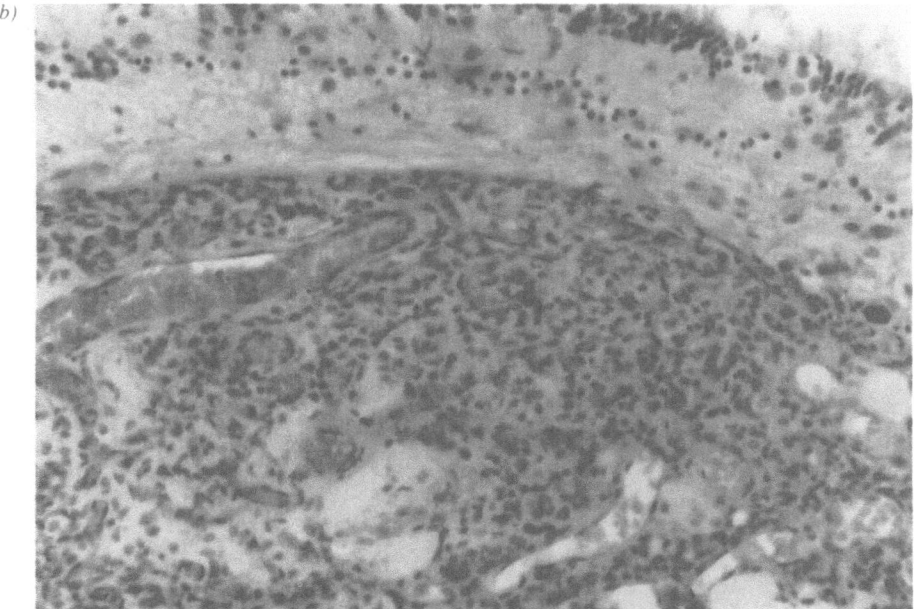

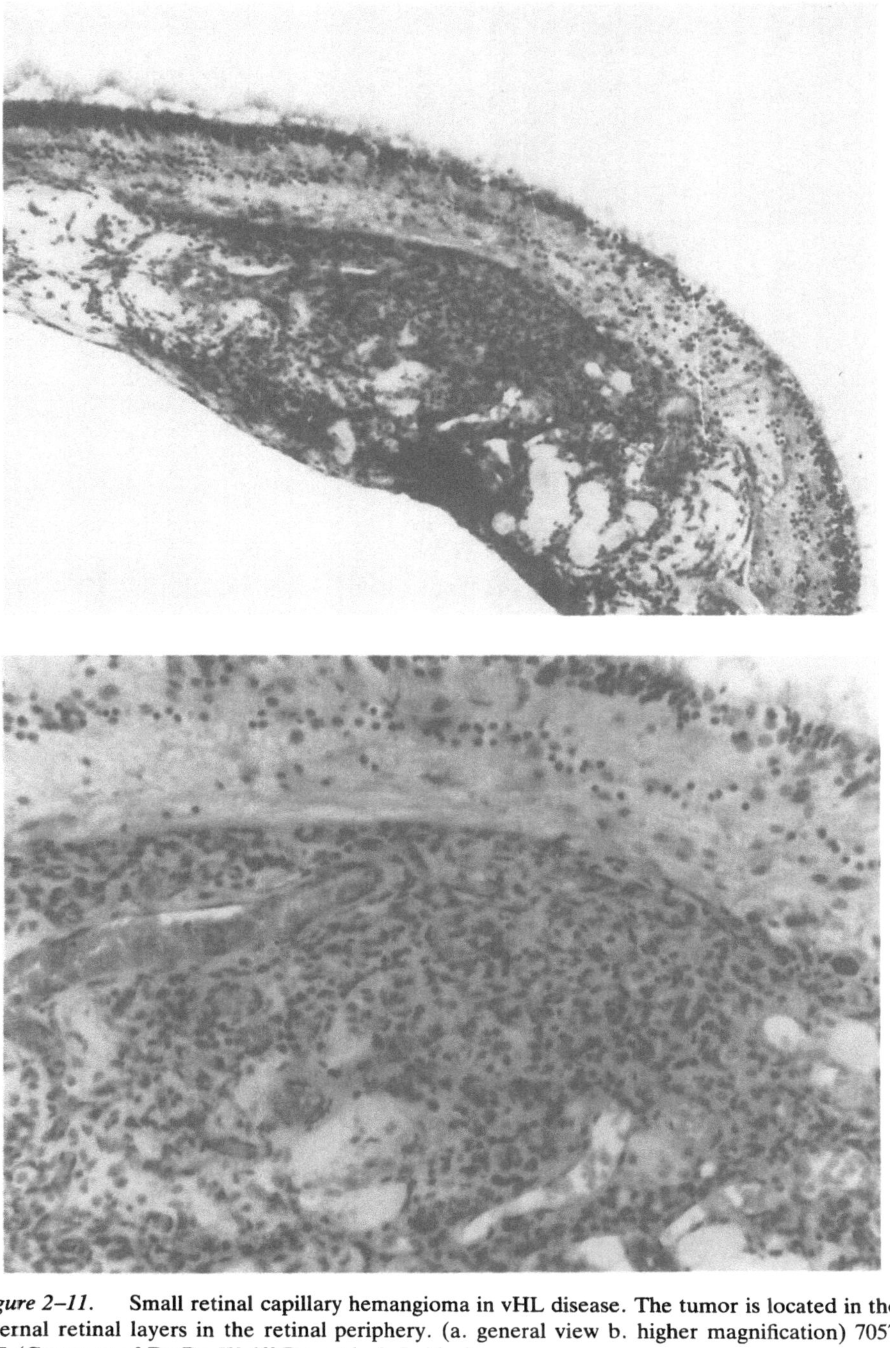

Figure 2–11. Small retinal capillary hemangioma in vHL disease. The tumor is located in the internal retinal layers in the retinal periphery. (a. general view b. higher magnification) 7057 HE (Courtesy of Dr De Wolff-Rouendaal, Leiden).

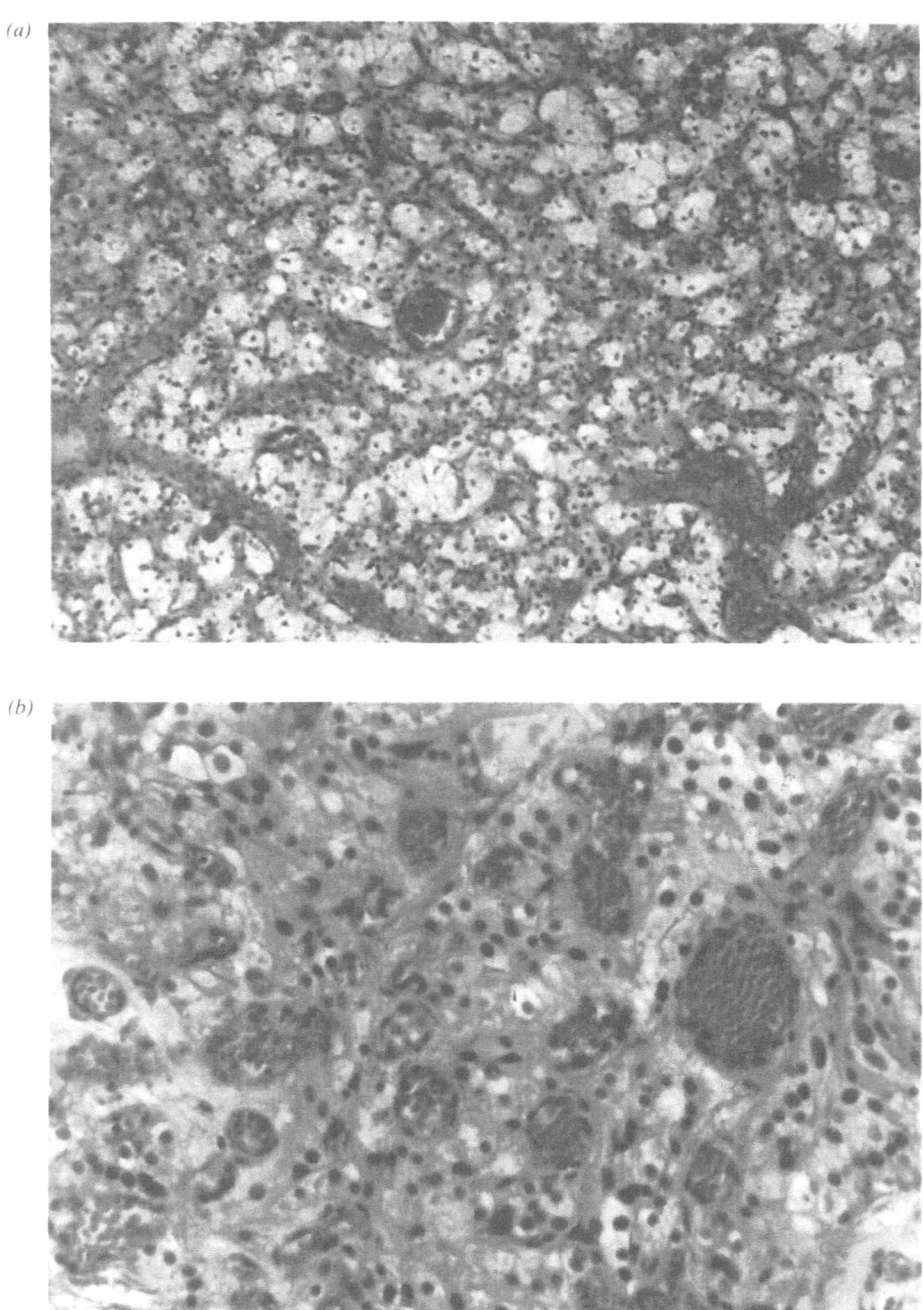

Figure 2–12.   Angiomatosis retinae (vHL disease). The vascular elements of the tumor are separated by nests of interstitial cells with foamy cytoplasm. 3299 HE (Courtesy of Dr P. C. Donders, Groningen)

Peripheral angiomas may be large or small [67], involving partial of full retina thickness [30, 43, 64, 67, 89] and obliterating the normal histological structure [89].

Communications between the angiomas and the retinal and choroidal circulation have been described [34, 64].

The lesions are built up by clusters of capillaries and small blood vessels, forming a network or anastomosing plexiform pattern [28, 43, 64, 89, 92] (Figs 2–9, 2–10, 2–11). The vessels of the tumor proper may be of varying diameter [5, 31, 61] with narrow lumina. Generally they are tortuous, densely packed capillaries [5, 64, 67] surrounded by reticulin [61, 64]. The structure of the walls of the larger feeder vessels does generally not allow differentiation between artery and vein [67], as they are generally markedly sclerosed with narrowed or occluded lumina [5] and chronic inflammatory infiltration [5, 67].

The vascular elements of the tumor are separated and compressed by nests of polyhedral interstitial cells [44] and embedded in a scanty, fibroglial matrix [5, 31, 61, 68, 89] with sometimes scattered foamy and inflammatory cells, erythrocytes, exudate, cystic spaces, cholesterol crystals and other hemorrhagic debris [5, 43, 61, 67, 89] (Fig. 2–12, 2–13). The tumor may become hyalinized by spontaneous sclerosis and fibrosis [68] and replaced by glial overgrowth [5], while calcification and ossification occur less frequently [5, 89] (*Fig. 2–14).

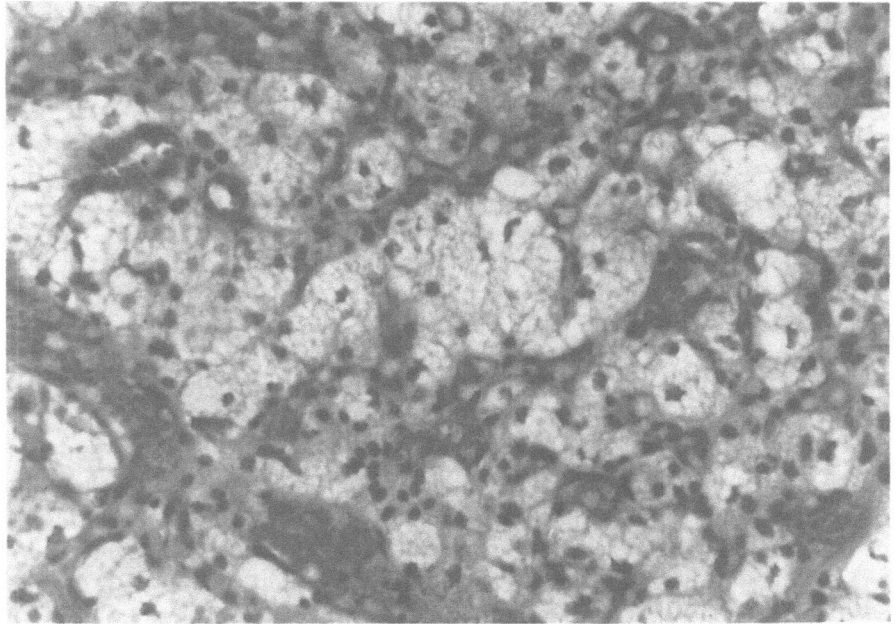

Figure 2–13. Angiomatosis retinae (vHL disease). Nest of interstitial cells with foamy cytoplasm. 3299 HE (Courtesy of Dr P. C. Donders, Groningen)

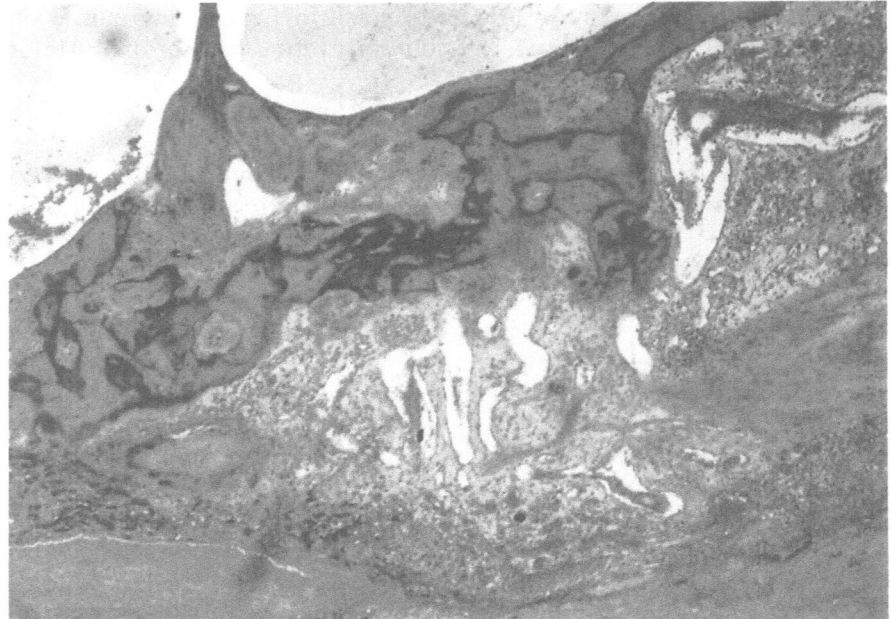

Figure 2–14.   Phtisis bulbi and marked ossification in a case of vHL disease. 3299 HE (Courtesy of Dr P. C. Donders, Groningen)

Typical features of the tumor are also nests of endothelial cells [5, 31, 67, 89] or a plaque composed of solid sheets of poorly canalized, endothelial cells and pericytes with lipidized, stromal cells. The vascular lumina in the plaque are lined by flattened, endothelial cells and ensheated by three to four layers pericytes. Over the plaque, a mixture of lipidized cells and fibrous astrocytes with PTAH-positive fibrils can occur [14].

On electron-microscopic level the cellular elements of the tumor include endothelial cells, pericytes, lipidized stromal cells and fibrous astrocytes in different stages of lipidization [44].

1. The endothelial cells

They have oval or fusiform nuclei [44] and may be normal, flattened or present focal hydropic degeneration [61, 64]. They have a thick, continuous basement membrane [44], with sometimes focal reduplications [61] and do not present evidence of interconversion with pericytes or stromal cells [44, 61]. Their definite cytoplasmic attenuations or fenestrations are bridged by small diaphragms [44, 61, 69, 92].

It has been suggested that these fenestrated, leaky and incompetent capillaries could be responsible for the exudate and fibrin in the retina and subretinal space [44, 97], as well as for the endothelial hydropic degeneration [61]. They also may allow the passive inbibition by plasma lipid of the fibrous astrocytes, which leads to their progressive transformation into fully lipidized stromal cells [44].

They may also lend a clue to the etiology of the focally thickened basement membrane as thickened or reduplicated basement membrane has been postulated to reflect repeated cycles of cell death and regeneration [87]. On the other hand, the thickened basement membrane could affect flow dynamics [62]. It is tempting to speculate that the reduplication process may also either directly compromise the lumen, or limit diffusion of nutrients to adjacent cells with attendant exudation and cellular degeneration.

2. *The pericytes*

The pericytes may be normal [64], sparse or show degenerative necrotic changes [61]. They are completely surrounded by a well-developed basement membrane which may focally be multilaminar [44, 61]. They show no significant lipidization [44], but some of the multilaminar pericytes may present evidence of early smooth muscle differentiation [44, 69]. No evidence could be found of interconversion with endothelial or stromal cells [44, 61].

3. *Nests of round to polyhedral cells*

Nests of round to polyhedral cells (described as interstitial cells [64], stromal cells [44, 61, 92], foam cells [89] or pseudo-xanthoma cells [5, 69]) can be found between the vascular elements. They have a clear [64, 92], foamy [44, 69, 43, 92], vacuolated [64], honeycombed [69] or heavily lipidized cytoplasm [5, 44, 69, 89] with positive fat-staining of the vacuoles [64]. On electron microscopy the vacuoles contain either lipid consistent with saturated, neutral lipid [64] or nonosmophilic lipid [61]. Lipid extracted from these cells is mostly cholesterol stearate, together with a hitherto uncharacterized, PAS-positive diastaseresistant material [44].

Organelles [44, 61, 64], intracytoplasmic glycogen granules [64] and filaments with granular degeneration [44, 61, 64] are scattered between the vacuoles. Membranous lamellar material, suggestive of complex lipids [64] and focal cytoplasmic densification along the plasma membrane, are also present [64]. The cells generally have no definite basement membrane [61, 64], although spotty basement membrane formation may be found where the cells abut on vascular elements [44].

The nuclei are oval and vesicular, sometimes indented by the vacuoles [44, 62]. There is no evidence of interconversion of these cells with endothelial cells or pericytes [44], but transformation of fibrous astrocytes into stromal cells has been observed [44].

The origin of these cells has been debated for a long time: neuroglial, microglial, neuro-epithelial, endothelial, pericytic, macrophagic, meningeal

[78], from primitive reticulum-cells or fibrous astrocytes [47], from angiogenic mesenchyme [47, 78] or degenerating cells, or arising from a common, vasoformative stem-cell under hypoxic stress [61]. Some favour the differentiation of a pluripotential, vasoformative stem-cell toward both an 'immature' stromal cell and its more mature but functionally limited endothelial cell counterpart [61].

As a matter of fact, they present no ultrastructural evidence of active phagocytosis [44]. The spotty formation of basement membrane could prove that they are not of primitive reticulum-cell or microglial origin [44], while the lack of definite basement membrane weakens the arguments for a pericytic origin [61]. Some state that as glial fibrillary acidic protein was not detectable in stromal foamy cells, this casts some doubt upon the theory of glial origin [61].

According to others however, electron microscopic findings permit positive identification of these cells as astrocytes [32, 64], while still others discovered their source in the early lipidization of fibrous astrocytes which could be identified in some portions of the tumor [44].

Secondary changes

1. The underlying *choroid* may be congested [61], infiltrated by chronic, inflammatory cells, atrophic or focally absent [44]. In later stages, subretinal and choroidal ossification may occur [16, 39].
2. The *retinal pigment epithelium* may be intact, proliferate [5, 44, 61, 67, 89] or disappear in late stages [67].
3. *In the retina*:
   - Retinal detachment by subretinal exudate and/or hemorrhage frequently occurs [5, 31, 67, 89, 92], while hemosiderin- and pigment-laden macrophages may be found scattered at the margins of the tumor [44].
   - A peripheral retinal tumor may secondarily give intra- or subretinal exudation in the macular area [93] and cause a subretinal, disciform scar in some instances [79].
   - There may be cystoid degeneration, hemorrhage, gliosis, exudate and degeneration of the neuro-epithelium [5, 67, 92].
   - The internal limiting membrane may be disrupted [61] or absent [64]. New vessels and fibroglial tissue may develop at the inner retinal surface and break into the subhyaloid space or vitreous in a fashion analogous to what is seen in proliferative retinopathy of other origin [5, 31, 61, 64, 89].
4. In the *vitreous*, fibrinous exudation [67] and hemorrhage [89] may occur in the later stages.
5. As ultimate secondary changes one may mention iridocyclitis, rubeosis iridis, secondary glaucoma or phtisis bulbi in the end stages of the

disease. In one particular case invasive growth has even been mentioned in the cornea [15].

X. Treatment

Although retinal angiomas may occasionally show spontaneous regression [74] or remain stable for prolonged period of times [49], retinal angiomas tend mostly to progress and provoke progressive exudation with ultimately loss of the eye. The purpose of the treatment should be to destroy the vascular anomaly. This can be performed by physical means.

1. Radiotherapy

Radiotherapy has been used in the past with limited success [84]. Ballantyne [8] published the histologic findings in an eye first treated with radon seeds, followed six months later by external radiation, with a total dosis of 4,750 rads. That eye lost vision two years later by a massive vitreous hemorrhage developed glaucoma and was eventually enucleated. Histology revealed more destruction of the normal retinal vessels than of the angioma or its feeders.

2. Transscleral diathermy

Diathermy was in fact the first successful treatment of retinal angiomas. The success, meaning a total destruction of the tumor with preservation or restoration of pre-operative vision, was obtained in up to 70% of the cases [84]. However, as attempts are made of destroying the tumor in a single procedure, this could result in excessive scleral and chorio-retinal damage [76]. Diathermy has actually been replaced in most instances by cryotherapy. However, perforating diathermy may still remain an effective method in the treatment of retinal angiomas larger than five papil diameters [13].

3. Cryotherapy

Cryotherapy is actually the treatment used for larger tumors, tumors situated beyond the reach of effective photocoagulation, in cases of associated retinal detachment or when the media are too hazy to permit correct photocoagulation [1, 2, 11, 38, 76, 88, 90].

A single application of cryotherapy is ineffective [53]. The method of choice is the triple freeze-thaw cycle [1], where the angioma is frozen transsclerally under close observation with the indirect ophthalmoscope, until it is completely white. The procedure is performed three times. In large tumors it is not always possible to freeze the entire angioma at once.

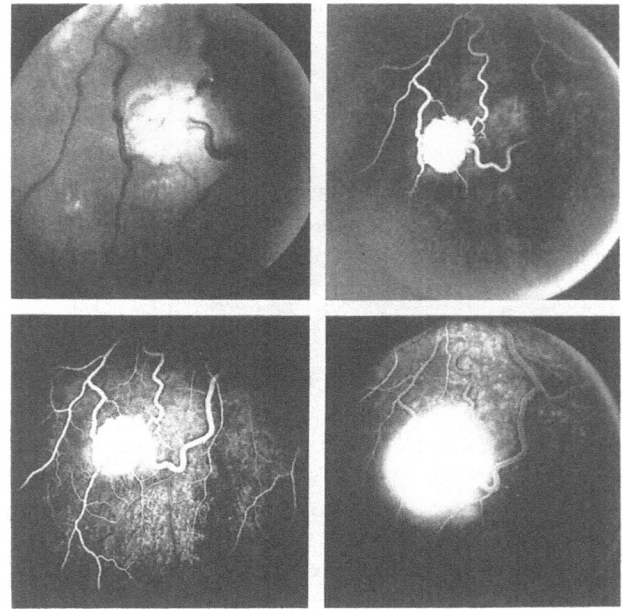

(a)

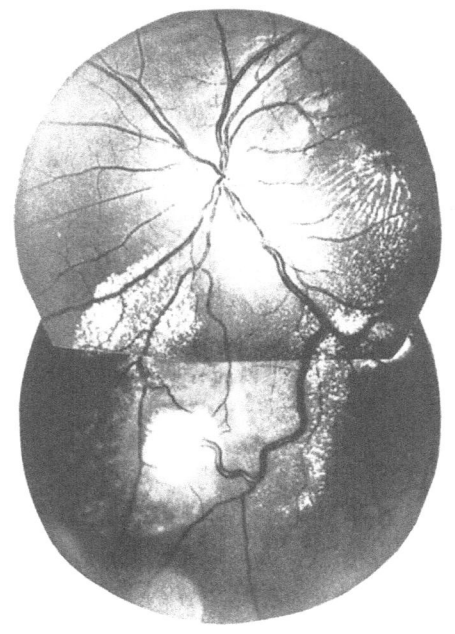

(b)

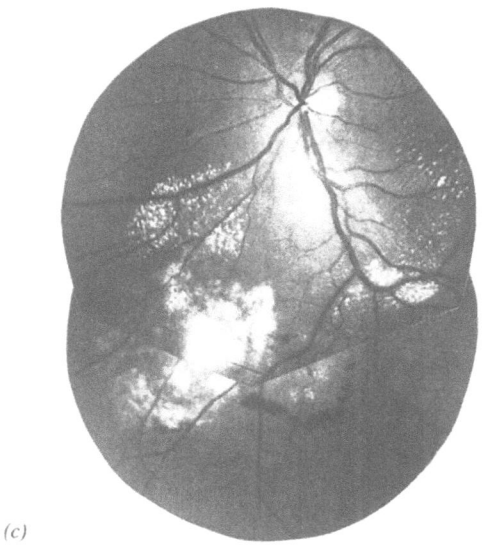

(c)

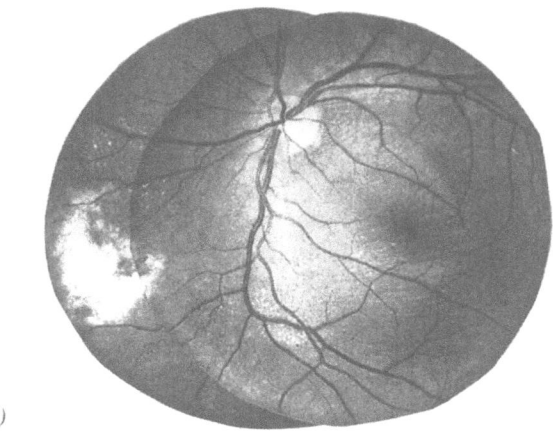

(d)

Figure 2–15.   a. retinal angioma before treatment, b. aspect after the first treatment (April 1983), c. aspect after the third treatment (September 1983), d. aspect one year later. Note the progressive normalization of the caliber of the feeder vessels and the regression of the lipoid exudates in the macular region.

The treatment must then be repeated with a six weeks to three months interval [88]. A successful treatment results in a progressive reduction in the size of the angiomas which are transformed into a chorioretinal scar. Even when on histologic examination the tumor proved to be completely destroyed and replaced by a fibrotic scar, the feeder vessels may still be patent [88]. Another disadvantage of the technique is that it usually produces extensive scars.

4. Photocoagulation

Photocoagulation can be performed with the Xenon arc or with the argon or dye laser. It is actually the best treatment when the lesion is smaller than two disc diameters and situated posterior to the equator [2, 4, 6, 9, 11, 30, 33, 76, 91]. Smaller lesions can be treated directly in a single session.

The technique we currently use is as follows: In a first session the tumor is surrounded by photocoagulation. Four to six weeks later the lesion itself is treated. Usually, several sessions are needed. When the treatment is sufficient a large scar remains, the feeder vessels normalize in size and are no more to be distinguished from normal retinal vessels and the exudative response around the tumor and in the macula gradually regresses (figs. 2–15, 2–16). In order to decrease the bloodflow into the tumor and thus to limit the risks of massive hemorrhages, it has been advocated to directly photocoagulate the arterial feeder. Because of the rapid flow, it is almost impossible to obtain a permanent occlusion of the feeder. A spasm is seen following the direct treatment of the feeder. However, the vessel reopens after a few seconds. Even after repeated photocoagulation the vessel may still remain patent. Even when using a suctioncup ophthalmodynamometer to increase intraocular pressure and reduce bloodflow [63], complete occlusion of the feeder is seldom obtained. The regression of the size of the blood vessels depends of the regression of the tumor.

Laser treatment is not always capable to destroy completely moderately large angiomas. Tissue destruction may be only superficial [4, 32]. Treated patients must be kept under surveillance, not only because they can develop new lesions but also because late recurrences of already treated angiomas are possible [32]. Fluorescein angiography is not always helpful in determining when retreatment is necessary, as even in the presence of viable lesion leakage is not always observed [32].

Photocoagulation of retinal angiomas may produce a number of complications [73, 91]:
1. Hemorrhages on top of the tumor are not unfrequent and usually regress easily. Massive hemorrhages are unusual and are often the result of too heavy treatment.
2. An increased exudation with resulting localized detachment is not uncommonly observed one day after photocoagulation. This may lead to a total retinal detachment which fortunately regresses spontaneously

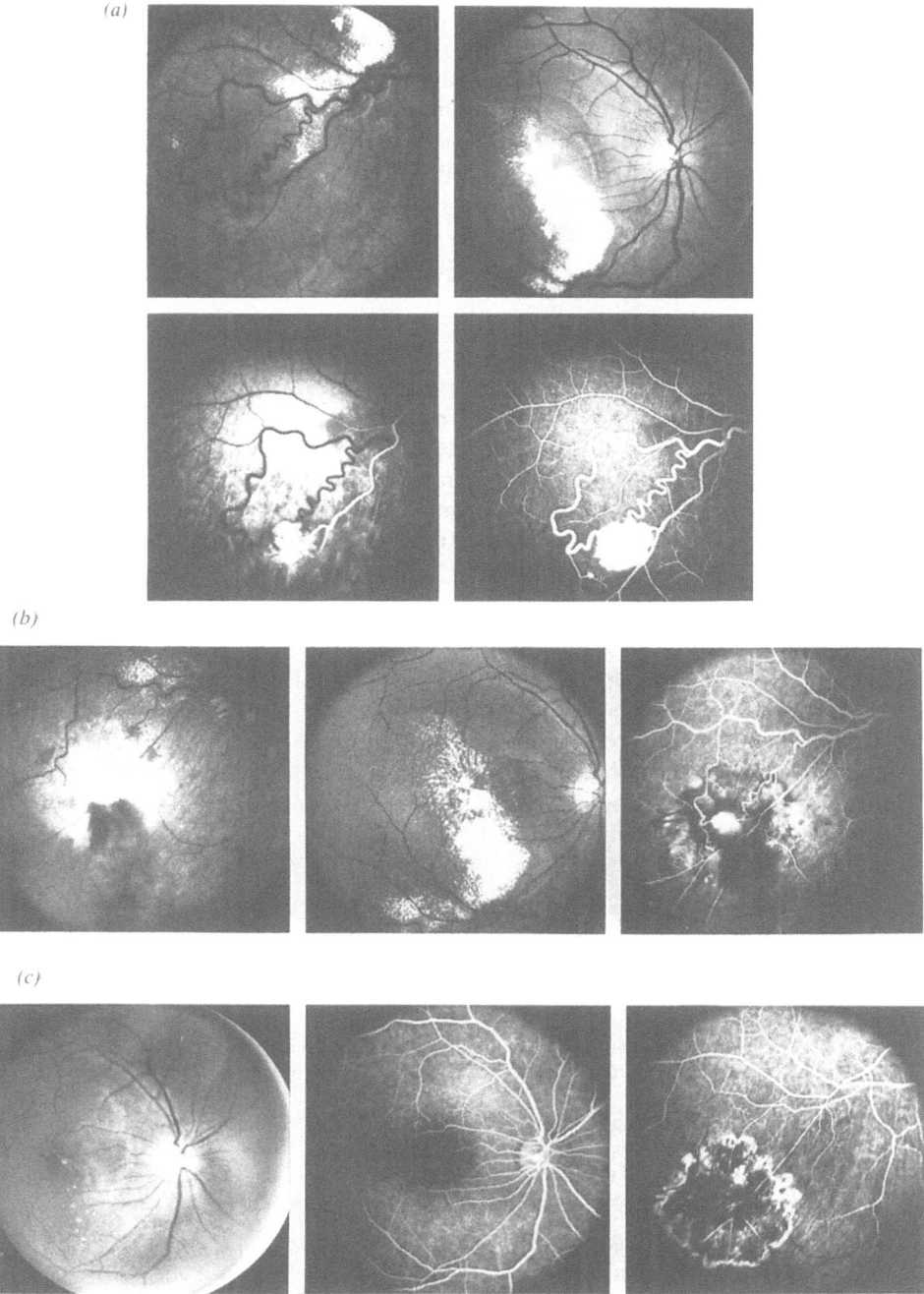

Figure 2–16.   a. retinal angioma with exudative detachment of the macula (April 1983), b. aspect after the third treatment (July 1983), c. situation 18 months after treatment. Total resorption of the exudative reaction. Note the presence of a chorioretinal anastomosis at the level of the coagulation scar.

(*ablatio fugax*). In order to avoid this complication it is better to treat in several sessions with less energy.

3. Proliferative vitreoretinopathy may be part of the evoluated form and may also be stimulated by an intensive treatment.

Annesley et al. compared the results of cryotherapy with that of photocoagulation in a series of 125 cases with a follow-up period ranging from 1 to 15 years. The results with both techniques were similar for lesions smaller than 2.5 disc diameter, whereas for larger lesions cryotherapy gave better results.

5. Surgery

Vitreoretinal surgery may be indicated in cases of vitreous hemorrhages, important fibrous strands or retinal detachment. In some cases a buckling procedure may have to be associated with subretinal fluid release and cryotherapy of an angioma. Peyman et al. [66] treated two patients with large angiomas by eye wall resection. The surgery was well tolerated and resulted in improved vision in one case and stable vision of 20/25 in the other.

The choice of the treatment mainly depends on the size and site of the lesion and on the associated findings such as retinal detachment, vitreous hemorrhage or fibrous strands. Photocoagulation is to be preferred in angiomas up to two disc diameters, provided the tumor can be reached and there is no associated retinal detachment. In the other cases cryocoagulation, possibly associated with vitreoretinal surgery, is the method of choice. Most important is that even after a successful treatment the patient must be followed regularly for the rest of his life.

References

1. Amoils S P and Smith TR (1969): Cryotherapy of angiomatosis retinae. *Arch Ophthalmol* 81: 689–691.
2. Annesley W H Jr, Leonard B C, Shields J A and Tasman W S (1977): Fifteen year review of treated cases of retinal angiomatosis. *Trans Am Acad Ophthalmol Otolaryngol* 83: 446–453.
3. Appelmans M, Verbruggen W, Fosse G and Reiter M (1972): La maladie de von Hippel-Lindau, hamartome, maladie tumorale multiple héréditaire. *Arch Ophthalmol*, 32: 521–530.
4. Apple D J, Goldberg M F and Wyhinny G J (1974): Argon laser treatment of von Hippel-Lindau, hamartome, maladie tumorale multiple héréditaire. *Arch Ophtalmol*, 32: 521–530. 92: 126–130.
5. Archer D B and Nevin N C (1977): The phakomatosis III. von Hippel-Lindau disease, pp. 1249–1274 in: Krill A E and Archer D B (eds), *Krill's hereditary retinal and choroidal diseases* Vol II Hagerstown: Harper and Row.
6. Augsburger J J, Shields J A, and Goldberg R E (1981): Classification and management of hereditary retinal angiomas. *Int Ophthalmol*, 4/1–2, 93–106.
7. Babel J (1972): Angiomatoses et malformations rétiniennes. *Bull Soc Ophtalmol Fr.* 72: 65–74.

8. Ballantyne A J (1942): Angiomatosis retinae: account of a case including histological results of X-ray treatment. *Proc Roy Soc Med*, 35: 345, cited by Vail D.

9. Baras I, Harris S and Galin M A (1964): Photocoagulation treatment of angiomatosis retinae *Am J Ophthalmol*, 58: 296–299.

10. Berblinger W (1922): Zur Auffassung von der sogenannten v. Hippelschen Krankheit der Netzhaut. *von Graefe's Arch Ophthalmol* 110: 395–413.

11. Bonnet M and Garmier G (1984): Traitement des angiomes capillaires rétiniens de la maladie de von Hippel. *J Fr Ophtalmol*, 7: 545–555.

12. Brandt R (1921): Zur Frage des Angiomatosis Retinae *von Graefe's Arch Ophthalmol*, 106: 127–165.

13. Cardoso R D and Brockhurst R J (1976): Perforating diathermy coagulation for retinal angiomas *Arch Ophthalmol*, 94: 1702–1715.

14. Chapman R C, Kempt V E and Taliaferro I (1959): Pheochromocytoma associated with multiple neurofibromatosis and intracranial hemangioma. *Am J Med*, 26: 883–890.

15. Collins E T (1894): Intra-ocular growths. I. Two cases, brother and sister, with peculiar vascular new-growth probably primarily retinal, affecting both eyes. *Trans Ophthalmol Soc U.K.*, 14: 141–149.

16. Czermak W (1905): Pathologisch-anatomisches Befund bei der von E. v. Hippel beschriebenen sehr seltenen Netzhauterkrankung. *Ber Dtsche Ophthalmol Ges*, 32: 184–195.

17. De Jong P T V M, Wiegel A R, Verkaart R J F and Majoor-Krakauer O F (1987): Twin vessels. A symptom of retinal angiomatosis (von Hippel-Lindau disease). *Ophthalmologica*, 193–3–86: 171–172. *Int Ophthalmol*. 10: 108.

18. Ditroi G (1923): Weitere Angaben zur Entwicklung der Angiomatosis Retinae. *Klin Mbl Augenheilk*, 71: 670–674.

19. Duke-Elder S and Dobree J H (1967): System of ophthalmology Vol X, *Diseases of the Retina*, London: Henry Kimpton, pp. 738–754.

20. Elliott R (1957): A case of von Hippel-Lindau syndrome. *Trans Ophthalmol Soc N.Z.*, 9: 18–24.

21. Fishbein F I, Schub M and Lesko W S (1972): Incontinentia pigmenti, pheochromocytoma and ocular abnormalities. *Am J Ophthalmol*, 73: 961.

22. Frenkel M (1967): Retinal angiomatosis in a patient with neurofibromatosis. *Am J Ophthalmol*. 63: 804–808.

23. Fuchs E (1887): Aneurysma arterio-venosum retinae. *Arch Augenheilk*, 11: 440–444.

24. Gamper F (1918): Ein klinischer und histologischer Beitrag zur Kenntnis der Angiomatosis Retinae. *Klin Mbl Augenheilk*, 61: 525–551.

25. Gass J D M (1977): Treatment of retinal vascular anomalies. *Trans Am Acad Ophthalmol Otolaryngol*, 83: 432–442.

26. Gass J D M (1987): Stereoscopic atlas of macular diseases. Diagnosis and treatment. The C V Mosby C°, St. Louis, 3rd edition.

27. Ginsberg S and Spiro G (1914): Uber Angiogliomatosis retinae (sog. v. Hippelsche Krankheit). *von Graefe's Arch Ophthalmol*, 88: 44–59.

28. Glushien A S, Mansuay M M and Littman D S (1953): Pheochromocytoma: its relationship to the neuro-cutaneous syndromes. *Am J Med*, 14: 318–327.

29. Go R C P, Lamiell J M, Hsia Y E and Y Paik (1984): Segregation and linkage analyses of von Hippel-Lindau disease among 220 descendants from one kindred. *Am J Hum Genet*, 36: 131–142.

30. Goldberg M F (1977): Clinico-pathologic correlation of von Hippel angiomas after Xenon arc and Argon laser photocoagulation. Chapt. 16, Peyman G A, Apple D J, Sanders D R eds, Intra-ocular Tumors, Appleton, Century Crofts, New York, 219–234.

31. Goldberg M F and Duke J R (1968): von Hippel-Lindau disease. Histopathologic findings in a treated and an untreated eye. *Am J Ophthalmol* 66: 693–705.

32. Goldberg M F and Koenig S (1974): Argon laser treatment of von Hippel-Lindau retinal angiomas. I. Clinical and angiographic findings. *Arch Ophthalmol* 92: 121–125.

33. Dupont-guerry D III, Wiesinger H and Ham W T (1958): Photocoagulation of the retina: report of a successfully treated case of angiomatosis retinae *Am J Ophthalmol* 46: 463–466.

34. Guzmann E (1915): Zur Histologie der Gliosis retinae diffusa. *von Graefe's Arch Ophthalmol*, 89: 323–336.
35. Hagler W S, Hyman B N and Waters W C (1971): von Hippel's angiomatosis retinae and pheochromocytoma. *Trans Am Acad Ophthalmol Otolaryngol*, 75: 1022–1034.
36. Haining W M and Zweifach P H (1967): Fluorescein angiography in von Hippel-Lindau disease. *Arch Ophthalmol*, 78: 475–479.
37. Hardwig P and Robertson D M (1984): von Hippel-Lindau disease: a familial often lethal, multisystem phakomatosis. *Ophthalmology*, 91: 263–1270.
38. Haut J, Limon S, Dhermy P, Marre J M (1974): Cryothérapie des angiomes rétiniens de la maladie de von Hippel-Lindau. *Bull Soc Ophtalmol Fr* 74: 1125–1129.
39. Heine L (1923): Uber Angiogliosis retinae mit Hirntumor (Capilläres Hämangiom) *Ztschr. Augenheilk*, 81: 1–14.
40. Horowitz P (1981): cited by Wing G L et al., *Ophthalmology*, 88: 1311–1314.
41. Horton W A, Wong V and Eldridge R (1976): von Hippel-Lindau disease. Clinical and pathological manifestations in 9 families with 50 affected members. *Arch Intern Med*, 136: 769–777.
42. Hubschmann O R, Vijayanathan T and Countee R W (1981): von Hippel-Lindau disease with multiple manifestations: diagnosis and management. *Neurosurgery*, 8: 92–95.
43. Jackson J H (1872): A series of cases illustrative of cerebral pathology. Case 1. *Med Tms Gaz*, II, 541.
44. Jakobiec F A, Font R L and Johnson F B (1976): Angiomatosis retinae. An ultrastructural study and lipoid analysis. *Cancer*, 38: 2042–2056.
45. Jesberg P O, Spencer W H and Hoyt W F (1968): Incipient lesions of von Hippel-Lindau disease. *Arch Ophthalmol* 80: 632–640.
46. Joe S and Spencer W H (1964): von Hippel-Lindau disease. *Arch Ophthalmol*, 71: 508–509.
47. Kawamura J, Garcia J H and Kamiyo Y (1973): Cerebellar hemangioblastoma: histogenesis of stromal cells. *Cancer* 31: 1528–1540.
48. Kawasaki K, Yanagida T, Yonemura D, Morita Y, Matsuda T, and Shiraishi Y (1975): Chromosomal study in a family with von Hippel disease. *Jap J Ophthalmol*, 19, 175–183; *Rinsho Ganka* 29: 287–292.
49. Keith C G (1973): Angiomatosis retinae. *Br J Ophthalmol*, 57: 593–594.
50. Kobayashi M and Shimada K (1966): Chromosomal aberrations in von Hippel-Lindau's disease. Report of two cases. *Jap J Ophthalmol*, 10: 186–192.
51. Kollarits C R, Mehelas T J, Shealy T R and Zahn J R (1982): von Hippel tumors in siblings with retinitis pigmentosa. *Ann. Ophthalmol*, 14: 256–259.
52. Kupersmith M J and Berenstein A (1981): Visual disturbances in von Hippel-Lindau disease. *Ann Ophthalmol*, 13: 195–197.
53. Lincoff H J, Mc Clean J and Long R (1967): The cryosurgical treatment of intra-ocular tumors *Am J Ophthalmol*, 63: 389–399.
54. Lindau A (1926): Studiën über Kleinhirnsystem: Bau, Pathogenese und Beziehungen zur Angiomatosis Retinae. *Acta Pathol Microbiol Scand Suppl I*, 1.
55. Lindau A (1927): Zur Frage der Angiomatosis Retinae und ihrer Hirnkomplikationen. *Acta Ophthalmol*, 4: 193–226.
56. Lowden B A and Harris G S (1976): Pheochromocytoma and von Hippel-Lindau's disease. *Can J Ophthalmol*, 11: 282–289.
57. Macrae H M and Newbigin B (1968): von Hippel-Lindau disease: a family history. *Can J Ophthalmol*, 3: 28–34.
58. Magnus H (1874): Aneurysma arterio-venosum retinalis *Virchows Arch Path Anat*, 60: 38.
59. Magnusson L and Tornquist R (1973): Incipient lesions in angiomatosis retinae. *Acta Ophthalmol* 51: 152–158.
60. Meller J (1913): Uber das Wesen der sog. Hippelsche Netzhauterkrankung. *von Graefe's Arch Ophthalmol* 85: 255–272.
61. Mottow-Lippa L, Tso M O M, Peyman G A and Chejfec G (1983): von Hippel angioma-

tosis. A light, electron-microscopic and immunoperoxydase characterization. *Ophthalmology*, 90: 848–855.

62. Murphy M E and Johnson P C (1975): Possible contribution of basement membrane to the structural rigidity of blood capillaries *Microvasc Res*, 9: 242–245.

63. Nicholson D H (1983): Induced ocular hypertension during photocoagulation of afferent artery in angiomatosis retinae. *Retina*, 3: 59–61.

64. Nicholson D H, Green W R and Kenyon K R (1976): Light and electron-microscopic study of early lesions on angiomatosis retinae. *Am J Ophthalmol*, 82: 193–204.

65. Panas F and Remy A (1879): Anatomie pathologique de l'oeil. Adrien Delahaye et Cie, Paris.

66. Peyman G A, Rednam K R V, Mottow-Lippa L and Flood T (1983): Treatment of large von Hippel tumors by eye wall resection. *Ophthalmology*, 90: 840–847.

67. Pulhorn G and Fauth E (1975): Klinik und Histopathologie der von Hippel-Lindauschen Erkrankung. *Klin Mbl Augenheilk*, 167: 884–891.

68. Reese A B (1976): Tumors of the eye. Harper and Row Publ., 3rd edition, New York, 266–269.

69. Reich H and Hollwich F (1984): Zum von Hippel-Lindau syndrom. *Klin Mbl Augenheilk* 184: 513–519.

70. Ridley M, Green J and Johnson G (1986): Retinal angiomatosis: the ocular manifestations of von Hippel-Lindau disease. *Can J Ophthalmol*, 21: 276–283.

71. Rumbaur W (1941): Uber Angiomatosis retinae (von Hippel-Lindausche Krankheit) *Klin Mbl Augenheilk*, 106: 168–198.

72. Salazar F G and Lamiell J M (1980): Early identification of retinal angiomas in a large kindred with von Hippel-Lindau disease. *Am J Ophthalmol*, 89: 540–545.

73. Schieck F (1912): Das Peritheliom der Netzhautzentralgefässe, ein bislang unbekanntes Krankheitsbild. Auf Grund einer klinischen und pathologisch-anatomischen Beobachtung dargestellt. *von Graefe's Arch Ophthalmol*, 81: 328–339.

74. Schmidt D and Neumann H P H (1987): Atypische retinale Veränderungen bei Hippel-Lindau Syndrom. *Fortschr. Ophthalmol.*, 84: 187–189.

75. Seidel E (1932): Anatomische Frühstadien der Angiomatosis retinae (v. Hippelsche Erkrankung) *Ber Dtsche Ophthalmol Ges*, 49: 535–541.

76. Sellors P J H and Archer D (1969): The management of retinal angiomatosis *Trans Ophthalmol Soc U.K.*, 89: 529–543.

77. Shields J F (1983): Vascular tumors of the retina and optic disc. in Diagnosis and management of intra-ocular tumors, the C V Mosby C°, St Louis, Toronto, London, 534–568.

78. Spence A H and Rubinstein L J (1975): Cerebellar capillary hemangioblastoma: its histogenesis studied by organ culture and electron microscopy. *Cancer*, 35: 326–341.

79. Spencer W H (1985): *Ophthalmic Pathology. An Atlas and Textbook*, Vol. 2, pp. 631–643, 3rd ed., W B Saunders and C°; Philadelphia, London, Toronto.

80. Thomas J V. Schwartz P L and Gragoudas E S (1978): von Hippel's disease in association with von Recklinghausen's neurofibromatosis. *Br J Ophthalmol*, 62: 604–608.

81. Tishler P V (1975): A family with coexistent von Recklinghausen's neurofibromatosis and von Hippel-Lindau's disease. Diseases possibly derived from a common gene. *Neurology*, 25: 840–844.

82. Tuppurainen K and Tersvirta M (1985): von Hippel-Lindau's angiomatosis. A disease with multiple manifestations. *Acta Ophthalmol*, 63: (suppl. 173), 57–59.

83. Uehara M and Ichinomiya T (1975): A case of intraorbital optic nerve hemangioblastoma associated with von Hippel's disease (Japanese). *Folia Ophthalmol Jap*, 26: 1219–1226.

84. Vail D (1958): Angiomatosis retinae 11 years after diathermy coagulation. *Am J Ophthalmol*, 46: 525–534.

85. Van Der Hoeve J (1932): Doyne Memorial Lecture: Eye Symptoms in Phakomatosis *Trans Ophthalmol Soc U.K.*, 52: 380–401.

86. von Hippel E (1911): Die anatomische Grundlage der von mir beschriebenen 'sehr seltenen

Erkrankung der Netzhaut'. *von Graefe's Arch Ophthalmol*, 79: 350–377.

87. Vracko R (1974): Basal lamina layering in diabetes mellitus, evidence for accelerated rate of cell death and cell regeneration. *Diabetes*, 23: 94–104.

88. Watzke R C (1974): Cryotherapy for retinal angiomatosis: a clinicopathologic report. *Arch Ophthalmol*, 92: 399–401.

89. Watzke R C, Weingeist T A and Constantine J A (1977): Diagnosis and management of von Hippel-Lindau disease. Chapt. 15 in Peyman, Apple, Sanders Eds., Intraocular tumors, Appleton, Century Crofts, New York, 199–217.

90. Welch R B (1970): von Hippel-Lindau disease: the recognition and treatment of early angiomatosis retinae and the use of cryosurgery as an adjunct to therapy. *Trans Am Ophthalmol Soc*, 68: 367–424.

91. Wessing A (1967): Ten years of light-coagulation in retinal angiomatosis *Klin Mbl Augenheilk*, 150: 57–71.

92. Wing G L, Weiter J J, Kelly P J, Albert D M and Gonder J R (1981): von Hippel-Lindau disease. Angiomatosis of the retina and central nervous system. *Ophthalmology*, 88: 1311–1314.

93. Wise G N, Dollery C T and Henkind P (1971): The retinal circulation. Harper and Row, New York.

94. Wise G N and Wangvivat Y (1966): The exaggerated macular response to vascular disease. *Am J Ophthalmol*, 61: 1459–1463.

3   Capillary Hemangioma of the optic disc

The diagnosis of an angioma of the optic disc is not always easy. Up to the 1970's these cases were usually diagnosed after removal of the eye either because of secondary complications or because the lesion was considered clinically as a malignant melanoma. In 1972 Oosterhuis and Rubinstein [38] described the clinical and fluoroangiographic characteristics of hemangiomas of the disc and predicted that improved diagnostic methods would bring to light more cases.

I. Classification of angiomatous tumors of the optic disc

Three main types of angiomatous tumors of the optic disc may be considered [3]:
1. *Capillary angioma.* Capillary angiomas of the optic disc may or may not be associated with retinal angiomatosis and are considered as a peculiar form of von Hippel's disease.
2. *Cavernous angioma.* Cavernous angiomas of the optic disc are very rare. They may also be associated with a cavernous hemangioma of the retina.
3. *Angioma racemosum.* In such cases the involvement of the optic disc is only part of the fundus lesion.
   In this chapter the discussion will be limited to capillary angiomas of the disc. Cavernous angiomas will be dealt with in chapter 4 and angioma racemosum in chapter 5.

II. Incidence

Schindler et al. [45] traced 58 cases of hemangiomas of the disc published from 1912 to 1975 and added seven additional cases. Since then at least 30 other cases were published [1, 3, 7, 12–14, 21, 26, 27, 35–37, 41, 47, 50, 52].

59% of the patients are males and 41% are females. In 52% only the right eye is affected, in 40% only the left eye and in 8% bilateral involvement was noticed [45]. Bilateral cases were described by a number of authors [9, 18, 20, 21, 30, 48].

III. Clinical features

Capillary hemangiomas of the optic disc are usually diagnosed during the third decade, in 53% of the cases because of visual loss and in 30% on routine examination in patients without subjective signs. The other cases were found after enucleation for secondary glaucoma or leucocoria or during a systematic investigation of members of families with von Hippel-Lindau's disease. The earliest clinical aspect is probably that of a flat vascular lesion, better detected by fluorescein angiography [26]. An angioma of the disc was even an incidental finding during autopsy in a patient with von Hippel-Lindau, where the retina and optic nerve had been clinically considered as normal [35].

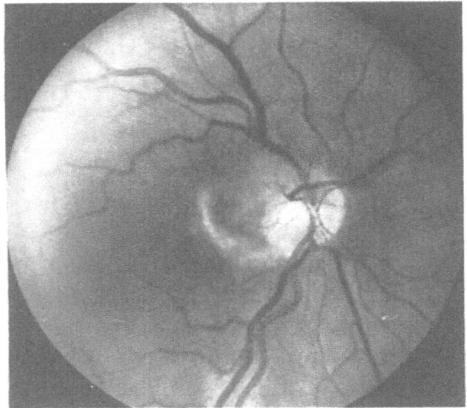

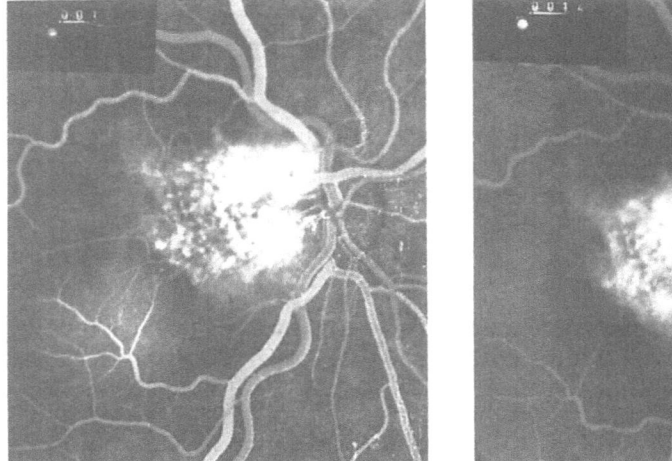

Figure 3–1.   Optic disc hemangioma on the right optic disc in a 62 year old woman. a. aspect in redfree light. b, c. fluoroangiography. The uninvolved part of the optic disc does not stain in the late sequence of the fluoroangiography.

The clinical aspect of capillary angiomas of the optic disc and of the juxtapapillary retina is determined by their location. They can be endo-phytic, sessile or exophytic [18, 20, 21]. Endophytic tumors are the most characteristic. The lesion is usually small (about 1/2 to 1 DD) and slightly elevated. Its color is pink or grayish [3, 12, 45]. The tumor involves a portion of the optic disc and of the juxtapapillary retina. The unaffected part of the disc may appear completely normal. Fluorescein angiography indicates a cluster of dilated capillaries. They fill simultaneously with the retinal circulation and leak fluorescein profusely. The unaffected part of the disc does however not show abnormal late staining (Figs 3–1, 3–2).

Whereas endophytic tumors protrude from the inner surface of the papilla or peripapillary retina, sessile or exophytic angiomas develop in the middle and outer layers of the juxtapapillary retina [18, 20, 21]. They appear as an ill-defined thickening of the disc and surrounding retina [2]. Even with fundus biomicroscopy it is not always possible to define the angiomatous nature of the tumor and it is therefore not surprising that these lesions are often misdiagnosed. Fluorescein angiography shows an increased fluorescence of the affected part of the disc and of the juxtapapillary retina (Fig. 3–3). The angioma may be associated with disc edema (Fig. 3–4), which may possibly subside spontaneously.

The ophthalmoscopic aspect as well of endo- as of exophytic tumors may be modified by secondary phenomenons such as glial proliferation, preretinal fibrosis, hemorrhages, lipoid exudates or exudative localized or diffuse retinal detachment (Figs 3–5, 3–6, 3–7).

In capillary angiomas of the optic disc, feeder vessels are almost always missing. However, we did observe a typical feeding arteriole in a patient with a von Hippel of the disc (Fig. 3–7). Some of these tumors have little tendency to grow even for periods of ten years or more [12, 27]. The tumor may however progress. Visual loss is usually the result of an exudative response with lipoid exudates in the macular region or with an exudative retinal detachment [3, 21, 45]. The chronic exudation is probably also a stimulus to fibroglial proliferation resulting in preretinal fibrosis and macular

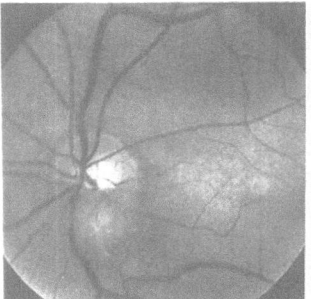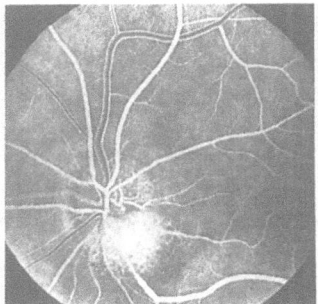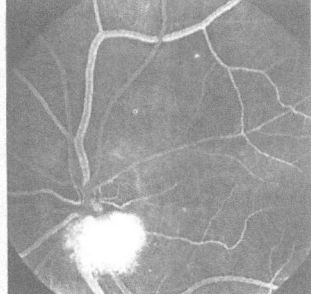

Figure 3–2. Capillary hemangioma of the optic disc (endophytic) in the left eye of a 65 year old woman.

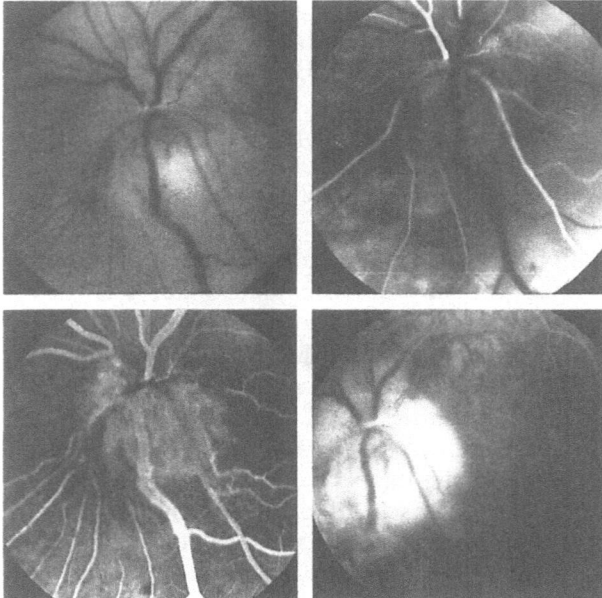

Figure 3–3.   Exophytic angioma of the left optic disc of a 32-year old woman. The redfree picture shows a tumoral mass mainly affecting the inferior half of the optic disc. Note the dilated retinal veins and the intense staining on fluoroangiography.

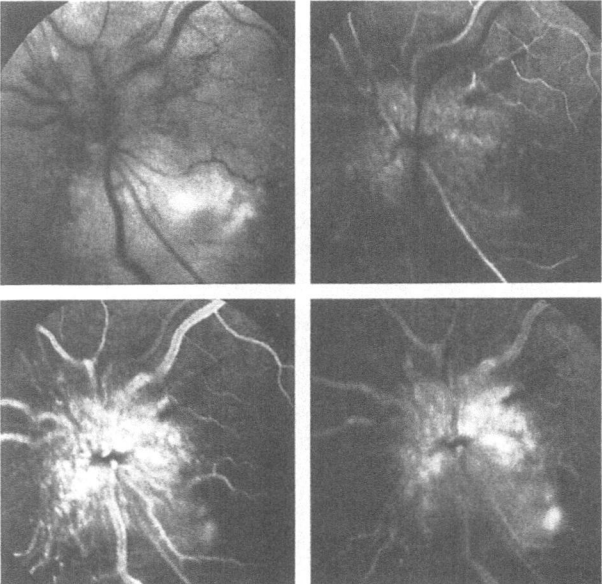

Figure 3–4.   Same eye as Fig. 3–3 two months later. Massive associated papiledema. The edema will gradually regress spontaneously and six months later the fundus had regained the initial appearance.

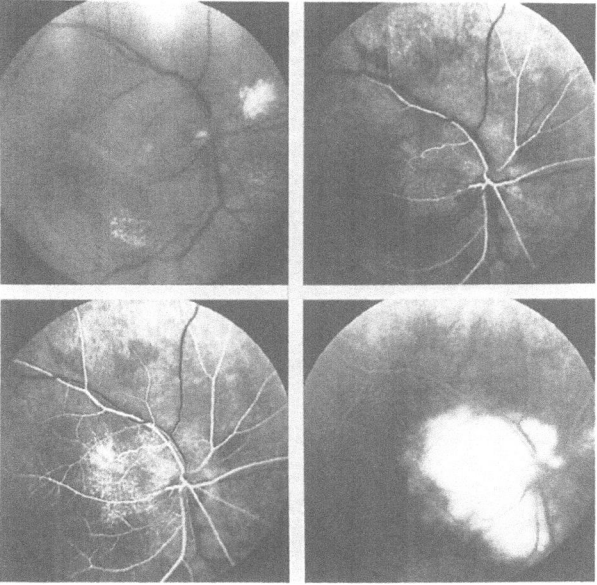

Figure 3–5. Capillary angioma of the disc complicated by a serous detachment of the macular region.

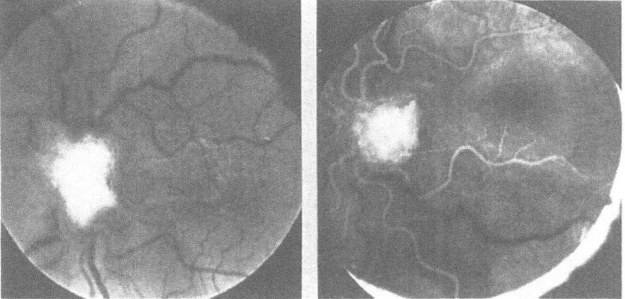

Figure 3–6. Optic disc angioma covered by glial tissue and associated with preretinal fibrosis resulting in macular distortion.

traction (Figs 3–6, 3–8). The exudative reaction is sometimes only temporary, so that the fundus aspect or the vision may improve again [12, 49]. Spontaneous sclerosis of an angioma has been observed [38]. But repeated vitreous bleeding [38], chronic exudation, exudative retinal detachment and secondary glaucoma may be the cause of the functional loss of the affected eye [7, 21, 28, 32, 48, 54].

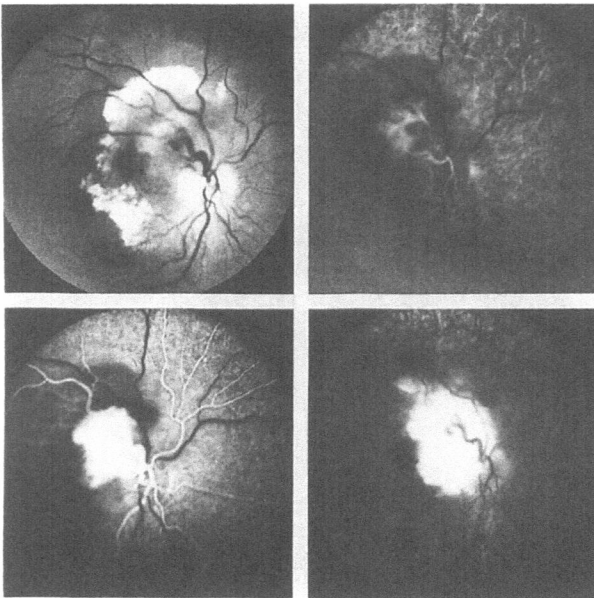

Figure 3–7.   Capillary angiomas of the optic disc and the peripapillary retina. Note the distinct arterial feeder as well as the marked exudative response.

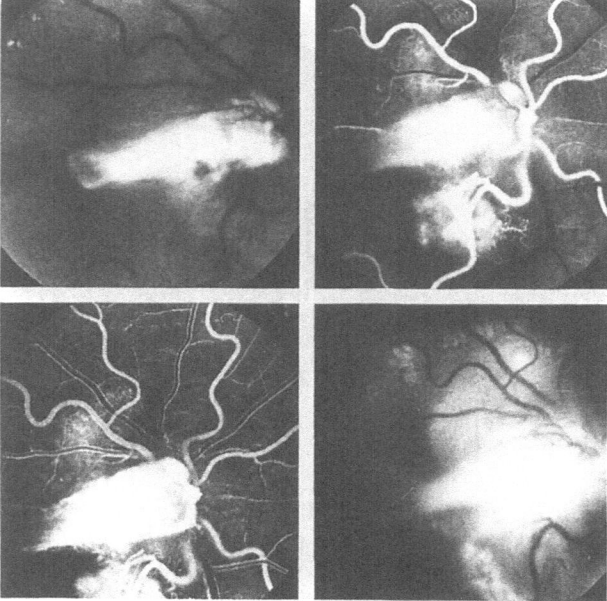

Figure 3–8.   Capillary angioma of the disc and the juxtapapillary retina in a 52 year old man who had been operated on at the age of 34 years for a cerebellar hemangioblastoma. The right eye shows dense, glial tissue extending from the optic disc towards the macula and covering three angiomas which are only revealed by fluorescein angiography.

IV. Relationship with von Hippel-Lindau's disease

Franceschetti and Babel [16] were the first to consider the hemangioma of the optic disc as a form of von Hippel's disease. Almost 50% of patients with retinal capillary angiomas may present with hemangiomas of the disc or of the juxtapapillary retina and 43% of the patients with optic disc angiomas have also retinal angiomas [21, 45]. However, as Gass and Braunstein [21] pointed out, the true incidence of solitary hemangiomas of the optic disc is probably higher than reported in the literature as a large number of cases may have been misdiagnosed or have not been published.

A number of cases of angioma of the disc has been found in families with vHL disease or associated with its neurological or systemic complications [7, 9, 12, 14, 25, 26, 30, 35, 38, 45, 46].

V. Diagnosis

The diagnosis of capillary hemangioma of the optic disc is mainly based on the ophthalmoscopic, biomicroscopic and fluoroangiographic appearance of the lesion [12, 21, 36, 38]. A careful examination permits to define the extent of the lesion and to appreciate the secondary phenomenons.

In doubtful cases echography may be of some help in differentiating a hemangioma from a malignant melanoma, provided the lesion has an elevation of more than 1 mm. In contrast with the low reflectivity of malignant melanoma on A-scan, hemangiomas are characterized by a tissue reflectivity of 60 to 100% [22].

VI. Differential diagnosis

Hemangiomas of the optic disc have to be differentiated from other tumoral or pseudotumoral conditions of the optic disc [45].

1. Papiledema
Papiledema may sometimes be confused with angiomas of the disc. On the other hand papiledema may complicate the clinical appearance of a capillary angioma of the disc (Fig. 3–4).

In hemangiomas of the disc the vascu   anomalies, as seen on fluorescein angiography, are usually confined to one sector of the disc and of the juxtapapillary region, whereas in papiledema all the epipapillary capillaries are affected. In ischemic optic neuropathy however, a sectorial dilatation of optic disc capillaries can be observed [11]. In such cases nevertheless, the late fluorescence is not limited to the sector of the disc, but affects the whole optic disc, whereas the late fluorescence of hemangiomas is usually confined to the tumor. Also the clinical context and the functional signs are quite different, so that the differential diagnosis between ischemic optic neuropathy and angiomas of the disc does not present major difficulties.

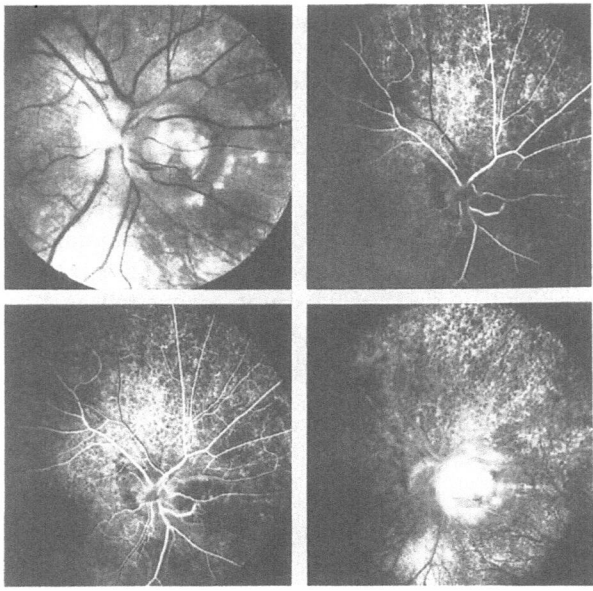

Figure 3–9.

2. Drusen of the optic disc

Drusen of the optic disc may present diagnostic difficulties when they are buried. The absence of marked late staining on fluorescein angiography and sometimes echography may be helpful. As drusen of the disc may be dominantly inherited, it makes sense to also examine the parents when there is still doubt.

3. Peripapillary, choroidal neovascularization

A peripapillary, disciform response may be found as a consequence of drusen of the optic disc or of previous inflammatory conditions such as Harada's disease or presumed histoplasmosis choroiditis. It may also be found in degenerative condition, angioid streaks or age-related changes.

We observed a bilateral case with pseudotumoral aspect in a young Tunesian woman who had been treated a few years before for Harada's disease from which she completely recovered (Figs 3–9, 3–10). According to her Tunesian ophthalmologist no tumor was seen at the optic discs during the acute phase of the disease.

4 Arterial macro-aneurysms

Although the clinical aspect of an arterial macro-aneurysm is very typical, the marked exudative reaction may lead to confusion [4].

5. Inflammatory conditions

Inflammatory conditions such as sarcoid may mimic a vascular tumor.

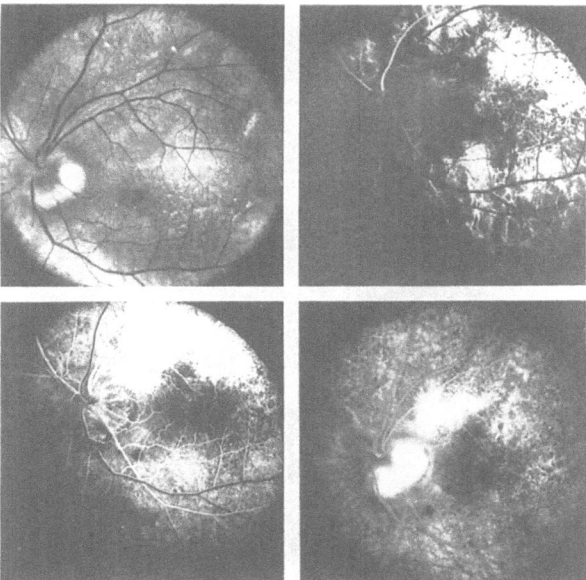

Figure 3–10. Patient who was previously treated for Harada's disease. The optic disc lesions are probably not angiomatous lesions but rather choroidal neovascularization as a complication of the previous chorioretinal inflammation.

6. Congenital lesions

Congenital lesions such as persistant hyperplastic primary vitreous can be sometimes mistaken for an angiomatous tumor.

7. Tumors

Hemangiomas of the optic disc have to be differentiated from other tumors. As seen in a following chapter, the astrocytic hamartoma of tuberous sclerosis may be markedly vascularized, which makes the differentiation with an hemangioma more difficult. The diagnosis will partly depend on the pink color of the angioma as compared to the more pearly white aspect of an astrocytic hamartoma.

Angiomas of the disc have been mistaken for other tumors such as choroidal hemangiomas, metastatic tumors or malignant melanomas. In most cases of angioma of the optic disc, described in the literature before 1970, the diagnosis was only made after the eye was removed for suspicion of a malignant melanoma.

Hyperplasia of the retinal pigment epithelium can also be confused with angiomas to the disc [45]. One of the patients we previously described in a series of patients with angiomas of the disc [12, case 4] was probably a hyperplasia of the disc. This patient was first seen by us in 1973. Ten years

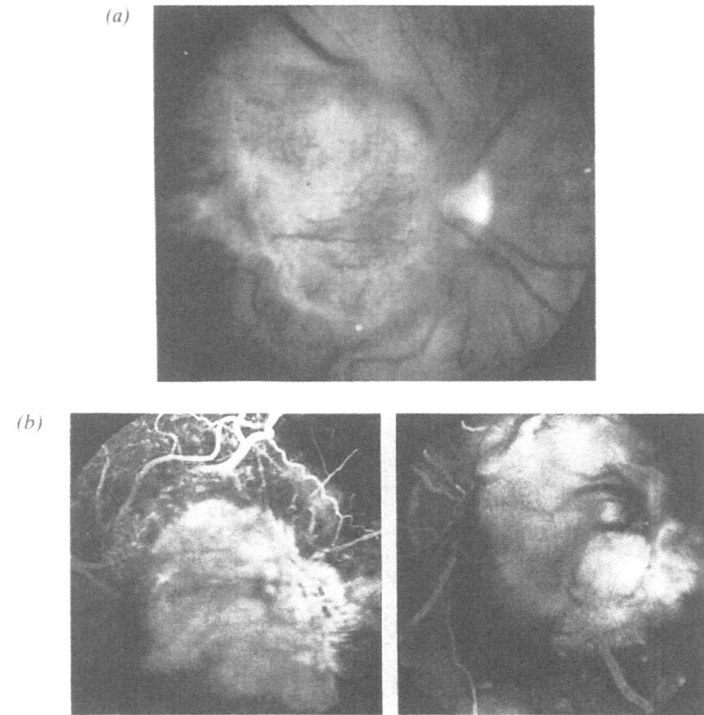

Figure 3–11.   a. ophthalmoscopic aspect b. fluoroangiography of a lesion which was clinically diagnosed as an angioma of the optic disc.

before a lesion was found in the left papillo-macular area and diagnosed as cicatricial chorioretinitis. When we saw her for the first time the right eye was normal, whereas the left eye presented a highly vascularized mass on the temporal site of the disc extending towards the macula (Fig. 3–11a). The lesion was 3 d elevated and 3 DD large. Fluorescein angiography showed large vessels in the lesion and extensive late diffusion (Fig. 3–11b). Treatment with the argon laser resulted in some reduction of the lesion, which from then on remained stable for almost ten years.

In July 1984 a serous detachment was noted in the upper temporal quadrant of the left eye and in October 1985 the eye developed secondary glaucoma and was subsequently enucleated. Much to our surprise, on histologic examination there was no evidence of an angiomatous tumor but an aspect suggestive of hyperplasia of the retinal pigment epithelium (Figs. 3–12, 3–13, 3–14) [23].

VII. Histopathology

Wallner and Moorman [53] found in the literature 8 cases with pathological examination: six of them were diagnosed as von Hippel's tumors and two as

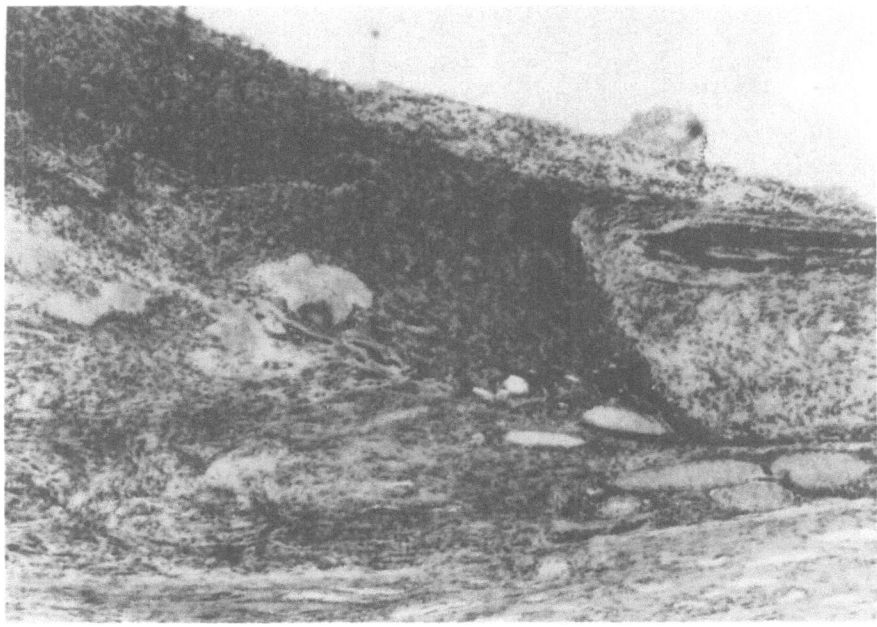

Figure 3–12.   Histopathology of the eye seen in Fig. 3–11. Sharp transition between the altered retina at the periphery of the lesion and the tumor. Continuity between the superficial tumor and the RPE.

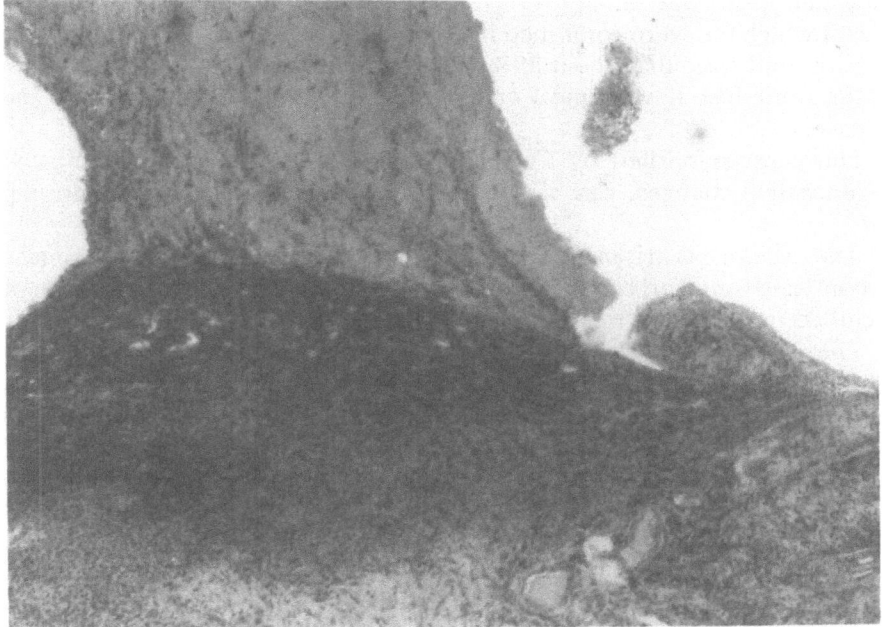

Figure 3–13.   Prepapillary and pretumoral granulation tissue extending into the vitreous (same eye as Fig. 3–11).

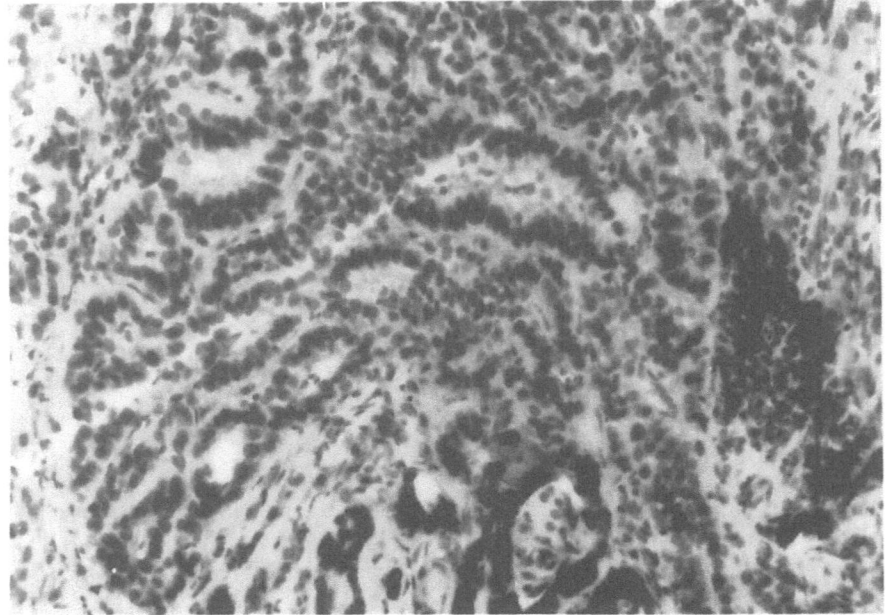

Figure 3-14.   Tubular or pseudo-acinar arrangement of the tumor cells (same eye as Fig. 3-11).

endotheliomas. Darr et al. [9] reported 14 cases of von Hippel tumors at the disc of which ten were confirmed histologically. Schindler et al. [45] reviewed 55 cases and state that about 25% of the patients with capillary hemangioma of the optic disc have clinical or hereditary features of von Hippel-Lindau disease.

The case, published by Carr and Stallard [6] as angiogliomatosis with degenerative changes, can be considered as von Hippel's angiomatosis [42, 53].

The case of Nastri and Basile [32], published as angio-endothelioma – as it consisted only of capillaries and endothelial cells –, was later on also included in the group of von Hippel's disease [42].

The case of Souders [49] was first diagnosed as mixed type glioma, but later reclassified as hemangio-endothelioma or von Hippel's disease [42, 53].

Finally, Weisse's case [54] was diagnosed as capillary angioma or angioma simplex.

Several pathologically confirmed cases of von Hippel's disease were reported [5, 8, 9, 16, 29–31, 34, 39, 42, 51, 55]. In practically all cases, both the disc and the peripapillary retina were involved. There seems to be a predilection for the temporal portion [9].

In one case [51] only the disc was involved, in one only the peripapillary retina but in both eyes, while in another the optic nerve was also invaded [8].

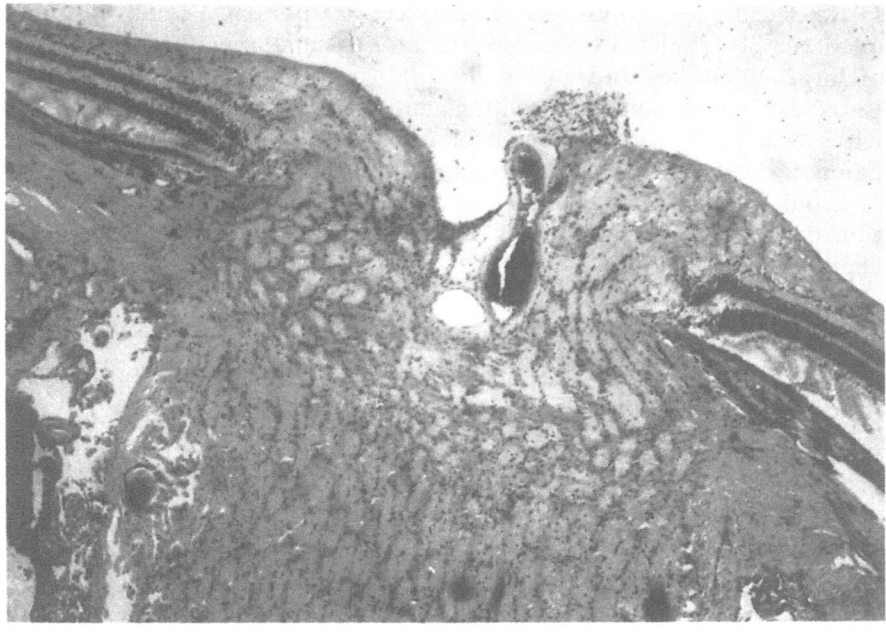

(a)

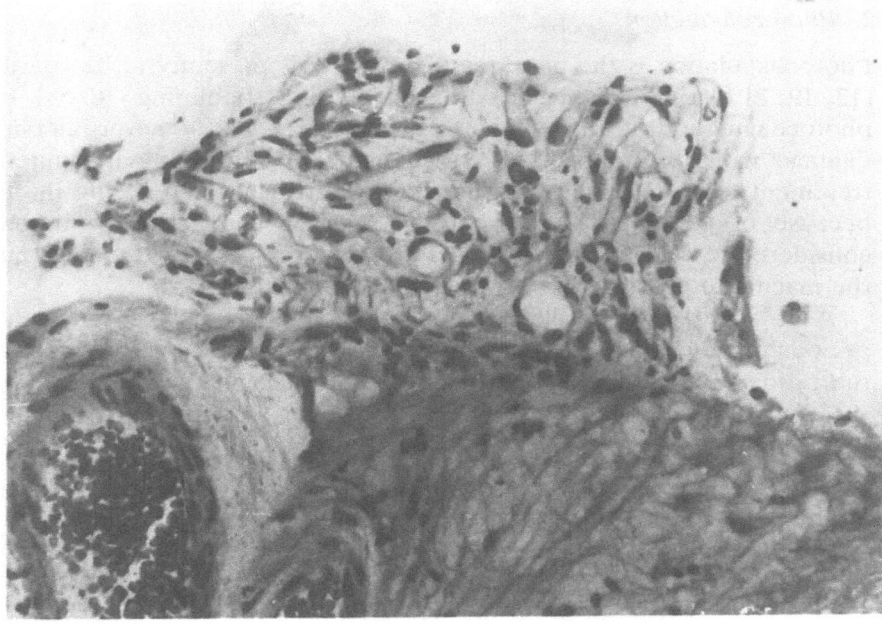

(b)

Figure 3–15. von Hippel-Lindau's disease. Capillary hemangioma of the optic disc. a. general view b. higher magnification 6820 H & E (Courtesy of Dr D. De Wolf-Rouendaal, Leiden).

Histologically, the optic disc lesions consist of many small endothelium-lined vessels, similar in size and structure to capillaries (Fig. 3–15), clusters of large capillaries and glial tissue [35], or proliferating small vessels [9]. Large astrocytes, sometimes with gigantiform nuclei and large cystoid spaces with watery or proteinaceous exudate can be found (9). In the optic disc laminated calcific masses may be found anterior to the lamina cribrosa [9].

Lipid deposits or foam cells may be absent and there may be communication between the angioma and the capillaries of the optic disc and choriocapillaris [35].

VIII. Treatment

As these lesions tend to grow and may provoke extensive exudative reaction resulting ultimately in functional loss of the eye, treatment has to be considered.

1. Radiotherapy

Radiotherapy has been used in two cases. One [33] treated with radon seeds developed cataract, whereas in the other [43] the lesion was not reduced in size after radiotherapy, although it appeared stabilized.

2. Photocoagulation

Photocoagulation is the only treatment which is presently to be considered [13, 19, 21, 38, 45]. The results are sometimes disappointing [36, 56]. Heavy photocoagulation of an angioma of the disc may lead to severe nerve fibre damage with resulting loss of visual field [13]. In exophytic tumors the treatment has little chance to succeed in destroying or reducing the tumor because of the deep location of the vascular anomaly [21]. It may be considered to place a barrier of photocoagulations between the angioma and the macula to prevent central spread of the exudate.

As a number of capillary angiomas may remain stable for prolonged periods of time, the risks of treating such cases should only be taken when the exudative reaction undoubtly jeopardizes macular function.

References

1. Appelmans M, Decock G and Van Opstal R (1949): Traitement de l'angiome rétinien par diathermocoagulation. *Bull Soc Belge Ophtalmol* 92: 326–340.
2. Augsburger J J, Shields J A and Goldberg R E (1981): Classification and management of hereditary retinal angiomas. *Int Ophthalmol* 4: 93–106.
3. Brown G C and Shields J A (1985): Tumors of the optic nerve head. *Survey Ophthalmol*, 29: 239–264.
4. Brown G A and Weinstock F (1985): Arterial macro-aneurysm on the optic disc presenting as a mass lesion. *Ann Ophthalmol*, 15: 519–520.

5. Calmettes L, Deodati F and Bec P (1957): Tumeurs de la papille. *Bull Soc Ophtalmol Fr*, 10: 704–706.
6. Carr T A and Stallard H B (1933): A case of angiogliomatosis retinae with pathological report. *Br J Ophthalmol*, 17: 525–528.
7. Cordier J, Aflalo J and Raspiller A (1978): Angiome de la papille et maladie de von Hippel-Lindau. *Bull Soc Ophtalmol Fr*, 73: 973–983.
8. Cross A G (1943): Angioma of the retina. *Br J Ophthalmol*, 27: 372–373.
9. Darr J L, Hughes R P and Mc Nair J (1966): Bilateral peripapillary retinal hemangiomas. *Arch Ophthalmol*, 75: 77–81.
10. Davies W and Thumin M (1956): Cavernous hemangioma of the optic disc and retina. *Trans Am Acad Ophthalmol Otolaryngol*, 60: 217.
11. De Laey J J (1982): Sémiologie fluorescéïnique de la papille. *J Fr Ophtalmol*, 5: 639–648.
12. De Laey J J and Leys A (1978): Haemangiomas of the optic disc. *Doc Ophthalmol Proc Series* 17: 205–213.
13. Deutman A F and Aan De Kerk A L (1987): Diagnosis and therapy of parapapillary hemangioma. *Ophthalmologica*, 193: 170–171.
14. Dhoine G, Constantinides G and Madelain Fr (1977): Les angiomatoses papillaires. *Bull Soc Belge Ophtalmol* 190: 87–97.
15. Feig I (1938): A case of angioma retinae. *Br J Ophthalmol*, 22: 295–300.
16. Franceschetti O and Babel J (1954): Microangiome avec dégénérescence kystique de la rétine (forme monosymptomatique d'une maladie de von Hippel-Lindau ?) *Ophthalmologica*, 128: 23–29.
17. Frandsen A D (1950): A case of hemangioma retinae. *Acta Ophthalmol*, 28: 97–102.
18. Gass J D M (1974): Differential diagnosis of intra-ocular tumors. A stereoscopic presentation. The C V Mosby C°, St. Louis.
19. Gass J D M (1977): Treatment of retinal vascular anomalies. *Trans Am Acad Ophthalmol Otolaryngol*, 83: 432–442.
20. Gass J D M (1987): Stereoscopic atlas of macular diseases. Diagnosis and treatment. The C V Mosby C°, St. Louis, 640–648.
21. Gass J D M and Braunstein R (1980): Sessile and exophytic angiomas of the juxtapapillary retina and optic nerve head. *Arch Ophthalmol*, 98: 1790–1797.
22. Goes F. and Benozzi J (1980): Ultrasonography of haemangiomas of the optic disc. *Bull Soc Belge Ophtalmol* 190: 87–97.
23. Hanssens M and De Laey J J (1987): Haemangioma of the optic disc or hyperplasia of the retinal pigment epithelium. A clinico-pathological correlation. *Bull Soc Belge Ophtalmol* 224: 67–76.
24. Hartridge G (1901): Naevoid condition of the vessels of the disc, with naevus of the eyelid and face. *Trans Ophthalmol Soc U.K.*, 21: 83.
25. Hogan M J and Zimmerman L E (1962): Ophthalmic Pathology. 2nd Ed., W B Saunders C°, Philadelphia, London, 527–531.
26. Imes R K, Monteiro M L O R and Hoyt W F (1984): Incipient hemangioblastoma of the optic disc. *Am J Ophthalmol*, 98: 116.
27. Landbo K (1972): A case of optic disc angioma. With fluorescein angiography. *Acta Ophthalmol (Kbh)*, 50: 431–435.
28. Larsen H W (1969): Manual and color atlas of the ocular fundus. Ed. Munksgaard, Copenhagen, 172–173.
29. Litricin O (1972): Angiomatosis of the retina and optic disc. Lecture before the 6th meeting of the EOPS, Rotterdam, 1967, not published. Cited by Oosterhuis and Rubinstein.
30. McMichael I M (1970): Von Hippel-Lindau's disease of the optic disc. *Trans Ophthalmol Soc U.K.*, 90: 877–885.
31. Manschot W A (1968): Juxtapapillary retinal angiomatosis. *Arch Ophthalmol*, 80: 775–776.
32. Nastri F and Basile G (1939): Su di un raro caso di tumor primitivo (angio-endotelioma) della papilla ottica. *Boll Oculist*, 18: 797–810.
33. Neame H (1948): Angiomatosis retinae with report of pathological examination. *Br J Ophthalmol* 32: 677–689.

34. Niccol W and Moore R F (1934): A case of angiomatosis retinae. *Br J Ophthalmol*, 18: 454–457.
35. Nicholson D H, Green W R and Kenyon K R (1976): Light and electron-microscopic study of early lesions in angiomatosis retinae. *Am J Ophthalmol* 82: 193–204.
36. Nielsen P G (1979): Capillary haemangioma of the optic disc. *Acta Ophthalmol*, 57: 63.
37. O'Connor P R and Kaiser R J (1975): Atypical angiomatosis retinae. *Arch Ophthalmol*, 93: 1368–1369.
38. Oosterhuis J A and Rubinstein K (1972): Hemangioma at the optic disc. *Ophthalmologica*, 164: 362–374.
39. Pau H (1979): Angiomatosis Retinae (et Papillae). *Von Graefe's Arch Klin Exp Ophthalmol*, 210: 229–234.
40. Paufique L, Ravault M P and Durand L (1986): Maladie de von Hippel à localisation papillaire. *Bull Soc Ophtalmol Fr*, 66: 755–787.
41. Pinkerton O D (1970): Papillary hemangioma (von Hippel's disease) of the optic papilla. *J Ped Ophthalmol*, 7: 157.
42. Reese A B (1978): Tumors of the Eye. 3rd Edition, Harper and Row, New York.
43. Rosen F (1969): Vascular malformations in the human retina. *Am J Ophthalmol*, 67: 501–511.
44. Schieck F (1912): Das Peritheliom der Netzhautzentralgefässe, ein unbekanntes Krankheitsbild. *Von Graefe's Arch Ophthalmol* 81: 328–339.
45. Schindler R R, Sarin L K and Mc Donald P R (1975): Haemangioma of the optic disc. *Can J Ophthalmol*, 10: 305–318.
46. Sellors P J and Archer D (1969): The management of retinal angiomatosis. *Trans Ophthalmol Soc U.K.*, 89: 529–543.
47. Shields J A (1983): Diagnosis and Management of Intraocular Tumors. The C V Mosby C°, St. Louis, Toronto, London, 534–568.
48. Sidler-Huguenin H (1920): Ein Endotheliom am Sehnervenkopf. *Von Graefe's Arch Ophthalmol*, 101: 113–122.
49. Souders B F (1949): Juxtapapillary hemangio-endothelioma of the retina. Report of a case. *Arch Ophthalmol*, 41: 178–182.
50. Takahashi T, Wada H, Tani E, Nakamura A. and Hiramatsu K (1984): Capillary hemangioma of the optic disc. *J Clin Neuro-Ophthalmol*, 4: 159–162.
51. Vogel M (1965): Angiogliomatosis der Papille. *Klin Mbl Augenheilk*, 147: 44–50.
52. von Winning C H O M (1976): Haemangiomas of the fundus. *Doc Ophthalmol*, 40: 361–381.
53. Wallner E F and Moorman L T (1955): Hemangioma of the optic disc *Arch Ophthalmol*, 53: 115–117.
54. Weisse V (1965): Tumor der Papilla nervi optici. *Klin Mbl Augenheilk*, 146: 65–69.
55. Wilder H C (1946): Intraocular Tumors in Soldiers, World War II. *Mil Surgeon*, 99: 459.
56. Yimoyines D J, Topilow H W. Abedin S and Mc Meel J W (1982): Bilateral peripapillary exophytic retinal hemangioblastomas. *Ophthalmology*, 89: 1388–1392.

4 Cavernous hemangioma of the retina and of the optic disc

Cavernous hemangiomas of the retina and the optic disc are rare and some authors have even questionned their existence as a separate entity [11, 37]. They have been considered as localized vascular tumefactions, partly isolated from the normal retinal vascular tree [14, 16], as hamartomas part of a neurophakomatosis with probable autosomal dominant inheritance [15] or even as congenital venous malformations with a growth potential like that of von Hippel's disease [30]. Up to now, about 80 cases have been published [1–3, 5, 7–21, 23–53]. Cavernous hemangiomas of the retina and of the optic disc are probably congenital non-progressive tumors, which may be part of an oculo-neuro-cutaneous syndrome.

I. Incidence

Of the 81 cases we could trace in the literature, 39 were found in males and 40 in females, of two cases the sex was not mentioned. This contradicts the impression of Reese [37] and of Lewis et al. [29] that the tumor is probably more common in females. All patients but one black male [24] were caucasians. The tumor usually affects only one eye with no predilection for the right or the left eye. Bilateral cases have been described [12, 19, 21, 37, 41].

II. Clinical features

1. Age at presentation

The youngest patient at diagnosis was 48 hours old and was seen for a bluerubber naevus syndrome [8].

Another child was seen with an unilateral leucocoria at the age of 6 months [30]. The eye was enucleated and histopathological examination revealed a total retinal detachment, associated with a widespread cavernous hemangioma of the retina.

A diagnosis of cavernous hemangioma of the retina was however also made in patients over 70 years of age [19, 24], either during a routine examination or because of neurological signs. Two third of the cases are detected before the age of 30 years.

71

2. Presenting symptoms

A large number of cases of cavernous hemangiomas of the retina or the optic disc were found during a routine examination or during an examination for reasons unrelated to the fundus lesion. Strabismus and amblyopia were the presenting symptoms in a number of patients [14, 26, 27, 36, 44]. Three patients consulted because of oculo-motor palsy [21, 47, 53]. Other patients were seen because they presented convulsions or 'grand mal' seizures [12, 14, 49]. These neurological signs were possibly the consequence of cerebral manifestations of the disease. Other cases were detected during a familial survey [12, 21, 35]. A number of patients sought medical advice for blurred vision, metamorphopsia or visual loss [9, 19, 28, 31, 36, 37, 41, 52]. Some patients complained of headaches or retro-orbital pain [5, 14, 37].

3. Subjective signs

In a large number of cases the vision is either normal or only slightly affected. The visual acuity may be reduced when the lesion affects the

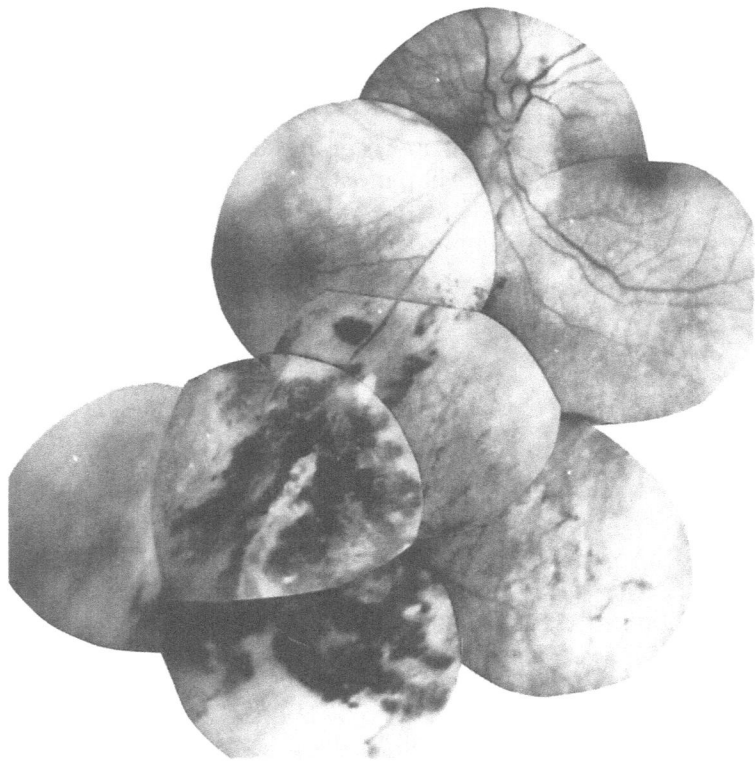

Figure 4–1.   Photomontage of the red-free prints of a cavernous hemangioma in the left eye of a 13 year old girl.

macula directly [24, 37, 39, 41, 47] or indirectly. This may be the result of traction [36] or of preretinal fibrosis [31]. A perimetric examination reveals a relative or absolute scotoma corresponding to the retinal anomaly or an enlargement of the blind spot when the optic disc is involved.

4. Ophthalmological aspect

Cavernous hemangiomas of the retina and the optic disc were described by Gass [17] as sessile tumors composed of clusters of thin-walled saccular aneurysms filled with dark venous blood that gives the appearance of a cluster of grapes projecting from the inner retinal surface (Figs. 4–1, 4–2). The dark red color of the tumor is especially striking. The lesion may be associated with isolated aneurysms (Fig. 4–4). There is no preferential location of the tumor. It may be solitary or multiple. These tumors may even be randomly distributed over large areas of the fundus [31] or follow large veins. The vein that drains the vascular lesion, is often massively dilated. This lead Messmer et al. [31] to suggest that cavernous hemangiomas

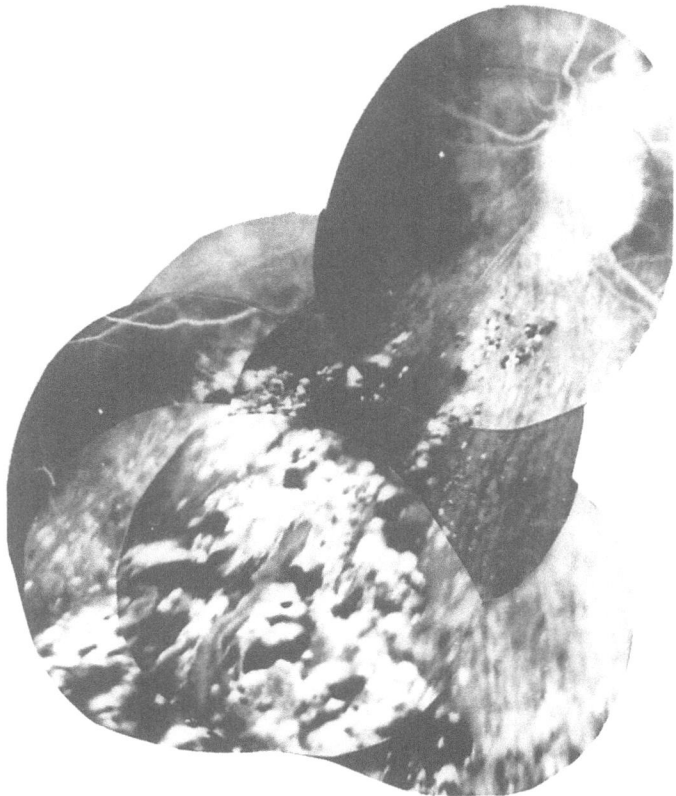

Figure 4–2.   Photomontage of the fluoroangiography corresponding to Fig. 4–1.

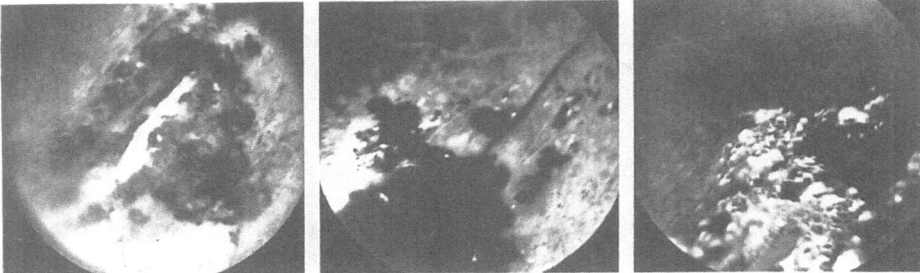

Figure 4–3.   Fluoroangiographic sequence of the same eye as fig. 4–1. Note the delayed filling (b) and the plasmaerythrocytic separation on late stages (c). The late staining is limited to the aneurysms.

are to be considered as a venous malformation rather than as a vascular hamartoma, such as von Hippel's disease.

The hemangiomas may be associated with retinal, preretinal or even vitreous hemorrhages. However, exudates are uncommon. In the first case of Klein et al. [24] few small deposits of yellow material were seen at presentation. Preretinal fibrosis is not uncommonly seen at the surface of the lesion and may even be a prominent component of the malformation [29].

Fluorescein angiography indicates a delayed and sometimes incomplete filling of the abnormal vascular structures (Figs. 4–3, 4–4). The plasma-erythrocytic separation which is especially manifest in larger aneurysms is well seen in late angiograms. The upper part of the aneurysm presents an intensive late fluorescence, whereas the bottom remains dark. This gives an aspect which has been compared to snow on coals. The blood-retinal barrier appears normal as no extravascular leakage of dye is observed. This of course corresponds also to the absence of exudates.

5. Evolution

In most cases the tumor appears to change very little during prolonged follow-up periods of up to 34 years [16, 24, 29, 31, 37]. Sometimes however

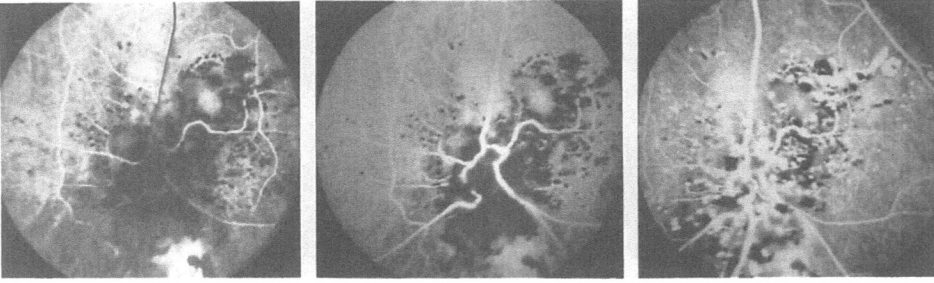

Figure 4–4.   Fluoroangiography of a cavernous angioma (courtesy Dr C. Verougstraete). Note the association of the lesion with isolated aneurysm.

progression has been documented [18]. Spontaneous sclerosis of some of the aneurysms has been seen [7, 19, 31], as well as increase of the preretinal glial tissue [35]. The most common complication is recurrent vitreous hemorrhages [19, 31, 47]. This complication is still relatively rare. We followed for more than 5 years a young girl with amblyopia and strabismus. She presented a large cavernous angioma in the inferonasal quadrant of the left eye. The lesion was associated with preretinal fibrosis. She was treated with argon laser photocoagulation because of recurrent vitreous hemorrhages. The treatment could not be completed and the eye developed a total traction retinal detachment.

III. Systemic manifestations – Gass' syndrome

Weskamp and Cotlier [49, 50] reported as first the association of cavernous angioma of the retina with cerebral angioma. Their patient, a young girl, presented angiomas of the scalp and was operated for a cavernous angioma in the pre-rolandic region. Her father had epilepsy. Gass [14] noted the association of vascular tumors on the face and legs, of a cavernous angioma of the retina and of 'grand mal' seizures in a 33 year old patient. Her father had a history of seizures and died from cerebral complications. Multiple angiomas of the retina with Briton-type hypogammaglobulinemia. The family was further investigated 18 years later by Pancurak et al. [35]. The sister, who also had cavernous hemangioma of the retina, later developed convulsions. A computed tomography showed subcortical parietal and frontal lobe lesions compatible with the diagnosis of cerebral cavernous hemangioma. Her daughter also presented a hamartoma of the left retina but did not show neurological signs. Her mother had an asymptomatic vascular lesion of the left frontal lobe, detected by CT-scan. That lesion was consistent with the diagnosis of cavernous hemangioma of the brain.
but did not show neurological signs. Her mother had an asymptomatic vascular lesion of the left frontal lobe, detected by CT-scan. That lesion was consistent with the diagnosis of cavernous hemangioma of the brain.

Colvard et al. [7] observed a 48 year old man with cavernous hemangiomas of the retina, congenital heart disease, severe polycythemia and neurologic defects. These neurological symptoms were considered to be unrelated to intracerebral hemorrhages from CNS angiomas.

Turut and François [47] discovered a retinal cavernous hemangioma in a 38 year old man, who complained of diplopia related to a paresis of the right inferior oblique. This was related to a tumor in the brainstem which, according to the angiographic characteristics, was probably not an angioma.

Schwartz et al. [42] described the association of right sided retinal cavernous hemangiomas, cutaneous angiomas and cerebrovascular tumors confirmed by computed tomography and nuclear magnetic resonance in a 32 year old man.

Yen and Wu [53] observed a cavernous hemangioma of the left eye in an 18 year old man with bilateral oculomotor palsies since early childhood. Agenesis of the right carotid artery was found. The ocular palsies were of the nuclear type and could be related either to a small cavernous hemangioma in the rostral midbrain, not demonstrable by angiography, or to vascular insufficiency.

Crompton and Taylor [8] published a case of retinal cavernous angioma in an infant with blue rubber bleb naevus syndrome. This child presented multiple vascular skin lesions, multiple mucosal lesions of the ileum, angiomas of the mouth and lesions in the iris and conjunctiva.

A patient with progressive angiomas of the skin and progressive neurological symptoms, due probably to angiomatous lesions affecting the roots of C_3 to T_1, was described by Gautier–Smith et al. [18]. This woman had a typical cavernous hemangioma in the temporal periphery of the right fundus.

Goldberg et al. [21] discussed a large pedigree of 4 generations with neurocutaneous angiomas including one case of bilateral retinal involvement. One member had the triad: cutaneous angiomas, neurological signs and retinal angioma; another presented only retinal angiomas; 6 members had seizures without known ocular or cutaneous signs; one had cutaneous lesions and seizures and several family members were known to have cutaneous lesions but no other signs. This pedigree stresses the autosomal dominant pattern of inheritance and the marked variability of the expression of the disease.

The familial nature of cavernous hemangiomas of the CNS is well recognized and the various pedigrees indicate an autosomal dominant inheritance [4, 22]. In these families no mention is made however of possible retinal involvement.

Small cutaneous angiomas are not uncommon in a general population. Their presence in association with a cavernous hemangioma of the retina may be fortuitous [16]. However, it is striking that a number of patients with fundus manifestations also presented seizures. Although the neurological investigations were negative, the possibility of the presence of CNS lesions appears probable [9, 19]. The brain tumors may be situated in the prerolandic area [49, 50], the parietal or frontal lobe midbrain, pons, cerebellum [7, 14, 42, 47, 53], the brachial plexus or the nerve roots [18]. The localization of small lesions is however difficult as they may escape detection even with carotid angiography or computer tomography. Nuclear magnetic resonance may offer improved diagnostic possibilities in such cases [42].

IV. Differential diagnosis

The aspect of the fundus is sufficiently characteristic. However, the lesion may in some cases be mistaken for Coats' disease [46, 47]. Coats' disease is however most frequently found in boys and is characterized by the presence of telangiectasis mainly situated in the temporal periphery. These lesions are the cause of massive exudation, which may result in retinal detachment. Cavernous angiomas of the retina may be randomly distributed in the fundus and are not associated with exudative phenomenons.

V. Histopathology

Histopathological examinations of cavernous hemangioma of retina and optic disc remain extremely rare [2, 9, 13, 14, 23, 25, 30, 33, 34]. Some cases were incidentally found in eyes enucleated for suspected malignant melanoma of the choroid [2, 9] or retinoblastoma [23, 25, 30]. In one case there was a monocular hydrophthalmos with an intraretinal capillary and cavernous hemangioma connected by a stalk to a choroidal angioma [13], so that it could be assumed that the retinal cavernous hemangioma was secondary to the choroidal angioma [37].

Microscopy (Figs 4–5, 4–6, 4–7)
The tumor is generally located in the inner retinal layers [14, 16, 25, 30, 40, 43], but may involve the full retinal thickness [2, 9, 34]. In the optic nerve it can reach the level of the lamina cribrosa [9] or even occasionally extend behind it [2].
Invasion of choroid and sclera was exceptionally reported [2], but the tumor may be in contact with the vitreous [13, 14, 16, 25, 30, 40].

– The tumor is composed of thin-walled [3–5, 7–9, 12, 14] dilated [2, 14, 16, 30] and engorged [2, 9, 13, 30, 34] vascular spaces of various sizes [1, 2, 5, 10, 16, 34], which are often interconnected by small orifices [14, 16, 30]. Sometimes one finds also telangiectatic vessels [30] or vessels of varying caliber [33], while the cavernous angioma communicates with branches of the central retinal vessels [34], but generally not with the choroidal vessels [9].
– The walls of the spaces consist of endothelium [2, 9, 14, 16, 30, 33, 34] and eventually a thin layer of stroma [14, 16]. On electron microscopy they appear as a continuous layer of non-fenestrated flat endothelial cells, with terminal bars and a continuous basement membrane encasing occasional pericytes [30].
– The vascular spaces abut on each other or are separated by thin fibrous septa [30] or neuroglial tissue [2, 34]. Around telangiectatic vessels one may find elongated processes of fibrous astrocytes, invested by a basement membrane and abutting in connective tissue mainly in the perivascular region. Fine collagen fibrils are sandwiched between the basement membranes of the endothelial cells and the fibrous astrocytes [30].

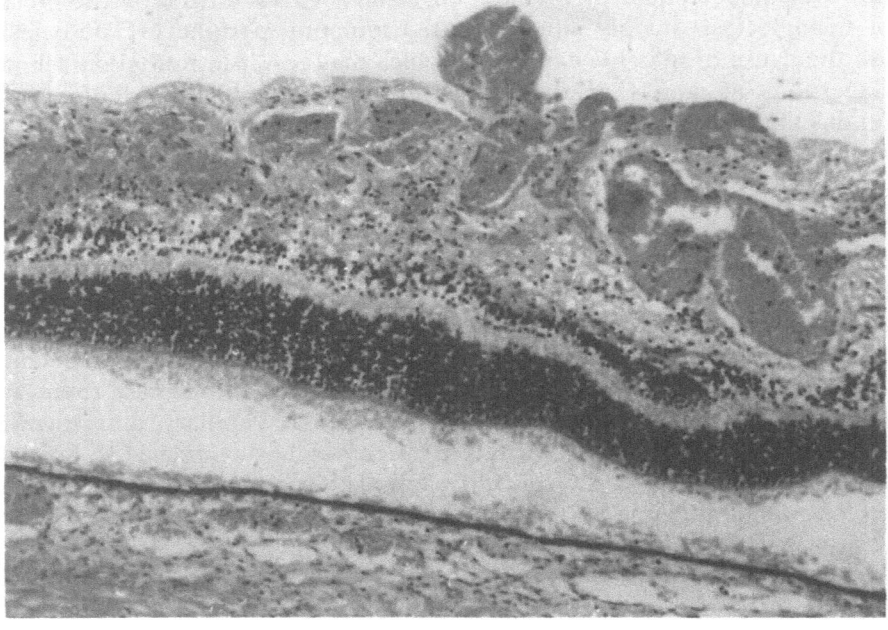

(a)

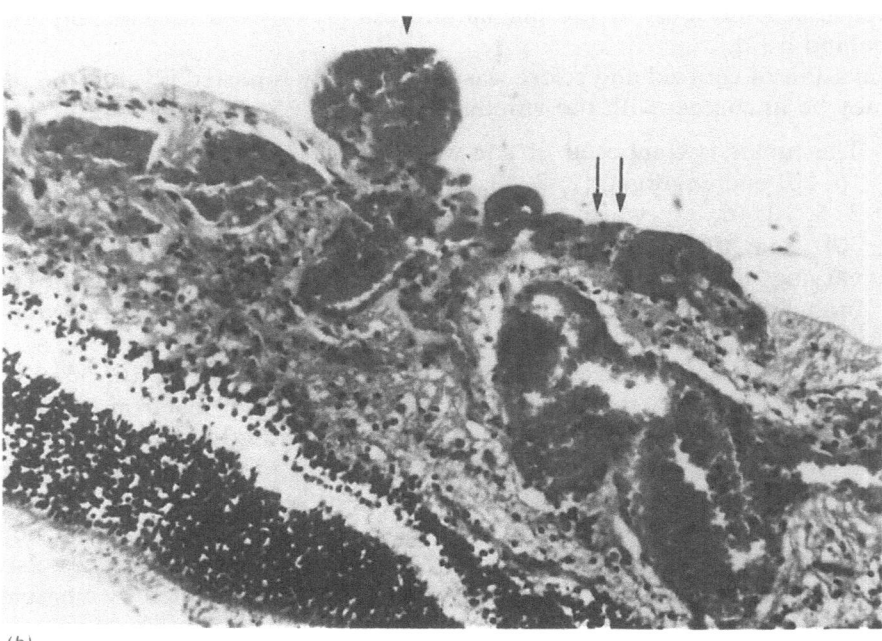

(b)

Figure 4-5.   Cavernous hemangioma of the retina in a case of sirenomelia and Peters' anomaly. H & E, P 716 656–265 (Courtesy of Prof. W. R. Lee, Glasgow). The tumor projects into the vitreous through breaks of the internal limiting membrane (arrows).

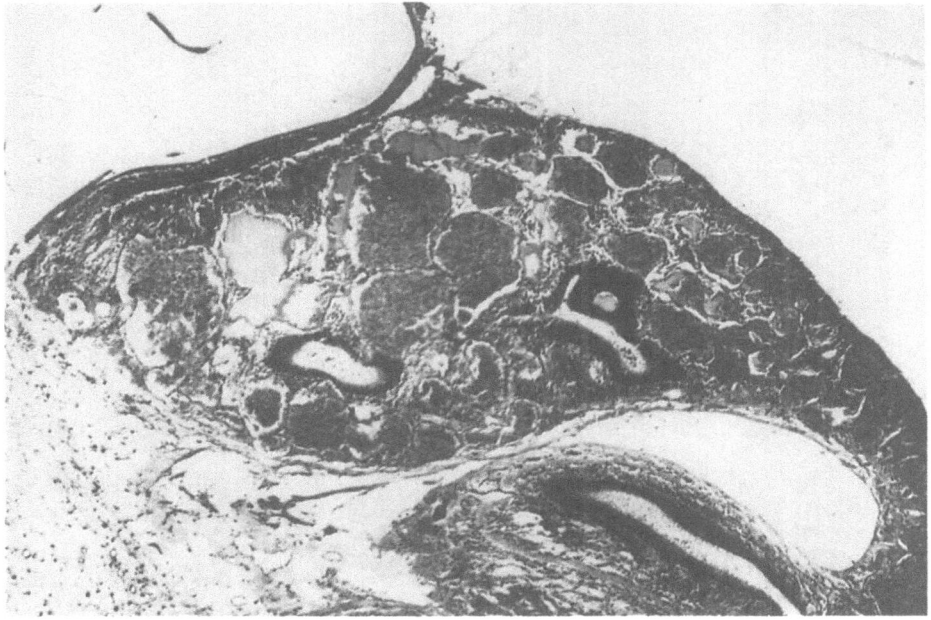

(a)

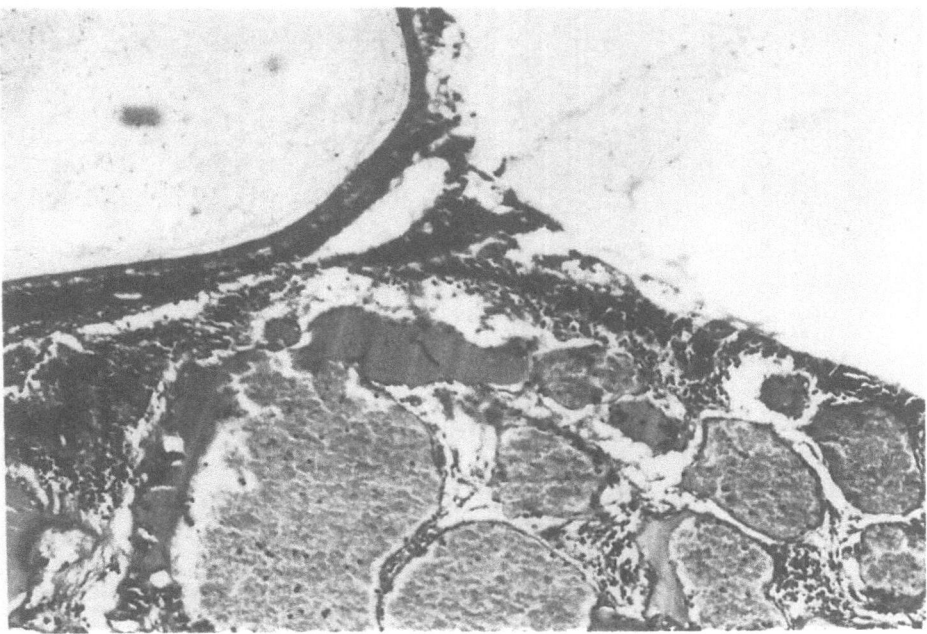

(b)

Figure 4–6. Cavernous hemangioma of the retina: interconnected blood-filled vascular spaces separated by thin septa. a. general view b. higher magnification 7442/80 PAS (Courtesy of Prof. Dr E. P. Messmer, Essen).

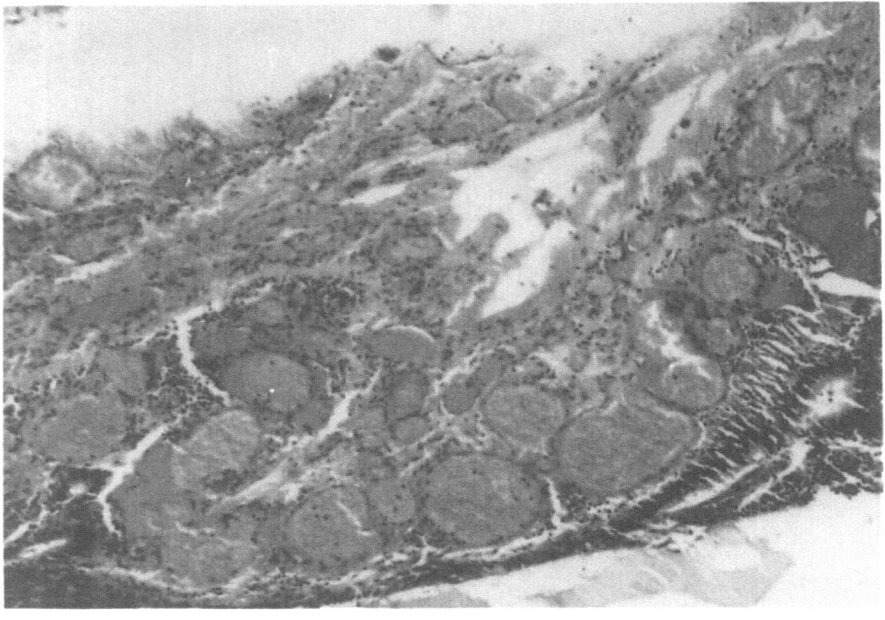

(a)

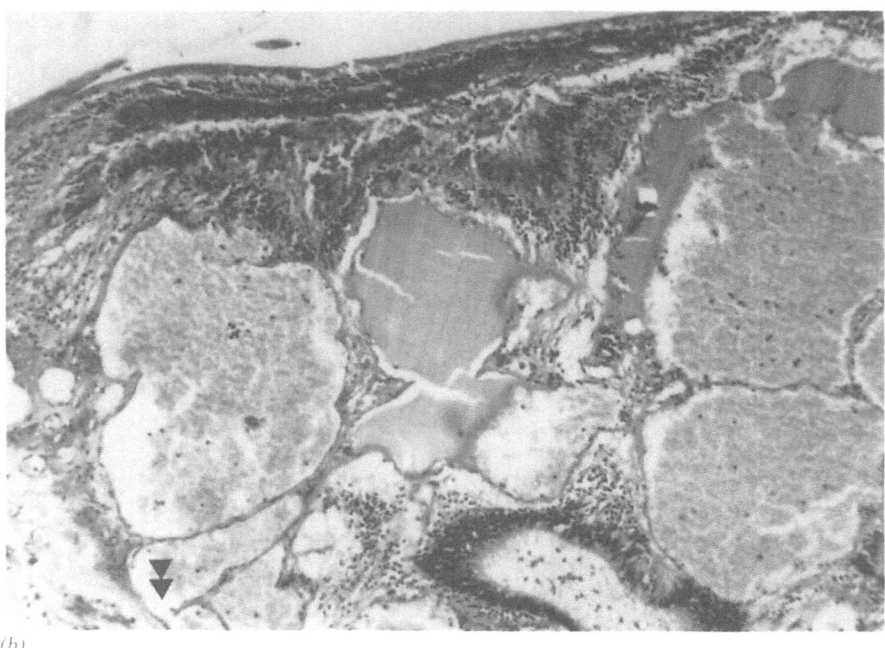

(b)

Figure 4–7.   Cavernous hemangioma of the retina: interconnected (arrowhead) blood-filled vascular spaces separated by thin septa. 7442/80 PAS (Courtesy of Prof. Dr E. P. Messmer, Essen).

Secondary changes

- In the choroid engorged vessels with interstitial round-cell infiltration can be found [33].
- The retina may be thickened [25, 43] with oedema [34], hyaline areas [34], migrated pigment epithelial cells [33], cystic degeneration near the tumor [9] or occasional hemorrhages [33, 34].
  Hemosiderin-loaden macrophages may be found perivascularly at the margin of the tumor as well as along the subretinal space [14].
- Flat or total retinal detachment may occur [9, 30, 33].
- Retinal exudates have only exceptionally been found [30, 33]. No sub-retinal cholesterol clefts or foamy histocytes were found [30] and the retina and the vessels appear normal outside the tumor [2, 14, 25].
  The relative isolation of the cavernous hemangioma from the retinal circulation may be an important factor in the rarity of exudation and hemorrhage from this tumor [16]. The fact that the vessels exhibit the anatomy of normal retinal vessels explains also the integrity of the blood-retinal barrier [30].
- The internal limiting membrane may be thinned over the tumor and present focal breaks [14, 16, 30]. Through this breaks:
a) The walls of the angioma may be in contact with the vitreous [14, 16]. The tumor may even project into the vitreous [34], which may contain scattered erythrocytes or small hemorrhages [14, 25, 34, 43] as well as hemosiderin-loaden macrophages [14, 30]. The hemorrhages may be due to the tumor in contact with the vitreous or to traction on the retina [43].
b) Nodular vascular proliferations may occur on the inner surface of the retina [25], as well as tufts of proliferated spindle cells originating from the inner retina and extending into the vitreous [30].
c) A preretinal membrane with hemosiderin-loaden macrophages and organized vitreous can in some places be continuous with glial cells in the inner retina [30].

VI. Treatment

As most cases of cavernous angiomas of the retina are non-progressive, photocoagulation is not advised, unless recurrent hemorrhages occur. Photocoagulation was successfully performed, either with the Xenon photocoagulator or with the Argon laser in a number of cases [1, 12, 24, 32, 38, 40, 47]. However, this treatment may precipitate a vitreous hemorrhage [14] and possibly played a role in the development of a tractional retinal detachment in our case.

References

1. Amalric P and Biau C (1968): L'angiographie fluorescéïnique chez l'enfant. *Arch Ophtalmol* 28: 55–60.
2. Appelmans M, Decock G and Van Opstal R (1949): Traitement de l'angiome rétinien par *diathermocoagulation. Bull Soc Belge Ophtalmol* 91: 326–340.
3. Atmaca S L and Kanpolat A (1983): Diagnosis and treatment of cavernous hemangiomatosis of the choroid and the retina. *Ann Ophthalmol*, 15: 210–212.
4. Bicknell J M, Carlow T J, Kornfeld M, Stovring J and Turner P (1978): Familial cavernous angiomas. *Arch Neurol*, 35: 746–749.
5. Blodi F C, Allen L and Frazier O (1970): 2: 94. *Stereoscopic manual of the ocular fundus in local and systemic disease*. The C. V. Mosby Co°: St. Louis.
6. Brown G C and Shields J A (1985): Tumors of the optic nerve head. *Survey Ophthalmol*, 29: 239–264.
7. Colvard D M, Robertson D M and Trautmann G C (1978): Cavernous haemangioma of the retina. *Arch Ophthalmol*, 96: 2042–2044.
8. Crompton J L and Taylor D (1981): Ocular lesions in the blue rubber bleb naevus syndrome. *Br J Ophthalmol*, 65: 133–137.
9. Davies W S and Thumim M (1956): Cavernous hemangioma of the optic disc and retina. *Trans Am Acad Ophthalmol Otolaryngol*, 60: 217–218.
10. Drummond W, Hall D L, Steen W H and Lusk E (1980). Cavernous hemangioma of the optic disc. *Ann Ophthalmol*, 12: 1017–1018.
11. Elwyn H (1940): The place of Coats' disease among the diseases of the retina. *Arch Ophthalmol*, 23: 507–521.
12. Frenkel M and Russe H P (1967): Retinal teleangiectasia associated with hypogamma-globulinemia. *Am J Ophthalmol*, 63: 215–220.
13. Garron A and Loewenstein A (1943): A case of monocular hydrophthalmia, with special reference to its possible relation to the Sturge-Weber syndrome. *Br J Ophthalmol*, 27: 335–354.
14. Gass J D M (1971): Cavernous hemangioma of the retina. A neuro-oculo-cutaneous syndrome. *Am J Ophthalmol*, 71: 799–814.
15. Gass J D M (1972): Cavernous hemangioma of the retina. *Int. Ophthalmol Clin*, 12: 116–118.
16. Gass J D M (1974): Differential diagnosis of intraocular tumours. The C. V. Mosby C°, St. Louis, 294–295.
17. Gass J D M (1987): Stereoscopic atlas of macular diseases. Third edition. The C. V. Mosby C°, St. Louis, 634–639.
18. Gautier-Smith P C, Sanders M D and Sanderson K V (1971): Ocular and nervous system involvement in angioma serpiginosum. *Br J Ophthalmol*, 55: 433–443.
19. Gislason I, Stenkula S, Alm A, Wold E and Walinder P E (1979): Cavernous hemangioma of the retina. *Acta Ophthalmologica*, 57: 709–717.
20. Giuffre G (1985): Cavernous hemangioma of the retina and retinal teleangiectasia. Distinct or related vascular malformations? *Retina*, 5: 221–224.
21. Goldberg E, Pheasant T R and Shields J A (1979): Cavernous hemangioma of the retina. Four-generation pedigree with neurocutaneous manifestations and an example of bilateral retinal involvement. *Arch Ophthalmol*, 97: 2321–2324.
22. Hayman L A, Evand R A, Ferrel R E, Fahr L M, Ostrow P and Riccardi V M (1982): Familial cavernous angiomas: natural history and genetic study over a 5-year period. *Am J Med Genet*, 11: 147–160.
23. Hogan M J and Zimmerman L (1962): Ophthalmic pathology. Second edition. Saunders, Philadelphia, p. 533.
24. Klein M, Goldberg M F and Cotlier E (1975): Cavernous hemangioma of the retina: report of four cases. *Ann Ophthalmol*, 7: 1213–1221.

25. Kogan L and Boniuk M (1962): Cause for enucleation in childhood with special references to pseudo-gliomas and unsuspected retinoblastomas. *Int Ophthalmol Clin*, 2: 507.
26. Krause U (1971): A case of cavernous haemangioma of the retina. *Acta Ophthalmologica*, 49: 221–231.
27. Larsen H W (1964): Atlas of the fundus of the eye. Blackwell, Oxford, p. 80.
28. Larsen H W (1969): Manual and color atlas of the ocular fundus. Munksgaard, Copenhagen, p. 38, 170.
29. Lewis R A, Cohen M H and Wise G N (1975): Cavernous hemangioma of the retina and optic disc. A report of three cases and a review of the literature. *Br J Ophthalmol*, 59: 422–434.
30. Messmer E, Font R L, Laqua H, Höpping W and Naumann G O H (1984): Cavernous hemangioma of the retina. Immunohistochemical and ultrastructural observations. *Arch Ophthalmol*, 102: 413–418.
31. Messmer E, Laqua H, Wessing A, Ruprecht K and Naumann G O H (1983): Nine cases of cavernous hemangioma of the retina. *Am J Ophthalmol*, 95: 383–390.
32. Mildner I (1971): Kavernöse Hämangiome der Retina als Symptom einer Phakomatose. *Ber Dtsche Ophthalmol Ges*, 71: 610–612.
33. Neame H (1948): Angiomatosis Retinae, with report of pathological examination. *Br J Ophthalmol*, 32: 677–689.
34. Niccol W and Moore R F (1934): A case of angiomatosis retinae. *Br J Ophthalmol*, 18: 454–457.
35. Pancurak J, Goldberg M F, Frenkel M and Crowell R M (1985): Cavernous hemangioma of the retina. Genetic and central nervous system involvement. *Retina*, 5: 215–220.
36. Piper H F (1954): Ueber kavernöse Angiome in der Netzhaut. *Ophthalmologica*, 128: 99–107.
37. Reese A B (1963): Tumors of the eye. Hoeber Inc., editors, 2nd edition, 384–385.
38. Robinson T R and Gitter K A (1974): Cavernous hemangioma of the retina. in K. Shimizu Ed., Fluorescein Angiography, Igaku Shoin, Tokyo, 107–110.
39. Rollin J P, Bonnet Y, Lyevre J J, Fabbing A and Andre Y (1981): Aspect angiographique d'un hémangiome caverneux de la rétine. *Bull Soc Ophtalmol Fr*, 81: 639–640.
40. Salvanet A, Cherifi M, Goudou C, Courson J P and Mawas E (1979): Un cas d'hémangiome caverneux de la rétine. *J Fr Ophtalmol*, 2: 45–48.
41. Scheyming H (1937): Ein seltenes Fall von Angiomatösen Veränderungen der Netzhaut *Klin Mbl Augenheilk*, 99: 362–367.
42. Schwartz A C, Weaver R G Jr, Bloomfield R and Tyler M D (1984): Cavernous hemangioma of the retina, cutaneous angiomas and intracranial vascular lesion by computed tomography and nuclear magnetic resonance imaging. *Am J Ophthalmol*, 98: 483–487.
43. Spencer W H (1985): Ophthalmic Pathology. An Atlas and Textbook. W. B. Saunders C°, Philadelphia, London, Toronto, ..., 3rd edition, vol. 1–2, 623–626.
44. Stucchi C A, Bianchi G, Commetta F and Faggioni R (1972): Angiome rétinien et toxoplasmose. *Ophthalmologica*, 165: 384–389.
45. Thiel R (1963): Atlas of diseases of the eye. Elsevier, Amsterdam, p. 546.
46. Turut P, Constantinides G and Woillez M (1978): Formes mixtes : hémangiome caverneux de la rétine-angiopathie de Leber-Coats. *Bull Soc Ophtalmol Fr*, 10: 663–667.
47. Turut P and Francois P (1979): Hémangiome caverneux de la rétine. *Jr Fr Ophtalmol*, 2: 393–404.
48. von Winning C H O M (1976): Haemangiomas of the fundus. *Doc Ophthalmol* 40: 361–381.
49. Weskamp C and Cotlier I (1939): Angioma del cerebro y de la retina con malformaciones capilares de la piel. *An Argent de Oftalmol*, 1: 71–79.
50. Weskamp C and Cotlier I (1940): Angioma del cerebro y de la retina con malformaciones capillares de la piel. *Arch Oftalmol*, (Buenos Aires), 15: 1.
51. Wessing A (1968): Fluoreszenzangiographie der Retina. Lehrbuch und Atlas. Georg Thieme Verlag, Stuttgart, 130–132.

52. Witmer R, Verrey F and Speiser R (1968): Retinal angiomatosis. A typical case of retinal angiomatosis and teleangiectasis. *Bibl Ophthalmol*, 76: 113.
53. Yen M Y and Wu C C (1985): Cavernous hemangioma of the retina and agenesis of internal carotid artery with bilateral oculomotor palsies. *J Clin Neuro-Ophthalmol*, 5: 258–262.

5 Congenital arteriovenous communications in the retina

Diseases characterized by abnormal arteriovenous communications in the retina have been described under various denominations: arteriovenous fistula [43], cirsoid aneurysm [11], varicose aneurysm, racemose aneurysm [43], racemose hemangioma [76], arteriovenous aneurysm [20, 39, 44, 65], arteriovenous malformation [60, 65, 76], venous angioma [39], congenital retinal macrovessels [17], Bonnet-Dechaume-Blanc syndrome and Wyburn-Mason syndrome or arteriovenous aneurysm of midbrain and retina associated with facial naevi and mental changes.

Arteriovenous retinal malformations were first described by Magnus in 1874 and were for many years considered as an ophthalmological curiosity. Yates and Paine [78] described probably the first case of association of arteriovenous anomalies in the fundus with vascular anomalies of the brain. Their patient, a man aged 32 years, presented lesions in the left fundus, a right homonymous hemianopsia and right hemiparesis. He died from cerebral hemorrhage. At autopsy numerous abnormal vessels were found in the left cerebral hemisphere, midbrain and above the left cavernous sinus.

The association of retinal arteriovenous anomalies with facial and cerebral vascular anomalies was first recognized as a separate clinical entity in 1943 by Bonnet-Dechaume-Blanc [11] and further characterized by Wyburn-Mason [77]. Since then the association is often referred to either as Bonnet-Dechaume-Blanc or as Wyburn-Mason syndrome.

I. Pathogenesis

The cause of the retinal vascular malformation is usually a congenital anomaly [61, 76]. Trauma has been implicated in some cases [76], whereas the etiology in other cases is still unknown [61].

Congenital and posttraumatic arteriovenous malformations may be very similar and are sometimes impossible to differentiate. A number of hypotheses have been formulated in order to explain these anomalies. They are mainly based on the work of Streeter [83], who divided the development of vessels of the head into 5 periods.

During the first stage (embryo of 3 to 4 mm) three primordial vascular plexusses are formed: the anterior, the middle and the posterior plexus.

In the second period (4 to 12 mm stage) the primordial vascular system is differentiated into arteries, veins and capillaries.

The third period (12 to 20 mm stage) is characterized by the cleavage of the vascular mesoderm in three layers, with respectively the external, the dural and the cerebral blood vessels.

During the fourth period (20–50 mm stage) the arteries and veins adjust to the site and form of the surrounding structures.

In the fifth period (larger than 50 mm stage) the histological differentiation of the vessel wall occurs with transformation into adult arteries, veins and various types of sinuses.

Wyburn-Mason [77] considered that a defect of the mesenchym in the anterior plexus would be likely to affect the retina as well and that this defect might extend caudally to involve the middle plexus. A primitive abnormal vascular tissue from the retina could extend via the optic stalk to the midbrain. As during the 12 to 20 mm stage the primordial vascular plexus is divided into three layers, a retinal and cerebral vascular malformation could also be associated with a vascular lesion of the skin.

Olivecrona and Ladenheim [50] underlined the importance of focal capillary agenesis in these arteriovenous malformations. They too suggested that the error in development had to occur in Streeter's second period when capillaries are formed. The modifications during the third period could determine if the malformation would be localized in the brain, the dura or the skin.

Arteriovenous malformations could thus be the consequence of failure of normal development of the mesoderm during the second month of gestation. This results in abnormal vasculature consisting of inappropriately arranged arteries and veins with a direct communication between the arterial and venous system via multiple vessels, but without interposed capillaries [22]. The factors, which may cause this abnormal vascular development, are however still unknown.

In cases of isolated retinal lesions a local defect in the maturation of the primitive retinal mesenchymal cells has been suggested [3]. The cells originate from the hyaloid vascular cells and differentiate into cords of endothelial cells, which gradually canalize in an elementary capillary network. This will be followed by the development of preferential flow pathways and focal capillary retraction and atrophy. In isolated AV communications extreme capillary atrophy may be present, with the development of large shunting vessels. This malformation possibly occurs at the 110 mm embryonic stage [35].

II. Heredity

Wyburn-Mason [77] considered the condition to be dominantly inherited. However, most authors agree that arteriovenous malformations are not familial. To the best of our knowledge no familial cases of retinal arterio-venous malformations of the fundus have ever been reported. We have observed a young woman with typical arteriovenous malformations in the fundus (Fig. 5–3), associated with cerebral vascular anomalies. Her son presented a peripapillary fundus lesion in the left eye, somewhat resembling a hamartoma of the retinal pigment epithelium.

III. Incidence

Arteriovenous malformations of the retina, associated or not with cerebral or cutaneous malformations are uncommon. In 1943 Wyburn-Mason re-viewing the literature, found 30 cases including his own cases. Nineteen were males and 12 females. In our survey of the literature we found 95 cases (97 eyes). The distribution is given in Table 1.

Table 1.

	Sex		Eye	
	M	F	R	L
Isolated ret. AVM	18	31	18	31
Ret. AVM and brain AVM	18	28	25	23
Total	36	59	43	54
		95		97

Retinal arteriovenous malformations, whether or not associated with cere-bral vascular anomalies, appear thus to be relatively more frequent in females and in left eyes. Bilateral cases are exceptional [18, 49]. Most patients are diagnosed before the age of 30 years. One of the youngest patients was 5 years old at diagnosis [69].

Arterio-venous malformations have also been described in monkeys [7, 33].

IV. Ocular manifestations

In a number of cases the retinal anomalies are discovered during a routine examination. Congenital retinal arteriovenous communications of the retina may thus be compatible with normal vision [1–3, 9, 17, 26, 31, 37, 42, 55, 62, 75]. However extensive AV malformations are usually associated with sometimes extremely poor vision or even blindness of the affected aye. Some patients presented with ill-defined symptoms, such as mist or flashes [26], visual disturbances with pulsating gradient [9] or because of local vascular complications such as vascular occlusions or retinal or vitreous hemorrhages. In cases of associated cerebral vascular malformations the diagnosis was made at the occasion of a systematic ocular examination. Midbrain lesions may indeed be the first to produce symptoms [77] sometimes related to subarachnoidal hemorrhages.

1. Ophthalmoscopic aspects

The fundus aspect depends on the extent of the AV anomalies. Usually a direct communication is seen between a dilated artery and vein. Arteries are sometimes indistinguishable from veins, except by fluorescein angiography. The temporal and especially the infero-temporal vasculature is most commonly affected. The abnormal vessels do not pulsate. Cilioretinal communications may be present [2]. Local retinal degeneration and pigmentation are sometimes observed. The optic disc is usually not atrophic but may be completely obscured by dilated retinal vessels. Vascular sheathing may be present [3]. Intraretinal hemorrhages [5] and lipoid exudates [74] are relatively rare and may be the result of secondary vascular complications. Fluorescein angiography shows a slowing down of the circulation in the affected vessels and sometimes indicates the presence of retinal capillary non-perfusion [17] or of telangiectatic changes in smaller vessels.

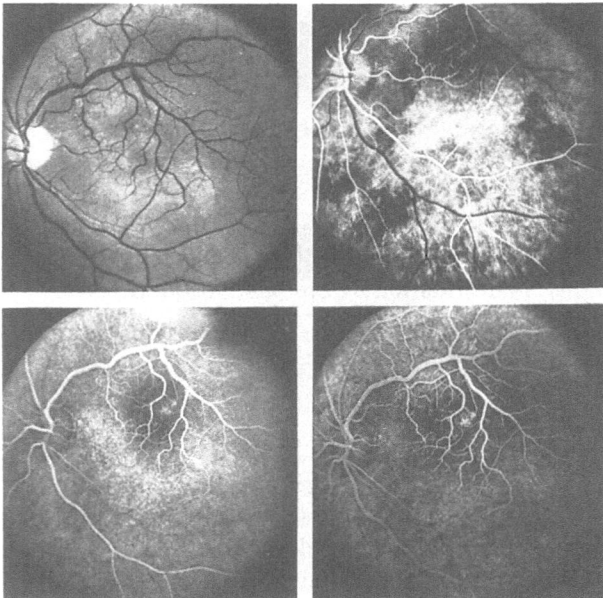

Figure 5–1.   Congenital arteriovenous malformation in the left eye of a man aged 32 years. He complained of a positive scotoma. Visual acuity was 9/10 in the left eye. The right eye was normal.

Archer et al. [3] divided congenital retinal arteriovenous communications into three groups:

- *Group 1.* Cases in this group are characterized by the presence of an arteriolar or abnormal capillary plexus interposed between the artery and the vein [Fig. 5–1). The communications are isolated or multiple and predominantly located in one quadrant of the fundus. The macular region is often affected. Fluorescein angiography does not reveal leakage of dye from the abnormal vessels and there are also no indications of early vascular sclerosis. This group is probably not associated with significant cerebrovascular anomalies.
- *Group 2.* In group 2 there is a direct arteriovenous communication, without interposition of capillary or arteriolar elements (Fig. 5–2). A hyperdynamic flow pattern develops. This may provoke beading of arteries, capillary non-perfusion in the vicinity and micro-aneurysm formation. Association with cerebrovascular anomalies are rare in group 2.
- *Group 3.* This group is characterized by the extent and complexity of the arteriovenous malformation (Fig. 5–3, 5–4). These vessels undergo sheating and sclerosis. A breakdown of the bloodretinal barrier may result in edema or exudates which may ultimately lead to pigmentary changes. The retina is often attenuated with cystic changes [39]. Visual acuity is usually poor and some eyes are even blind since birth. These patients fall into the category of associated retinal and cerebral vascular malformations described by Bonnet-Dechaume-Blanc and by Wyburn-Mason.

2. Anterior segment

Conjunctival vessels are sometimes dilated aspecially when the orbital vessels are also involved. The dilatation is usually not very marked and

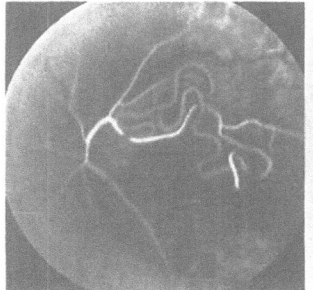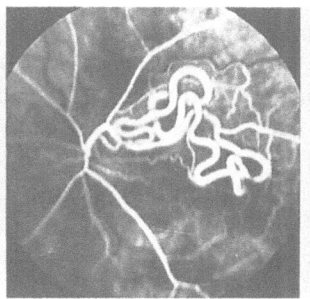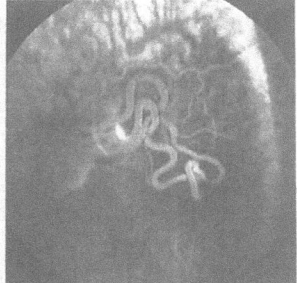

Figure 5–2. Congenital arteriovenous malformation in the left eye of a 45 year old woman, who complained of severe headache. The right eye was amblyopic (vision 3/10) but otherwise normal. Vision of the left eye was 9/10. A complete neurological and neuroradiological examination including CT-scan and carotid angiography was negative.

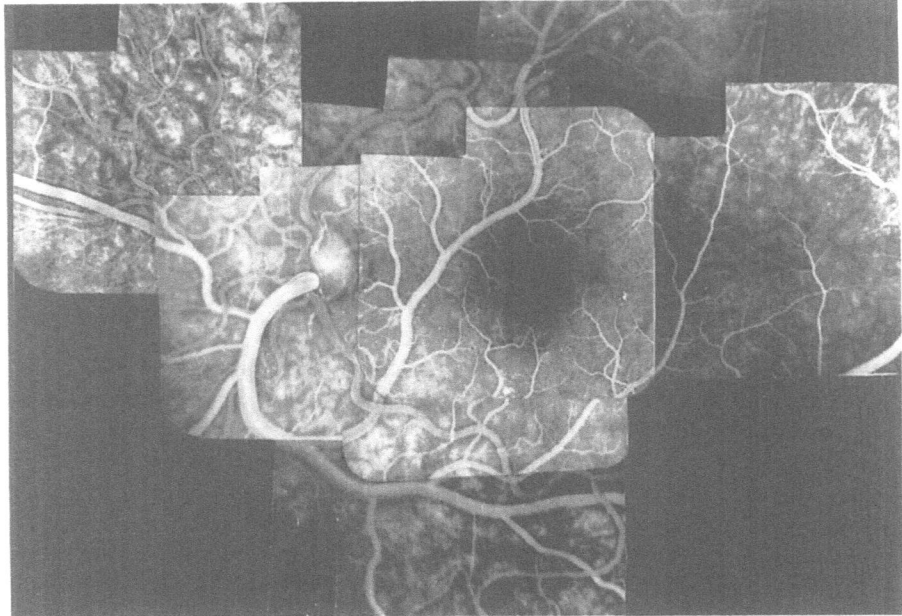

Figure 5–3.   Large arteriovenous malformation in the left eye of an otherwise healthy boy aged 11 years. Visual acuity was 10/10 in both eyes.

certainly not as pronounced as in cases of carotid-cavernous fistula. An AV malformation of the palpebral conjunctiva was described by Weve [73]. A discrete iris angiomatosis was also observed [18].

3. Orbit

Especially in extensive cases the orbit and the optic nerve are also affected [15, 22, 39, 41]. This may result in proptosis [19, 34, 38, 55, 58, 64, 69, 78]. The exophthalmos is usually not pulsating and a bruit, such as in carotido-cavernous fistula is only exceptionally noticed. In one case with AV malformation in the posterior aspect of the left orbit and in the suprasellar region a bruit was detected over the left mastoid and supraclavicular areas [25].

V. Wyburn-Mason syndrome

Congenital retinal AV malformations may be associated with cerebrovascular and dermatological anomalies. In such cases the disease is called Bonnet-Dechaume-Blanc or Wyburn-Mason syndrome.

Wyburn-Mason observed a high incidence of congenital retinal AV malformations associated with cerebrovascular anomalies. Such association

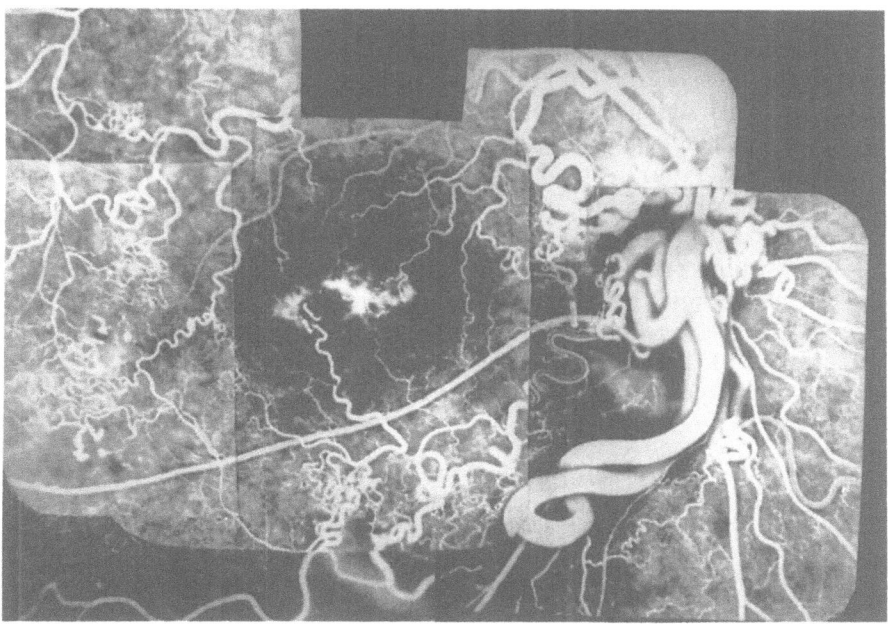

Figure 5–4. Left fundus of a 32 year old woman. That eye had only light perception. The patient complained of ptosis of the left eye. Twelve years later the patient developed a subarachnoidal hemorrhage and carotid angiography revealed the presence of two vascular malformations, one intra-orbital related to the ophthalmic artery, the other situated in the right frontal lobe and extending to the lateroventricular region.

was found in 22 of the 27 cases he reviewed. Although such a rate of associated cerebral involvement may appear too high this figure of over 80% becomes reasonable when only cases of group 3 of Archer's classification are considered [3].

1. Neurological signs

The neurological signs mainly depend on the extent and location of the cerebrovascular malformation. These are usually deeply located [65]. They are always unilateral and situated at the same site as the fundus lesions. Arteriovenous malformations most often involve the chiasm, hypothalamus, basal ganglia and mesencephalon. Extension into the vermis may be noted [39, 64, 65]. In one patient of Theron et al. [65] the vascular malformations extended from the retina along the optic nerve and geniculate bodies to the occipital cortex affecting thus the entire optic pathway. These malformations are vascularized from the carotid system, from the vertebral arteries or from both.

The resulting neurological signs may appear gradually or be acute. Acute symptoms are caused by a vascular accident (hemorrhage or thrombosis). In cases of hemorrhages, which have been classically been described at the level of the mesencephalon [77], blood will rapidly escape into the subarachnoid space provoking the typical symptomatology or subarachnoid hemorrhage: severe headache, vomiting, neck rigidity, associated or not to loss of consciousness. After recovery the patient may present signs of a midbrain lesion. Local edema may possibly be the cause of the obliteration of the aqueduct.

The resulting symptoms will thus be those of internal hydrocephaly with signs of intracranial hypertension. However, as the edema sometimes spontaneously regresses, the hydrocephaly can be intermittent in type.

Saraux et al. [57] reviewed the neurological signs in 35 cases of Wyburn-Mason's syndrome. These findings are summarized in Table 2.

Table 2.

Controlateral pyramidal deficit	22 cases
Homonymous hemianopsia	15 cases
Cranial nerve involvement	
III	11 cases
VI	4 cases
VII	3 cases
Parinaud syndrome	3 cases
Epilepsy	5 cases
Subarachnoid hemorrhage	13 cases
Mental disturbance	13 cases
Intracranial bruit	4 cases

Pupillary anomalies are nearly always present. A typical complication is Weber's syndrome [77] or the association of unilateral third nerve palsy with contralateral hemiplegia.

Visual field defects are also commonly found and are often homonymous. Bitemporal hemianopsia indicating chiasmal involvement is relatively rare [60, 65]. The association of pre- and postchiasmal localization may provoke important visual field loss [39].

Wyburn-Mason noticed intellectual and physical disturbances in the majority of cases. Mental symptoms may be temporary when they occur at the onset of the vascular accident in the midbrain. More permanent damage affects either intelligence or physical reactions. Mental retardation will be more severe when the vascular complications appear early in life. The mental disturbances are sometimes so severe that they lead to suicide.

Other neurological malformations are exceptional. Lakhanpal et al. [40] described a small frontal encephalocele in a 12 year old girl with mesencephalic AV malformation associated with retinal arteriovenous communications.

The question arises if intracranial AV malformations without associated retinal malformations should be considered as expressions of Wyburn-

Mason's syndrome [16, 22, 60]. This should only be the case if the patients also presents with at least facial or mucosal vascular malformations [47].

2. *Dermatological signs*

Bonnet-Dechaume-Blanc [11] noticed in their case an angioma of the lip at the side of the retinal AV malformation. Since then a large number of cases have been published with facial vascular involvement [3, 15, 29, 34, 35, 45, 48, 55, 57, 58, 64, 65, 70, 73, 77]. If present, these vascular malformations are situated in the trigeminal territory of the affected side. Usually they are rather discrete. Sometimes however, they may be the cause of dystrophic changes of the affected skin. The AV malformations may be so important as to provoke facial asymmetry.

3. *Mucosal involvement*

Arteriovenous malformations may also occur in the soft palate, the gums, the tonsillar fossa, the nasopharynx [4, 18, 29, 39, 54, 58]. This may be the cause of repeated bleedings which, in some cases, could only be stopped by ligating the carotid artery of the affected side [3, 39, 55].

VI. Evolution of the retinal lesions

A number of cases have been followed for up to 25 years [13]. In most cases the retinal lesion does not appear to change much in appearance [3, 10, 16, 53]. The lesion may sometimes regress spontaneously [4, 24, 74]. However, progression also occurs [69]. Complications such as retinal and vitreous hemorrhages [3, 8, 12, 18, 46] are not exceptional. Retinal arteriovenous malformations may be complicated by central or branch vein occlusion [3, 24, 30, 46, 79]. The progressive enlargement of the malformation may be associated with signs of retinal ischemia. Neovascularization of the iris and secondary glaucoma have been described [25, 46]. This can be explained by three possible mechanisms:
1. a partial thrombosis of the malformation supplying part of the retinal and choroidal circulation;
2. a steal phenomenon secondary to a change in hemodynamics following enlargement of the malformation;
3. a compression of the central retinal vein by the AV malformation resulting in ischemic central retinal vein occlusion [25, 68].

VII. Histopathology

An AVM represents a direct end-to-end anastomosis of the arterial to the venous system.

1. Extraocular AVM

Histopathologic descriptions have been obtained after autopsy [3, 14, 19, 39, 77] or craniotomy [22, 60].

When fully developed, the abnormal vessels extend as an unilateral tract of reddish vascular tissue from the retina, over the optic nerve, chiasm and optic tract, lying above the cavernous sinus [14, 39, 51, 77] and extending posteriorly to the brain [3, 5, 14, 19, 39, 59, 65, 77, 78].

The vessels appear extremely tortuous [5, 19, 51, 60, 77], variously sized [22, 60] and dilated [5, 51, 77] with much branching and intercommunication [77]. Between the vessels there is atrophic and gliotic nervous or fibrous tissue [5, 19, 77]. Many vessels have the appearance of arteries, some are venous and some resemble dilated capillaries [5, 22, 77]. In chronic cases the vessels may become arterialized [51]. The vessel wall may be thick with high content of fibrous tissue [19, 22], of uneven caliber with thick and thin portions [22, 77], or thinned [51, 77] and eventually rupture and bleed [5, 11, 18, 51]. The intima may be thickened, fibrosed, hyalinized or vacuolated [18, 77] with sometimes nodular ingrowth into the lumen. The internal elastic membrane may be well-marked [77] or hypertrophic [18], distorted [22], fragmented, reduplicated [77] or even absent [22, 77]. The media may be irregular and of varying thickness [22, 77] or thinned [7, 18] and susceptible to aneurysm formation [22]. The adventitia may be of varying thickness [77].

Sometimes there is marked fibro-hyalinosis and vacuolization [22, 77] with atheromatous plaques and calcification [22]. All these changes may lead to thrombosis or hemorrhage [11, 18, 22, 51].

2. Ocular lesions

Histopathology has been described in only a small number of cases [4, 6, 8, 9, 15] and concerns essentially the retina and optic nerve [14, 19, 27, 39, 76].

In the *retina* there is anteriorly an unusually well-developed system of larger-than-normal blood vessels [14, 39]. Posteriorly large tortuous blood vessels occupy the entire thickness of the retina even extending for some distance into the vitreous and locally touching the pigment epithelium and Bruch's membrane [14, 19, 27, 39, 61]. It is often not possible to distinguish arteries from veins [19, 61] since both have fibromuscular medial coats of varying thickness and wide, almost acellular, fibro-hyaline adventitial coats [19, 61].

For others however the aneurysmal vessels have the same structure as normal vessels, but with a markedly enlarged lumen [27]. Between the blood vessels the retina may be attenuated [14, 39, 61] or show cystic degeneration [14, 22, 39, 61], marked loss of nerve fibres, some diminution in the number of ganglion cells [19, 61] and proliferation of the pigment epithelium [4, 9, 14, 39].

The *choroid* is normal [19, 61] or may show some condensation under the vascular growth [14, 39]. Wolter [76] however described a choroidal lesion closely resembling a choroidal hemangioma, but without epichoroidal membrane or capillary network between large arteries and veins. Although considering it as belonging to the group of the so-called choroidal hemangiomas, he classified it as an arteriovenous fistula of the choroid, probably originating in a congenital vascular malformation.

The *optic nerve* is involved by a mass of large thin-walled and distended blood channels. So, the nerve stem is converted in a tangle of blood channels [14, 39], or grossly distorted by numerous abnormal blood vessels, such as endothelium-lined venous channels, with thick fibro-hyaline walls [19] or channels with thin atypical walls similar to cavernous tissue [39]. Large thick-walled muscular arteries, some of which show nodose thickenings of their medial muscle coats, may also be found [19]. There was a regular septum system between the vascular channels, with compressed and distorted islands of glial cells, a few axons, cells resembling foam-cells, but absence of myelin [4, 6, 9, 14, 19, 39].

VIII. Diagnosis

The ophthalmologist may be the first physician to diagnose a Wyburn-Mason's syndrome. The patient may be referred for problems related to amblyopia or squint. The finding of an AV malformation in the fundus does however not necessarily mean that the patient might also harbour cerebral vascular anomalies. Considering Archer's classification, group -1 almost never present cerebral vascular malformations. In group 2 they remain exceptional, whereas they are quite common in group 3.

Therefore extensive neuroradiologic examination, including CT-scan, NMR and sometimes carotid and vertebral angiography should be reserved to the major forms of retinal AV malformations, unless neurological symptoms are manifest. In cases of group 3 systematic neuroradiological examination is advisable as the extent of the vascular malformation in the brain or in the facial tissues cannot be predicted from the clinical signs or symptoms [65].

IX. Differential diagnosis

1. Other phakomatoses

The main differential diagnosis will have to be made with other phakomatoses:
1. von Hippel-Lindau's disease: see chapter 2
2. Sturge-Weber disease: see chapter 1. It is noteworthy that Ward and

Katz [70] described the association of Wyburn-Mason syndrome with Sturge-Weber disease in the same individual.

3. Ataxia teleangiectasia. This is an autosomal recessive disease characterized by progressive cerebellar changes, repeated pulmonary infections and skin problems. In this disease the capillaries are not scarce but on the contrary they are dilated and tortuous.

2. *Arteriovenous fistula*

When the AV malformation involves the orbit, proptosis and episcleral vascular dilatation is seen, which can be mistaken as a carotido-cavernous fistula. However, the exophthalmos is seldom pulsating and is not accompanied by a murmur. Also the episcleral vasodilatation is less marked. In doubtful cases a carotid angiography will provide the exact diagnosis.

3. *Secondary vascular retinal changes*

A number of cases in the literature are possibly not genuine arteriovenous malformations but rather secondary changes after a retinal vascular accident such as opticociliary anastomoses [30] or arteriovenous communications after a retinal vascular occlusion [30]. As however, AV malformations are sometimes complicated by branch or central vein occlusion, the differential diagnosis is not always so evident.

X. Treatment of the fundus lesions

Asymptomatic retinal AV malformations do not require treatment. In cases of recurrent hemorrhages or of progressive exudation, photocoagulation has to be considered [5, 39]. The fundus lesions are however sometimes so diffuse that treatment is almost impossible. Also most blind eyes have lost vision at an early age, already before they were seen by an ophthalmologist [3].

References

1. Adenis J P, Lebrand J and Einholtz F (1982): Anévrisme cirsoïde rétinien isolé. *Bull Soc Ophtalmol Fr*, 82: 403–405.
2. Amalric P and Bessou P (1962): Anastomose artérioveineuse rétinienne et ciliorétinienne bien compensée. *Bull Soc Ophtalmol Fr*, 62: 367–369.
3. Archer D B, Deutman A, Ernest J T and Krill A E (1973): Arteriovenous communications of the retina. *Am J Ophthalmol*, 75: 224–241.
4. Augsburger J J, Goldberg R E, Shields J A, Mulberger R D and Magargal L E (1980): Changing appearance of retinal arteriovenous malformation. *Von Graefe's Arch Klin Exp Ophthalmol*, 215: 65–70.

5. Baurmann H, Meyer F and Oberhoff P (1968): Komplikationen bei der arteriovenösen Anastomose der Netzhaut. *Klin Mbl Augenheilk*, 153: 562–571.
6. Bech K and Jensen O A: (1958): Racemose Haemangioma of the Retina. Two additional cases, including one with defects of the visual fields as a complication of arteriography. *Acta Ophthalmol*, 36: 769–781.
7. Bellhorn R W, Friedman A H and Henkind P (1972): Racemose (cirsoid) hemangioma in rhesus monkey retina. *Am J Ophthalmol*, 74: 517–522.
8. Bernth-Petersen P (1979): Racemose haemangioma of the retina: report of three cases with long-term follow-up. *Acta Ophthalmol*, 57: 669–678.
9. Billson F A, Taylor H R and Hoyt C S (1977): Unilateral arterio-venous malformation of the retina. *Austr. J Ophthalmol*, 5: 125–128.
10. Biro I (1951): Racemose retinal aneurysm. *Ophthalmologica*, 121: 201–207.
11. Bonnet P, Dechaume J and Blanc E (1938): L'anévrysme cirsoïde de la rétine (anévrysme racémeux ses relations avec l'anévrysme cirsoïde de la face et l'anévrysme cirsoïde du cerveau). *Bull Soc Fr Ophtalmol*, 51: 521–524.
12. Brihaye M, Preaux C and Brihaye J (1965): L'anévrysme cirsoïde de la rétine, dysplasie oculo-cérébrale. *Rev, Oto-Neuro-Ophtalmol*, 37: 354–370.
13. Brihaye M, Tassignon M J, Van Langenhove L and Demol S: (1987) Anastomose artério-veineuse, isolée et unilatérale de la rétine avec follow-up de 25 ans. *Bull Soc Belge Ophtalmol*, 225, II, 71–78.
14. Brock S and Dyke C (1932): Venous and arteriovenous angiomas of the brain: clinical and roentgenographic study of 8 cases. *Bull Neurol Inst N.Y.*, 2: 247.
15. Brodsky M C, Hoyt W F, Higashida R T, Hieshima G B and Halback V V (1987): Bonnet-Dechaume-Blanc syndrome with large facial angioma. *Arch Opthalmol*, 105: 854–855.
16. Brown D G, Hilal S K, Tenner M K (1973): Wyburn-Mason syndrome: report of two cases without retinal involvement. *Arch Neurol*, 28: 67–68.
17. Brown G C, Donoso L A, Magargal L E, Goldberg R E and Sarin L K (1982): Congenital retinal macrovessels. *Arch Ophthalmol*, 100: 1430–1436.
18. Cagianut B (1962): Das arterio-venöse Aneurysma der Netzhaut. *Klin Mbl Augenheilk*, 140: 180–191.
19. Cameron M E (1958): Congenital arterio-venous aneurysm of the retina. *Br J Ophthalmol*, 42: 655–666.
20. Cameron M E and Greer C H (1968): Congenital arteriovenous aneurysm of the retina. A post mortem report. *Br J Ophthalmol*, 52: 768–772.
21. Cashell G T W (1948): A case of arterio-venous (racemose) aneurysm of the retina. *Trans Ophthalmol Soc U.K.*, 68: 245–249.
22. Danis R and Appen R E (1984): Optic atrophy and the Wyburn-Mason syndrome *J Clin Neuro-Ophthalmol*, 4: 91–95.
23. Defauchy M (1987): Anévrysme opto-chiasmatique et maladie de Blanc-Bonnet-Dechaume: vers un troisième cas mondial avec examen tomodensitométrique et artériographique. *Bull Soc Ophtalmol Fr*, 87: 995–1000.
24. Dekking H M (1955): Arteriovenous aneurysm of the retina with spontaneous regression. *Ophthalmologica*, 130: 113–115.
25. Effron L, Zakov Z N and Tomsak R L (1985): Neovascular glaucoma as a complication of the Wyburn-Mason syndrome. *J. Clin Neuro-Ophthalmol*, 5: 95–98.
26. Ehlers H (1924): Aneurysma racemosum arteriovenosum retinae. *Acta Ophthalmol*, 2: 374–387.
27. Francois J and Rabaey M (1951): Hémosidérose prérétinienne et anévrysme artério-veineux. *Ophthalmologica*, 122: 348–356.
28. Frandsen A D (1950): A case of hemangioma retinae *Acta Ophthalmol*, 28: 97–102.
29. Glees M (1954): Arteriovenöse aneurysma des Augenhintergrundes und des Gleichseitiges Grosshirnhemisphäre. *Klin Mbl Augenheilk*, 124: 457–460.
30. Gregersen E (1961): Arteriovenous aneurysm of the retina. A case of spontaneous thrombosis and healing. *Acta Ophthalmol*, 39: 937–939.

31. Gunn M (1884): Direct arteriovenous communication on the retina. *Trans Ophthalmol Soc U.K.*, 4: 156–157.
32. Hopen G, Smith J L, Hoff T J and Quencer R (1983): The Wyburn-Mason syndrome. Concomitant chiasmal and fundus vascular malformations. *J Clin Neuro-Ophthalmol*, 3: 53–62.
33. Horiuchi T, Gass J D M and David N J (1976): Arteriovenous malformation in the retina of a monkey. *Am J Ophthalmol*, 82: 896–904.
34. Junius P (1933): Venöse und arterio-venöse Angiome in Bereich des Gehirns; ihre Beziehungen zum Sehorgan. *Zentralbl Ges Ophthalmol*, 29: 673–684.
35. Kottow M H (1978): Congenital malformations of the retinal vessels with primary optic nerve involvement. *Opthalmologica*, 176: 86–90.
36. Kraft (1961): Zur Klinik des arteriovenöses Angioms. *Klin Mbl Augenheilk* 139: 94.
37. Kravitz D and Lloyd R I (1935): Dilated and tortuous retinal vessels. Report of a case of congenital arteriovenous communication. *Arch Ophthalmol*, 41: 591–598.
38. Krayenbuhl H and Yasargil M G (1958): Das Hirnaneurysma. *Docum Geigy Ser Chir*, 4.
39. Krug E F and Samuels B (1932): Venous angioma of the retina, optic nerve, chiasm and brain. A case report with post mortem observations *Arch Ophthalmol*, 8: 871–879.
40. Lakhanpal V, Krishna Rao C V G, Schockett S S and Salcman M (1980): Wyburn-Mason syndrome. *Ann Ophthalmol* 12: 694–699.
41. Lalonde G, Duquette P, Laflamme P and Vezina J L (1979): Bonnet-Dechaume-Blanc syndrome. *Can J Ophthalmol*, 14: 47–50.
42. Larmande A, Boyer R, Margaillan A and Dahan A (1961): A propos d'un anévrysme cirsoïde limité de la rétina *Bull Soc Ophtalmol Fr*, 61: 865–873.
43. Leber T (1915): Das Aneurysma racemosum der Netzhautgefässe, Vol VII A1: pp. 37–42 In: *von Graefe-Saemisch Handbuch der Gesammten Augenheilkunde*, Engelmann (ed). Leipzig.
44. Magnus H (1874): Aneurysma arterio-venosum retinale, cited by Speiser, 1978.
45. Mansour A M, Walsh J B and Henkind P (1987): Arteriovenous anastomoses of the retina. *Ophthalmology*, 94: 35–40.
46. Mansour A M, Wells C G, Jampol L M and Kalina R E (1989): Ocular complications of arteriovenous communication of the retina. *Arch Ophthalmol*, 11: 956–959.
47. Miller M R (1988): Wyburn-Mason syndrome. In Walsh and Hoyt's Clinical Neuro-Ophthalmology, 4th edition, Williams and Wilkins, Baltimore, 1816–1819.
48. Moutinho H and Silvio-Rebelo C (1946): Anévrysme cirsoïde de la rétine de la face et du cerveau. *Bull Soc Fr Ophtalmol*, 59: 48–55.
49. Mozzetti M (1939): Sulle anomalie di vasi retinici ed in particular sull aneurisma cirsoide della retina. *Boll Oculist*, 18: 455–468.
50. Olivecrona H and Ladenheim J (1957): Congenital arteriovenous aneurysm of the carotid and vertebral arterial systems. *Springer Verlag* Berlin.
51. Reese A B (1976): Tumours of the eye. 3rd Edition, Harper and Row, New York, 272–276.
52. Rentz (1925): Aneurysma racemosum retinale *Arch Augenheilk*, 95: 84–91.
53. Riffenburgh R S (1954): Arteriovenous aneurysm of the retina. *Am J Ophthalmol*, 37: 908–910.
54. Romanet J P, Mouillon M, Bonnet J L and Vasdey A (1984): Le syndrome de Bonnet, Blanc et Dechaume. A propos d'une observation associant anévrysme cirsoïde rétino-encéphalique et angiome naso-palatin. *Bull Soc Ophtalmol Fr*, 84: 195–203.
55. Rundles W Z Jr and Falls H F (1951): Congenital arteriovenous (racemose) aneurysm of the retina. Report of three cases. *Arch Ophthalmol*, 46: 408–418.
56. Ryan E P (1940): Angiomatosis Retinae *Arch Ophthalmol*, 23: 623–624.
57. Saraux H, Le Besnerais Y, Graveleau D, Janet L Q and Chatellier P (1967): Les formes atypiques du syndrome de Bonnet, Dechaume et Blanc. *Bull Soc Ophtalmol Fr*, 80: 326–333.

58. Savir H (1978): Arteriovenous hamartoma of the orbit, lids, face, soft palate and retinal vessels. *Metab Ophthalmol*, 2: 381–383.
59. Seydel (1898): Ein Aneurysma arterio-venosum (Varix aneurysmaticus) der Netzhaut. *Arch Augenheilk*, 38: 157–163.
60. Sibony P, Lessell S and Wray S (1982): Chiasmal syndrome created by arteriovenous malformations *Arch Ophthalmol*, 100: 438–442
61. Speiser P (1978): Das arteriovenöse Hämangiom der Netzhaut. *Adv Ophthalmol*. 36: 90–101.
62. Stokes W H (1934): Racemose arteriovenous aneurysm of the retina (aneurysma racemosum arteriovenosum retinae). *Arch Ophthalmol*, 11: 956–959.
63. Streeter G L (1918): The developmental alterations on the vascular system of the brain of the human embryo. *Contribut Embryol*, 8: 7. Cited by Rundles W Z Jr and Falls H GF (1951).
64. Tamaki N, Fujita K and Yamashita H (1971): Multiple arteriovenous malformations involving the scalp, dura, retina, cerebrum and posterior fossa. Case report. *J Neurosurg*, 34: 95–98.
65. Theron J. Newton T H and Hoyt W F (1974): Unilateral retinocephalic vascular malformations. *Neuroradiology*, 7: 185–196.
66. Thorkilgaard O (1963): Racemose haemangiomata of the retina. Two additional cases. *Acta Ophthalmol*. 41: 564–567.
67. Tornquist R (1949): On an anomaly of the retinal vessels (so-called aneurysma cirsoides) sometimes combined with symptoms from the central nervous system. *Acta Ophthalmol*, 7: 11–17.
68. Traboulsi E I (1986): Neovascular glaucoma and ischemia. *J Clin Neuro-Ophthalmol*. 6: 126–127.
69. Unger H H and Umbach W (1966): Kongenitales okulozerebrales Rankenangiom. *Klin Mbl Augenheilk*, 148: 672–682.
70. Ward J B and Katz N N K (1983): Combined phakomatosis. A case report of Sturge-Weber and Wyburn-Mason syndrome occuring in the same individual. *Ann Ophthalmol* 15: 1112–1116.
71. Werncke Th (1940): Angioma papillae nervi optici (Caput Medusae) *Klin Mbl Augenheilk*. 104: 434–436.
72. Wessely (1933): Ueber Beziehungen zwischen intrakraniellem Angioma Racemosum bzw. Aneurysma cirsoides und Tortuositas vasorum des Augenhintergrundes. *Klin Mbl Augenheilk*, 90: 95.
73. Weve H. (1923): Varix aneurysmaticus vicarians retinae (Pseudo-aneurysma arteriovenosum racemosum retinae). *Arch Augenheilk* 93: 1–63.
74. Wiedersheim O (1942): Ueber zwei seltene angiomatöse Veränderungen des Augenhintergrundes und ueber Erweiterung des Begriffes Angiomatosis Retinae. *Klin Mbl Augenheilk*, 105: 205–213.
75. Wisnia K and Toussant D (1976): Abnormal macular arterio-venous communication. *J Ped Ophthalmol*, 13: 196–197.
76. Wolter R J (1975): Arteriovenous fistulas involving the eye region. *J Ped Ophthalmol*, 12: 22–39.
77. Wyburn-Mason R (1943): Arteriovenous aneurysm of mid-brain and retina, facial nevi and mental changes. *Brain*, 66: 163–209.
78. Yates A G and Paine C G (1930): A case of arteriovenous aneurysm within the brain. *Brain*, 53: 38–46.
79. Zylbermann R, Rozenman Y, Silverstone B Z, Ronen S and Berson D (1984): Central retinal vein occlusion in a case of arteriovenous communication of the retina. *Ann Ophthalmol*, 16: 825–828.

6 Neurofibromatosis or von Recklinghausen's disease

At least four different forms of neurofibromatosis can be considered [76]:
1. von Recklinghausen's neurofibromatosis
2. bilateral acoustic neurofibromatosis, where the cutaneous lesions, typical of the first form, are often lacking
3. segmental neurofibromatosis, where the typical lesions are confined to one segment of the body and
4. cutaneous neurofibromatosis, which is probably to be considered as a 'forme fruste' of generalized neurofibromatosis.

As ocular involvement is mainly seen in von Recklinghausen's disease, only this form of neurofibromatosis will be discussed in this chapter.

Generalized neurofibromatosis was first described by Smith in 1849, but is usually associated with the name of von Recklinghausen [111]. The disease is characterized by cutaneous manifestations ('café au lait' spots, freckles and sessile tumors), multiple tumors of the central and peripheral nervous system, skeletal changes (scoliosis and congenital bone defects) and sometimes endocrine changes. The ocular manifestations have been reviewed in several studies [3, 5, 20, 28, 29, 58, 62, 76]. The disease may directly or indirectly affect the various tissues of the eye. In this chapter however the main emphasis will be laid on the fundus manifestations.

I. Pathogenesis

Bielschowski [9] associated as first tuberous sclerosis or Bourneville's disease with neurofibromatosis. In 1923 van der Hoeve [108] introduced the term phakomatosis (phakos = lens, motherspot or birth mark) to characterize these two diseases. Later Sturge-Weber [109] and von Hippel-Lindau diseases were included, followed by Wyburn-Mason's syndrome, ataxia teleangiectasia syndrome, Klippel-Trenaunay syndrome, Albright syndrome, incontinentia pigmenti [30], Gass syndrome and some others.

Phakomatoses are characterized by the appearance of multiple tumors or malformations in various organs of the body, mainly the skin, the central nervous system and the eye. The four cardinal features are [30]:
1. small spots in patches on the skin or mucous membranes
2. localized tumor-like hyperplastic formations (hamartomas)
3. true tumors arising from undifferentiated embryonic cells
4. other congenital malformations.

The relation between the involvement of diverse tissues in neurofibromatosis has remained enigmatic, up to the moment Pages (1955) pointed out that the cells involved originate from the neural crest. A genetically determined maldevelopment in the neural crest may result in the association of various lesions which at first have no obvious relationship one with the other [11]. When the cells are considered which derive from the neural crest, they all may give rise to the typical manifestations of von Recklinghausen's disease (Table 1). This disease may thus be considered as the most typical example of a neurocristopathy.

Table 1. Manifestations of von Recklinghausen's disease (after Brini, [14])

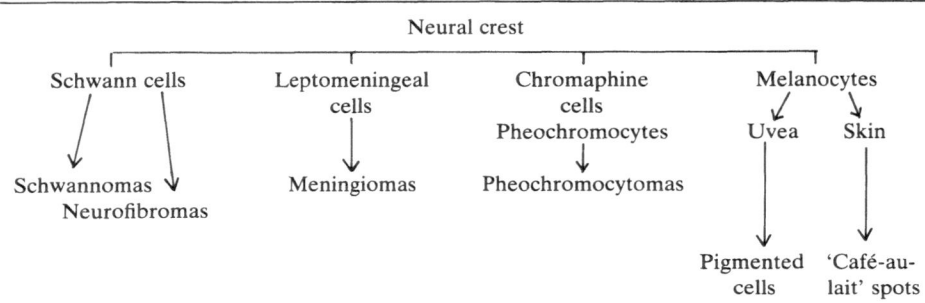

II. Incidence and heredity

The prevalence of von Recklinghausen's disease is estimated at 1 in 2,500 to 3,000 births [23]. Neurofibromatosis is inherited as an autosomal dominant disorder with incomplete penetrance. There is a great intrafamilial variability in the expression of the disease [63] and affected members may be missed, due to the difficulties in diagnosing 'forme fruste' cases [3].

Barker et al. [4] in a linkage analysis of 15 Utah kindreds could demonstrate that the gene responsible for von Recklinghausen neurofibromatosis is located near the centromere of chromosome 17. Their diagnostic criterion was the presence of at least two of the following signs:
1. five or more 'café au lait' spots, greater than 0.5 cm in diameter
2. one or more biopsy proven neurofibromas
3. multiple iris Lisch nodules
4. axillary or groin freckling
5. the presence of distinctive neurofibromatosis manifestations, either optic glioma or tibial pseudo-arthrosis and
6. the presence of neurofibromatosis in a first degree relative.

III. Pathognomonic lesions

Three major clinical signs are considered to be of diagnostic importance in von Recklinghausen's neurofibromatosis:
1. pigmentary changes of the skin
2. neurofibromas
3. Lisch nodules of the iris

1. Pigmentary changes of the skin

Pigmentary changes of the skin are found in over 99% of patients with von Recklinghausen's disease. The large yellowish-brown spots or 'café au lait' spots may reach several centimeters in diameter [77]. They present smooth regular borders and are mainly situated on the trunk, the neck or the axillary region. Their number varies, but six or more 'café au lait' spots, larger than 1.5 cm in diameter are considered as a criterion for the diagnosis [23]. This is sometimes called the six spots criterion. 'Café-au-lait' spots may be present at birth but they may also appear gradually until adulthood [77]. They increase in number and in size during the first ten years of life, especially during the first and second year. Histologically they are characterized by an increased formation of both melanocytes and of melanin.

Freckles or lentigines usually appear later than the 'café au lait' spots and may continue to develop during life. Axillary freckling is a clinical sign specific for neurofibromatosis [58]. Freckles may also be found in other intertriginous areas.

Less often than these pathognomic lesions, Addison's-like hyperpigmentation may be observed, sometimes associated with an underlying plexiform neurofibroma [77].

2. Neurofibromas

Cutaneous neurofibromas or fibroma molluscum are pedunculated pigmented nodules which may be distributed over the whole body. They are usually benign and asymptomatic [28]. Their number and size increase with the puberty and also during pregnancy. A fibroma molluscum is composed of enlarged cutaneous nerves with proliferation of Schwann cells and connective tissue [28]. Early tumors contain numerous nerve fibers, whereas older ones show mainly proliferation of the Schwann sheaths and in particular of the endoneural connective tissue [77]. This is the result of the degeneration and disappearance of the nerve fibers.

The plexiform neurofibromas consist of prominently enlarged nerves and the feeling on palpation has been compared to knotted cords, vermicelli or a bag of worms [28, 114]. The eyelids are a common site of neurofibromatous lesions [20]. The most characteristic lesion is a plexiform neurofibroma of the upper eyelid. This may already be present at birth, but usually appears between the ages of two and five years. The neurofibroma gradually increases and provokes elephantiasis of the eyelid (Fig. 6–1). The lesion is usually unilateral and may be accompanied by homolateral buphthalmos and homolateral hemihypertrophy of the face. This triad already described in 1925 [116] is pathognomonic of neurofibromatosis [32].

Massive neurofibromatosis may also cause a massive swelling of the limbs, sometimes called Virchow's elephantiasis neuromatosa [77].

3. Lisch nodules of the iris

Involvement of the iris in neurofibromatosis was already clinically mentioned in 1929 [78]. However, we owe to Lisch [69] the classical description of the

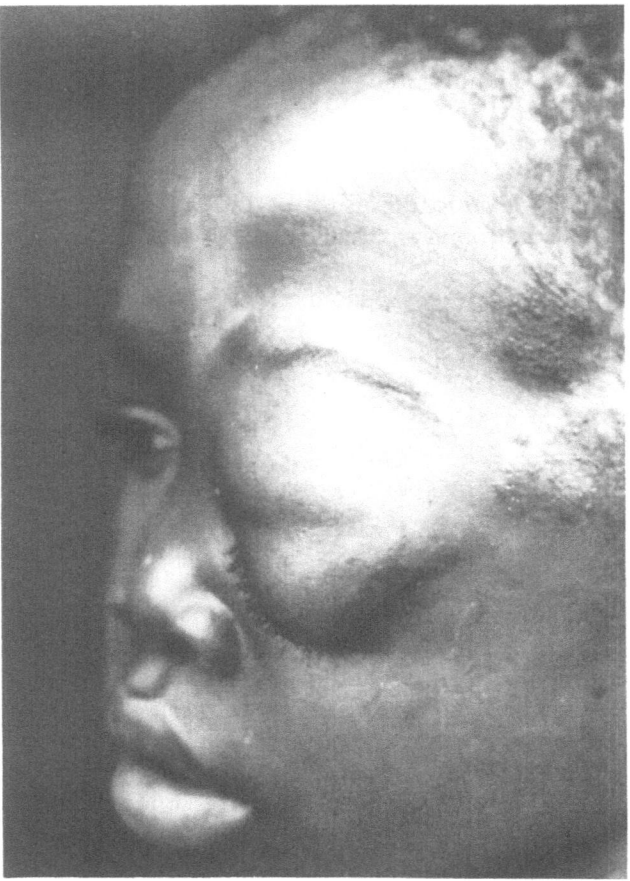

Figure 6–1.   Elephantiasis of the lids in a young boy with neurofibromatosis. (Case 3144.71)

nodules, which since Waardenburg [112] are considered as a major sign in the diagnosis of generalized neurofibromatosis. They have exceptionally been described in a patient with segmental neurofibromatosis [113].

Lisch described them as numerous round, more or less brown pigmented tumors [Fig. 6–2). Their elevation and translucency on biomicroscopy distinguish them from iris nevi [67]. Their size vary from being barely visible up to 2 mm in diameter [58]. They are a common manifestation of the disease [107] and their presence is correlated with the age of the affected individual, but not with the severity of the disease. Lewis and Riccardi [67] found Lisch nodules in 92% of subjects of 6 years of age or more and in 100% of affected individuals aged 16 years or more. Kilchhofer et al. [60] found Lish nodules in all patients aged 12 years or more and none in healthy controls. Most patients do not present iris hamartomas before the age of 6 years [67]. Huson et al. [58] consider that it is extremely unlikely that older children of a patient with neurofibromatosis have inherited the disease if they do not present either 'café-au-lait' spots or Lisch nodules.

Lisch nodules are considered as melanocytic hamartomas [28]. Electron microscopic studies of the iris nodules, obtained by iridectomy during cataract surgery in a 75 year old man with neurofibromatosis proved the spindle shaped cells within the nodules to be of melanocytic origin [81]. As expected, these nodules were also found in eyes with glaucoma [73, 120], although they are probably not the cause of glaucoma in such eyes.

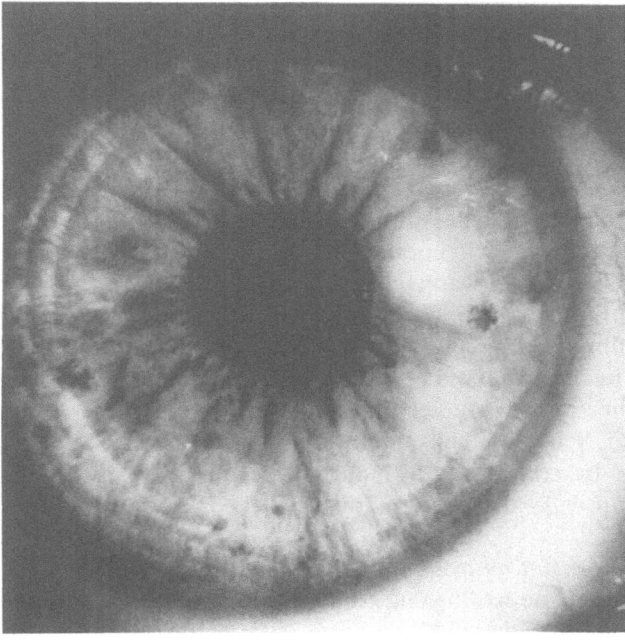

Figure 6–2.   Lisch nodules.

IV. Fundus examinations in von Recklinghausen's disease

1. Choroidal lesions

a. Choroidal nevi and nodules
Choroidal hamartomas are probably the most common fundus manifestation in ocular neurofibromatosis. Such lesions were found in 18 of 51 patients (29%) in the series of Huson et al. [58] and in 51% in the series of Lewis and Riccardi [67]. The lesions are discrete with pigmentation varying between yellow-white to light brown. Their number varies from one to twenty in the same fundus and their size is about two disc diameters. They are scattered around the posterior pole and behave like nevi on fluorescein angiography. Sometimes however they may present hyperfluorescence during fluorescein angiography [61, 89]. They are usually found during a systematic examination of neurofibromatosis patients and do not provoke visual disturbances [89]. Gass followed such lesions during a three years period and observed no change in fundus appearance [40]. These lesions, which are seen only in Caucasians and not in blacks [67], were called 'café-au-lait' spots of the fundus [22].

b. Larger choroidal tumors and diffuse neurofibromatosis of the choroid
Diffuse involvement of the uvea is rarely diagnosed clinically in neurofibromatosis as it is often associated with buphthalmos [16, 18, 62, 65, 74, 119] or with retinal detachment [86].

Histologically the choroid appears markedly thickened. The tumors seems to arise in the vicinity of ciliary nerves [18, 34, 74, 97] or from the perivascular nerve plexus [36]. In some cases it appears possible to demonstrate a direct connection with the ciliary nerves [18, 31, 34]. The tumor consists of nervous fibers, Schwann cells, ganglion cells, fibrocytes and variable amounts of melanocytes [51] (Fig. 6–3). The distinction between neurofibroma and neurilemmoma or schwannoma is not always very obvious, but the latter does not contain axons or neurites [34]. The typical ovoid bodies consist of Schwann cells arranged in whorls [18, 119] (Fig. 6–4). These ovoid bodies were considered as the result of the transverse section of the neurofibromatous bundles, which form the tumor [86]. Wolter [119] demonstrated that nerves entered the ovoid bodies. This was confirmed by electron microscopic studies [65] which showed that ovoid bodies consist of proliferated Schwann cells in intimate contact with axons. Ovoid bodies should thus be considered as enlarged peripheral nerves with hyperplasia of the Schwann cells and of the axons.

c. Malignant melanomas of the uvea
A number of neurofibromatosis patients have developed a malignant melanoma of the choroid or of the ciliary body [19, 29, 39, 45, 98, 117]. There is a possible relationship between the greater number of nevi of the

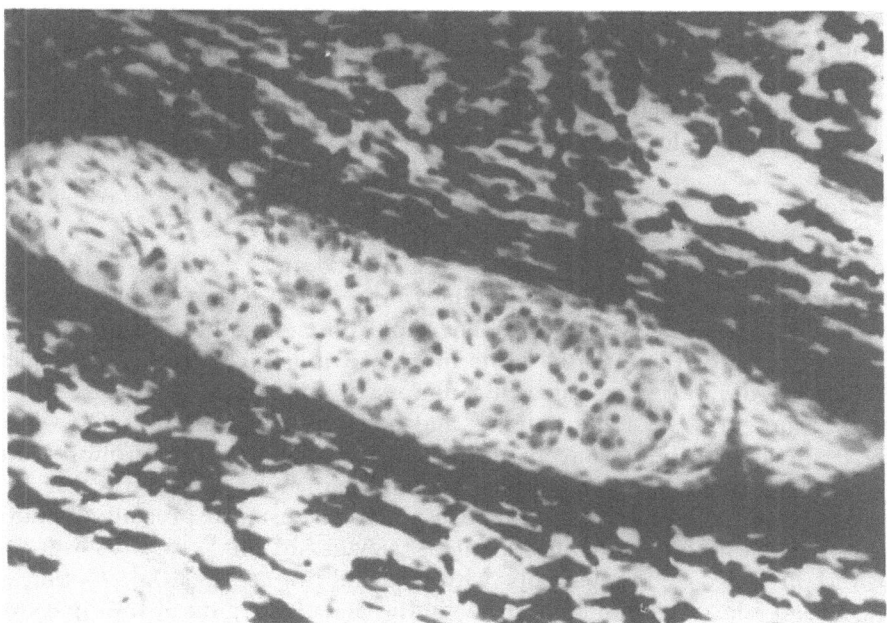

Figure 6-3.   Accumulation of ganglion cells in the choroid (case 3144.71, H. E., same case as Fig. 6-1).

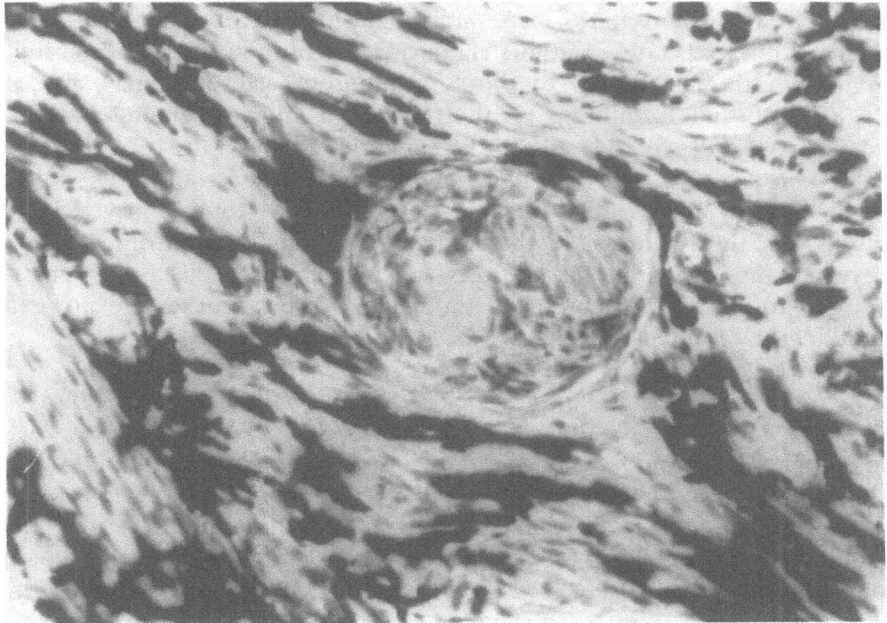

Figure 6-4.   Ovoid bodies in the choroid (case 3144.71, H. E., same case as Fig. 6-1).

choroid in patients with neurofibromatosis and the slightly increased incidence of uveal melanomas [117]. According to Nordmann and Brini [79] the association of a tumor of the optic nerve with a melanoma of the iris should be considered as von Recklinghausen's disease, even in the absence of cutaneous anomalies.

2. *Retina*

a. *Retinal tumors*

The presence of retinal tumors similar to the phakomas of tuberous sclerosis was described [10, 28, 73, 103]. They look like a mulberry mass and have little or no growth potential [10]. In 42 previously reported, histologically documented reports on astrocytic tumors of the retina, tuberous sclerosis was found in 52% of the patients and neurofibromatosis in 14%, whereas 29% appeared otherwise to be normal. The patients with neurofibromatosis as well as the apparently normal patients had more frequently disc based lesions, while patients with tuberous sclerosis usually presented multiple peripheral tumors containing giant astrocytes. Multiple tumors were also found in 50% of the patients with neurofibromatosis [106]. Cotlier [22] described a large retinal hamartoma in the macular region of the right eye of a patient with neurofibromatosis. A second retinal hamartoma was found more peripherically in the same eyes. These lesions were associated with 'café au lait' spots of the fundus.

From a histological point of view some state that the astrocytic hamartomas in neurofibromatosis are indistinguishable from those in tuberous sclerosis [28, 62]. Other authors claim that the retinal tumors of neurofibromatosis, although similar to those of tuberous sclerosis, may also show angiomatous malformations [103]. It is worthwhile to remember that van der Hoeve [109] already stressed the similarity between the retinal tumors in these two diseases. They are built up by the same fibers and cells, but some of them show also vessels, which are more like the tumors in von Hippel's disease. It thus seems as if the retinal lesions in neurofibromatosis stands between those in tuberous sclerosis and von Hippel's disease. It appeared evident to van der Hoeve that although the three diseases are not exactly similar, they are closely related.

a.1. *Neurogenic retinal tumors (Fig. 6–5)*. The first cases were reported by van der Hoeve [108, 109]. A case of Bloch [10] unfortunately lacks a histological examination. Hogan and Zimmerman [54] described a tumor of the optic nerve head, the peripapillary and peripheral retina with the appearance of an astrocytic hamartoma. Hales [50] described retinal gliomas composed of branching astrocytes and large ganglion-like cells, involving only the inner retinal layers. Martyn and Knox [73] observed an extensive glial hamartoma of the retina in a case of generalized neurofibromatosis. The tumor consisted of fine fibrils and cells, with round or oval nuclei, some

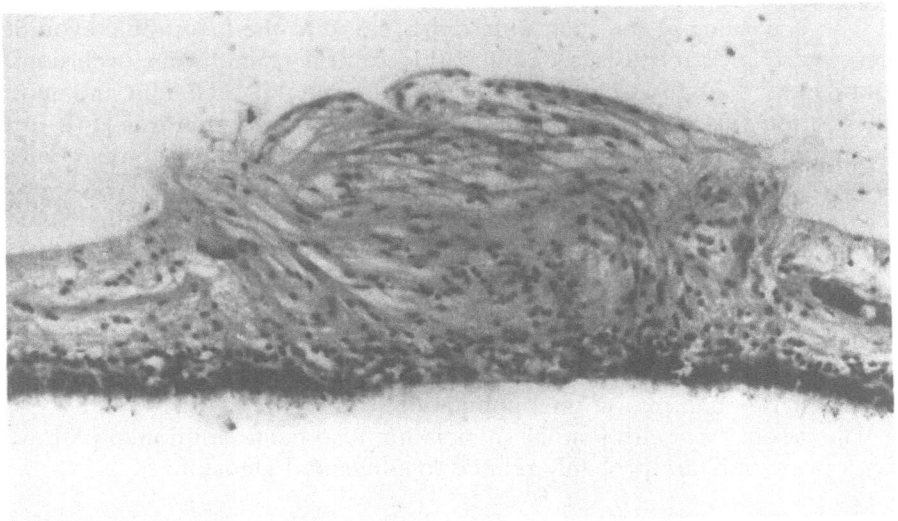

Figure 6–5. Retinal lesion in ocular neurofibromatosis (courtesy of Prof. W. Manschot, Rotterdam, case 0703).

arranged in swirl-like formation. Some cells had spindle-shaped or large pale nuclei and stellate cytoplasmic processes. Several foci of calcification and vascular channels were also present. Davis [25] noticed the association of an optic nerve glioma with an intraocular plexiform neuroma.

a.2. Angiomas. Retinal angiomas, usually solitary, with or without retinal neuromas have also been reported in patients with neurofibromatosis [15, 37, 108, 119].

a.3. Other tumors. Large retinal tumors, which were classified as retinal neuromas, were described by Mans [71] and von Papolczy [110]. In the case of Pieck [82] there was no relation with neurofibromatosis. Hansanreisoglu et al. [53] presented a young child with neurofibromatosis and unilateral retinoblastoma.

b. Non-tumoral retinal changes
Various retinal changes have been described in patients with neurifibromatosis, such as retinal detachment, atrophy, drusen or cystic degeneration [3]. There are two reports on sectorial retinitis pigmentosa [1, 66] in association with von Recklinghausen's disease.

Retinal vascular changes are also found. Hemorrhages, neo-vascularization [3] and hypertensive retinopathy may be the consequence of pheochromocytomas which are relatively more frequent in von Recklinghausen's disease [27, 57] as well as in von Hippel-Lindau's disease [93]. In twins with neurofibromatosis ophthalmic vein occlusion was reported [84].

In fact, according to the clinical description and to the favourable evolution, these were probably cases of idiopathic central retinal vein occlusions in young individuals. A Coats-like aspect, with retinal detachment and neovascularization was observed in association with neurofibromatosis [15]. In the patient of Frenkel [37] the so-called retinal angiomatosis looks clinically much more like retinal macro-aneurysms.

Gliosis is frequently reported in association or not with retinal tumors. The membraue extends upon the internal face of the retinal through breaks in the internal limiting membrane [83] (Figs 6–6, 6–7). A good clinical example is given by Cotlier's patient [22].

Medullated retinal fibers have been observed in neurofibromatosis [28, 44, 62, 114], but it is not clearly established if their frequency is greater in such patients than in a normal population [8].

The association with familial myopia has also been mentioned [90]. Most cases of myopia are probably related to congenital glaucoma.

3. Optic disc

a. Tumors of the optic disc

Tumors confined to the optic disc are extremely rare in neurofibromatosis [3, 42, 44, 88, 95] as they generally represent an anterior extension of a glioma of the much more frequently involved orbital portion of the nerve [3, 12, 72, 88]. It has indeed been stated that approximately one fourth of the gliomas of the optic nerve could be combined with von Recklinghausen's disease [33]. Also intraocular extension of optic nerve meningioma has been observed (Fig. 6–8), associated or not with neurofibromatosis [21].

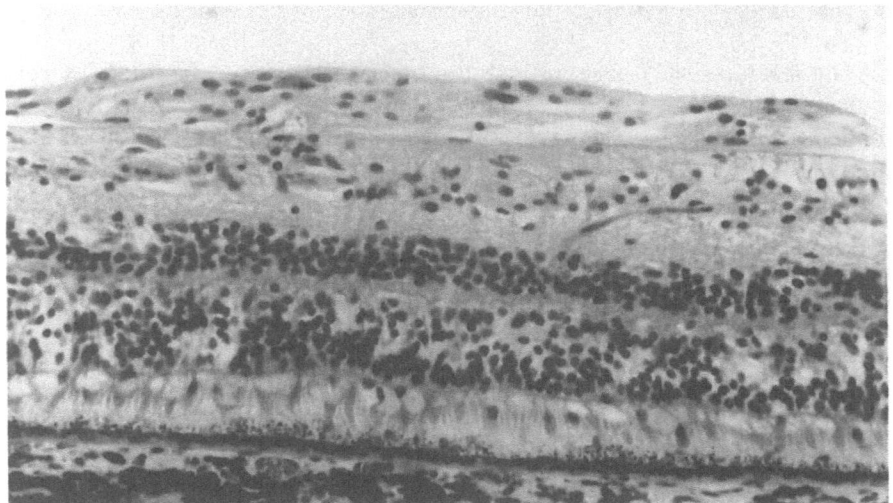

Figure 6–6.   Preretinal glial proliferation in neurofibromatosis oculi (courtesy of Prof. W. Manschot, Rotterdam, case 0703).

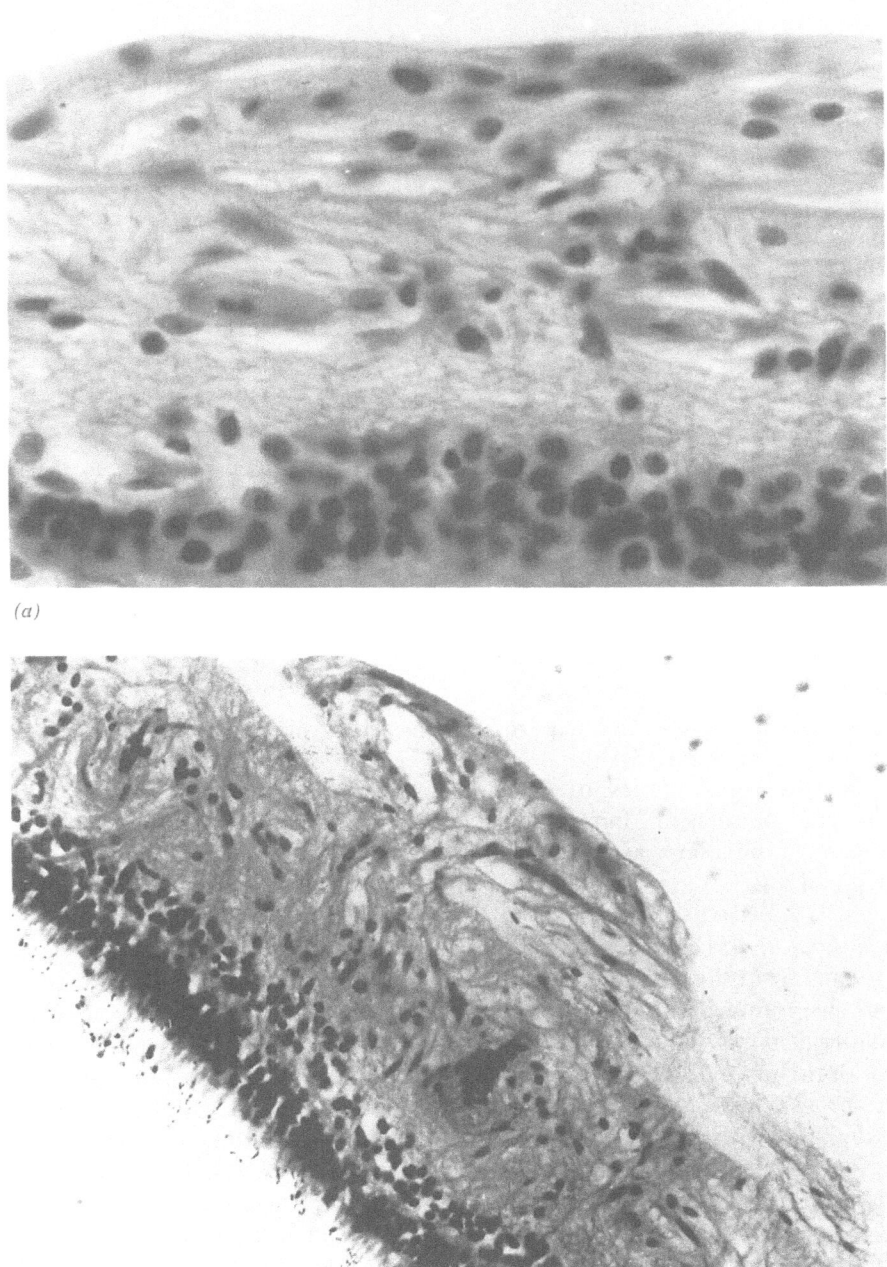

(a)

(b)

Figure 6–7. Ocular neurofibromatosis. Preretinal glial proliferation with breaks in the internal limiting membrane (courtesy of Prof. W. Manschot, Rotterdam, case 0703).

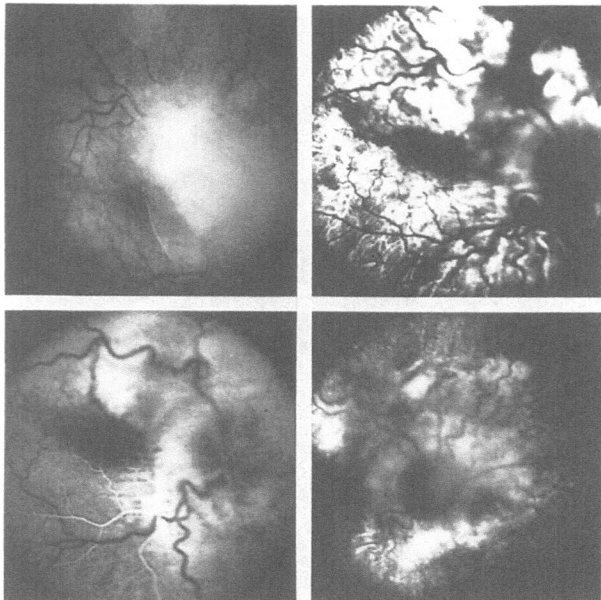

Figure 6–8.   Intra-ocular extension of a meningioma of the optic nerve. Ophthalmoscopic and fluoroangiographic aspect.

Lateral extension into the peripapillary retina occurs commonly but does not extend very far [7].

The mulberry masses involving the optic nerve head are histologically not true glial neoplasms, but rather a hamartomatous malformation composed mainly of fibrillary astrocytes with frequent secondary dystrophic calcifications [28].

a.1. Unilateral cases. Stallard [95] observed a hemispherical mass projecting forward from the disc and described it histologically as a neuroma of the disc and the retina. Trueman and Rubin [102] also reported a case but without histological examination. In Hogan and Zimmerman's case [54] the tumor of the optic nerve head, parapapillary and peripheral retina had the appearance of an astrocytic hamartoma. Hales [50] described a glioma of the disc associated with peripheral retinal gliomas and extending into the adjacent retina and behind the lamina cribrosa. Tincao et al. [101] reported a well-defined, richly vascularized astrocytic hamartoma of the optic disc and the peripapillary retina. Boles et al. [12] noticed in a young girl a mushroom shaped mass arising from the nerve head into the vitreous. The tumor extended into and underneath the retina. It was formed by spindle shaped structures, some arranged in whorls.

It may be remembered that White and Loewenstein [115] described an unpigmented tumor of the optic disc, which was composed of unusual large

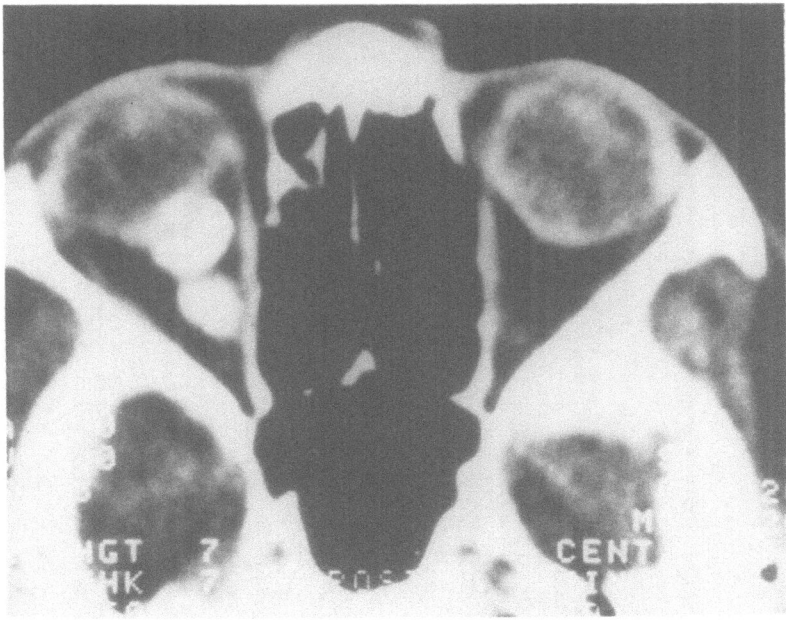

Figure 6-9.   CT-scan of the orbit in a case of intraocular extension of a meningioma of the optic nerve (same case as Fig. 6-8).

foamy cells. The tumor clinically resembled the disc lesions in von Reckling-hausen's disease, although there was no systemic evidence of neurofibro-matosis.

a.2. Bilateral cases. In Goldsmith's case there was no histological study of the ocular tissues [44]. In the case of Saran and Winter [88] the tumors also invaded the surrounding retina.

From a pathological point of view [3] the tumors are composed of bundles and whorls of slender fibers with oval or elongated nuclei. Fibrillary astro-cytes, ganglion cells and large polyhedral cells may be found. Calcification and cystic changes are common, as well as gliosis of the overlying nerve fiber layer. The tumors typically extend laterally to some degree into the retina, with the advancing edge forming a wedge between the nuclear layers. They may invade all layers and sometimes even destroy the photoreceptors and pigmentepithelial cells. The lamina cribrosa generally limits the posterior extension, although occasionally the tumor may invade the distal optic nerve [50].

b. Secondary changes of the optic disc
Papiledema [52, 91] or optic atrophy [92] may be the consequence of intracranial neurofibromas or secondary to the presence of a glioma of the

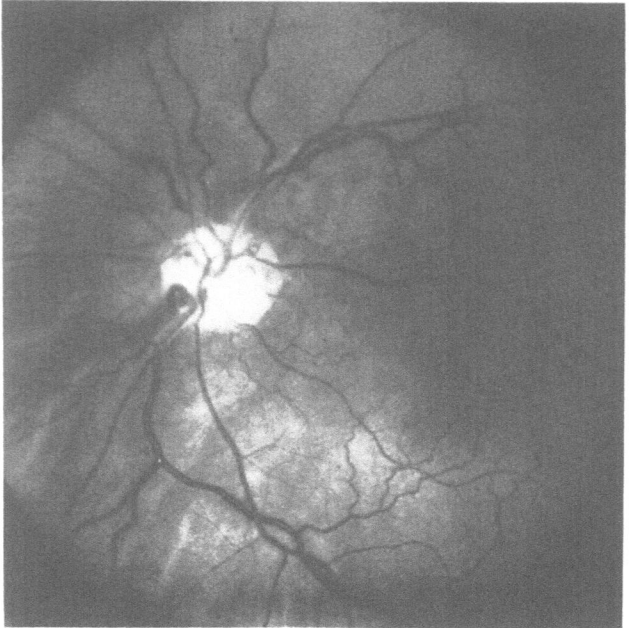

Figure 6–10.   Optico-ciliary shunt vessels and optic atrophy associated with optic nerve sheath meningioma in a patient with generalized neurofibromatosis.

optic nerve or of the chiasm.

The association of optic atrophy, poor vision and opticociliary veins may be related to the presence of primary optic nerve sheath meningioma [38, 122] (Fig. 6–10). These opticociliary veins probably result from a progressive obstruction of the central vein by the severe compression of the optic nerve [122] and they must be differentiated from opticociliary shunt vessels caused by central retinal vein occlusion from other causes.

c. Other manifestations
Cilio-optic veins have been noted in a patient with neurofibromatosis and in another with Sturge-Weber disease [124]. They probably represent a congenital anomaly unrelated to phakomatoses.

V. Other ophthalmological manifestations

1. Orbit

Proptosis may be the first sign of orbital involvement in neurofibromatosis [62] and may result from the presence of intra-orbital neurofibroma [64], optic nerve tumors or dysplasia of the orbital bones [20, 123]. The partial loss or absence of the orbital wall is usually not due to the destruction of the bone by the tumor but is congenital in origin [35]. The sphenoid is most commonly affected although involvement of the orbital floor has also been described [48].

An extensive deficit of the orbital wall may result in pulsating enophthalmos or exophthalmos [17, 40, 80, 89, 114].

2. *Tumors of the eye (except choroidal and retinal tumors)*

In neurofibromatosis tumors may affect the various parts of the eye with the exception of the lens. Neurofibromas have been described in ocular muscles [62], conjunctiva [2, 59], episclera [6], cornea [41, 62]. The corneal nerves may appear thickened [76, 118, 120]. The most important tumors however are gliomas of the optic nerve [24–27, 43, 56, 87, 96]. Their association with von Recklinghausen's disease is well established. In patients with neurofibromatosis, the diagnosis of optic nerve glioma is usually made at a younger age than in patients without neurofibromatosis [96]. It is important to realize that a large number of cases are not detected by ophthalmological examination [68]. Lewis et al. [68] found a 15% incidence of optic nerve or chiasmal gliomas in neurofibromatosis, whereas previous reports estimated it between 1 and 5%. This is largely due to improved diagnostic methods [24, 49, 55, 68, 123]. Optic gliomata may be associated with normal or nearnormal visual acuity [46, 56] and such tumor was even an autopsy finding in an older patient, who died from an unrelated cause [56].

Other optic nerve involvement includes meningiomas [91], gangliomata [7] and diffuse optic nerve hyperplasia [94].

3. *Congenital glaucoma*

Congenital glaucoma is frequently described in neurofibromatosis in association with neurofibromas of the eyelids and facial hypertrophy [38, 83, 114, 116, 121]. Bilateral buphthalmos has been reported [104]. Glaucoma in neurofibromatosis does not necessarily present with buphthalmos [120]. Grant and Walton [47] consider four possible mechanisms which may provoke glaucoma in such eyes:
1. invasion of the angle by tumor
2. thickening of the choroid and ciliary body by neurofibromas pushing the iris forwards
3. neovascularization of the iris
4. failure of the normal development of the angle structures with absence of Schlemm's canal. The last eventuality is possibly a secondary phenomenon.

4. Cataract

The presence of cataract in neurofibromatosis [13, 16, 52] is probably either coincidental or to be considered as a secondary phenomenon.

VI. Association with other phakomatoses

We already pointed out that van der Hoeve considered neurofibromatosis, von Hippel-Lindau's disease and tuberous sclerosis as closely related.

The coexistence of von Recklinghausen's disease and of von Hippel-Lindau's disease in a same family was reported by Tischler et al. [100]. The same family was further studied by Thomas et al. [99] and three of the family members were found to have retinal angiomas which had not been noticed three years previously. In three patients ocular and systemic signs of neurofibromatosis were also found.

Association of Sturge-Weber's syndrome and neurofibromatosis has also been described in a patient who died at the age of 36 years of an acute shock secondary to adrenal insufficiency. The patient presented a nevus flammeus and histologically proven neurofibromata in the flank and in the back. At autopsy bilateral phaeochromocytomas were found, as well as a capillary cavernous angioma of the choroid, hypertrophied nerves in the ciliary muscles and nodules on the anterior surface of the iris [85].

The association of an isolated choroidal hemangioma and neurofibromatosis has been reported [52] as well as the association of neurofibromatosis and retinal angioma [119].

VII. Treatment

Except when malignant melanomas are found, treatment is seldom needed for neurofibromatous lesions of the retina or of the choroid.

The management of optic nerve gliomas is still debated. According to Hoyt and Baghdassarian [56] as the optic glioma in neurofibromatosis does not markedly affect the prognosis for life, excision of such a tumor should only be considered when it provokes intracranial hypertension or if it is the cause of marked proptosis in a blind eye. Lloyd [70] however advocates a radical approach of tumors confined to one optic nerve and according to Rush et al. [87] the survival of patients with optic nerve tumors is significantly related to the completeness of surgical excision.

References

1. Agoston I (1968): Beidseitige symmetrische Sektorenförmige Pigmentveränderung der Netzhaut bei den Recklinghauschen Neurofibromatosis. *Acta Ophthalmol*, 46: 41–48.

2. Allende F P (1945): Diffuse neurofibromatosis (von Recklinghausen's disease) involving the bulbar conjunctiva. Report of a case with lesions of the skeletal system and skin, bodily asymmetry and intracranial involvement. *Arch Ophthalmol*, 33: 110–115.

3. Archer D B and Nevin N C (1977): The phakomatoses. I. Neurofibromatosis – von Recklinghausen's disease in *Krill's Hereditary retinal and choroidal diseases*, Harper and Row Publishers, vol. 2, 1193–1218.

4. Barker D, Wright E, Nguyen K, Cannon L, Fain P, Goldgar D, Bishop D T, Carey J, Baty B, Kiu Lin J, Willard H, Waye J S, Greig G, Leinwand L, Nakamura Y, O'Connell P, Leppert M, Lalouel J M, White R, and Skolnick M (1987): Gene for von Recklinghausen's neurofibromatosis is in the pericentrometric region of chromosome 17. *Science*, 236: 1100–1102.

5. Beck R W and Hanno R (1986): The phakomatose. *Int Ophthalmol Clin*, 25: 97–116.

6. Bengisu U, Tahsinoglu M, and Toker G (1973): La neurofibromatose associée au choristome cartilagineux de l' épisclère. *Ann Oculist*, 206: 401–403.

7. Bergin D J, Johnson T E, Spencer W H and McCord C D (1988): Gangliomata of the optic nerve. *Am J Ophthalmol*, 105: 146–149.

8. Bickler-Bluth M E, Custer P L, and Smith M E (1988): Neurilemmoma as a presenting feature of neurofibromatosis. *Arch Ophthalmol*, 106: 665–667.

9. Bielschowsky M (1914): Ueber tuberöse Sklerose und ihre Beziehungen zur Recklinghausensche Krankheit. *Z Ges Neurol Psychiatr*, 26: 133–155.

10. Bloch F J (1948): Retinal tumor associated with neurofibromatosis (von Recklinghausen's disease). Report of a case. *Arch Ophthalmol*, 40: 433–437.

11. Bolande R P (1974): The neurocristopathies. A unifying concept of disease arising in neural crest maldevelopment. *Hum Pathology*, 5: 409–429.

12. Boles W M, Naugle T C and Samson C L M (1958): Glioma of the optic nerve. Report of a case arising from the optic disc. *Arch Ophthalmol*, 59: 229–231.

13. Bonamour G and Leopold (1958): Cataracte de type syndermatotique et maladie de Recklinghausen. *Bull Soc Ophtalmol Fr*, 58: 592–593.

14. Brini A (1986): La neurofibromatose, l'oeil et ses annexes. Une synthèse. *Bull Soc Ophtalmol Fr*, 86: 335–337.

15. Bronner A, Roth A, and Fritz B (1959): Lésions oculaires au cours d'une neurofibromatose de von Recklinghausen. *Bull Soc Ophtalmol Fr*, 11: 723–729.

16. Brownstein S, and Little J M (1983): Ocular neurofibromatosis. *Ophthalmology*, 91: 1595–1599.

17. Bullock J D, and Bartley G B (1986): Dynamic proptosis. *Am J Ophthalmol*, 102: 104–110.

18. Callender G R, and Thigpen C A (1930): Two neurofibromas in one eye. *Am J Ophthalmol* 13: 121–124.

19. Cernea P, and Dobrescu G (1973): Mélanome malin uvéal, manifestation de la maladie de Recklinghausen. *Ophthalmologica*, 166: 161–171.

20. Charleux J (1960): Les manifestations palpébrales et orbitaires de la neurofibromatose de Recklinghausen. *Ann Oculist*, 193: 930–962.

21. Cibis G W, Whittaker C K, and Wood W E (1985): Intraocular extension of optic nerve meningioma in a case of neurofibromatosis. *Arch Ophthalmol*, 103: 404–406.

22. Cotlier E (1977): Café au lait spots of the fundus in neurofibromatosis. *Arch Ophthalmol*, 95: 1990–1992.

23. Crowe F W, Schull W J, and Neel J V (1956): A clinical, pathological and genetic study of multiple neurofibromatosis Charles C. Thomas (ed.): Springfield (III).

24. Curatolo P, and Cusmai R (1987): Optic glioma in children with neurofibromatosis. *Lancet*, 1: 1140.

25. Davis F A (1939): Plexiform neurofibromatosis (Recklinghausen's disease) of orbit and globe with associated glioma of the optic nerve and brain. Report of a case. *Arch Ophthalmol*, 22: 761–791.

26. Davis F A (1940): Primary tumors of the optic nerve (a phenomenon of Recklinghausen's disease). A clinical and pathologic study with a report of five cases and a review of the

literature. *Arch Ophthalmol*, 23: 735–821, 957–1018.

27. Fledelius H, and Eldrup Jorgensen P (1977): Optic nerve glioma and phaeochromocytoma associated with von Recklinghausen's disease: a case report. *Br J Ophthalmol*, 61: 240–243.

28. Font R L, and Ferry A P (1972): The phakomatoses. *Int Ophthalmol Clin*, 12: 1–50.

29. Francois J (1948): Les manifestations oculaires de la maladie de Recklinghausen. *Ann Oculist*, 181: 753–791.

30. Francois J (1972): A general introduction. in *Handbook of clinical neurology*, P J Vinken and G W Bruyn, vol. 14. The phakomotoses, North Holland Publishing C°, Amsterdam, 1–18.

31. Francois J, Hanssens M, and Evens L (1972): Ganglioneurome mélanique de la choroïde. *Bull Soc Belge Ophthalmol*, 162: 858–867.

32. Francois J, and Katz C (1961): Association homolatérale d'hydrophtalmie, de névrome plexiforme de la paupière supérieure et d'hémihypertrophie faciale dans la maladie de Recklinghausen. *Ophthalmologica*, 142: 549–571.

33. Francois J, Verriest G, and Deblond R (1963): Gliome du chiasma, manifestation d'une neurofibromatose de Recklinghausen. *Acta Neurol Belg*, 63: 545–550.

34. Freedman S F, Elner V M, Donev I, Gunta R, and Albert D M (1988): Intra-ocular neurilemmoma arising from the posterior ciliary nerve in neurofibromatosis. Pathologic findings. *Ophthalmology*, 95: 1559–1564.

35. Freeman A G (1987): Proptosis and neurofibromatosis. *Lancet* 1032–1033.

36. Freeman D (1934): Neurofibroma of the choroid. *Arch Ophthalmol*, 11: 641–645.

37. Frenkel M (1967): Retinal angiomatosis in a patient with neurofibromatosis. *Am J Ophthalmol*, 63: 804–808.

38. Frisen L, Hoyt W F, and Trengroth B M (1973): Optociliary veins, disc pallor and visual loss: a triad of signs indicating spheno-orbital meningioma. *Acta Ophthalmol*, 51: 241–249.

39. Gartner S (1940): Malignant melanoma of the choroid and von Recklinghausen's disease. *Am J Ophthalmol*, 23: 73–78.

40. Gass J D M (1974): Differential diagnosis of intraocular tumors. A stereoscopic presentation. The C V Mosby C°, St, Louis, 22–23.

41. Gasteiger (1938): Ueber seltene Augenveränderungen bei Neurofibromatose. *Ztschr Augenheilk*, 95: 167–168.

42. Gilly J P, Leguellec M, Cotineau J and Sorato M (1975): Les tumeurs primitives de la papille au cours de la neurofibromatose de Recklinghausen. *Ann Oculist*, 208: 13–28.

43. Goldmann H, and Grunthal E (1941): Ueber einen Tumor des Sehnerven und seiner Leptomeningen bei Recklinghausenscher Krankheit. *Ophthalmologica*, 102: 79–92.

44. Goldsmith J (1949): Neurofibromatosis associated with tumors of the optic papilla. Report of a case. *Arch Ophthalmol*, 41: 718–729.

45. Goldstein I, and Wexler D (1930): Melanosis uveae and melanoma of the iris in neurofibromatosis (Recklinghausen). *Arch Ophthalmol*, 3: 288–296.

46. Goldstein I and Wexler D (1932): Spongioneuroblastoma of the optic nerve in neurofibromatosis (Recklinghausen). *Arch Ophthalmol*, 7: 259–267.

47. Grant W M, and Walton D S (1968): Distinctive gonioscopic findings in glaucoma due to neurofibromatosis. *Arch Ophthalmol*, 79: 127–134.

48. Gurland J E, Tenner M, Hornblass A, and Wolintz A H (1976): Orbital neurofibromatosis: involvement of the orbital floor. *Arch Ophthalmol*, 94: 1723–1725.

49. Haik B G, Saint Louis L, Bierly J, Smith M E, Abramson D A, Ellsworth R M, and Wall M (1987): Magnetic resonance imaging in the evaluation of optic nerve gliomas. *Ophthalmology*, 94: 709–717.

50. Hales R H (1963): Glioma of the optic disc. *Arch Ophthalmol*, 70: 648–650.

51. Hanssens M (1973): Recklinghausen's disease with ocular involvement. Presented at EOPS' 12th annual meeting, Dublin.

52. Hartemann P, Dureux J B, and Martin J (1957): Considérations ophthalmologiques et électro-encéphalographiques sur 31 observations de sclérose tubéreuse de Bourneville et

de neurofibromatose de Recklinghausen. *Rev Oto-Neuro-Ophtalmol*, 29: 216–225.

53. Hasanreisoglu B, Or M, and Akbatur H (1988): Neurofibromatosis associated with retinoblastoma: case report. *Br J Ophthalmol*, 72: 139–141.
54. Hogan M J and Zimmerman L E (1962): Ophthalmic Pathology. 2nd Edition, W B Saunders, Philadelphia, 443–530.
55. Holman R E, Grimson B S, and Drayer B P (1985): Magnetic resonance imaging of optic gliomas. *Am J Ophthalmol*, 100: 596–601.
56. Hoyt W F, and Baghdassarian S A (1969): Optic glioma of childhood. Natural history and rationale to conservative treatment. *Br J Ophthalmol*, 53: 793–798.
57. Humble R M (1967): Phaeochromocytoma, neurofibromatosis and pregnancy. *Anaestesia*, 22: 296–303.
58. Huson S, Jones D, and Beck L (1987): Ophthalmic manifestations of neurofibromatosis. *Br J Ophthalmol*, 74: 235–238.
59. Insler M S, Helm C, and Napoli S (1985): Conjunctival hamartoma in neurofibromatosis. *Am J Ophthalmol*, 99: 731–733.
60. Kilchhofer A, Boltshauser E, and Flueler U (1986): Aspekt und Inzidenz der Irishamartome bei Neurofibromatosis von Recklinghausen. *Klin Mbl Augenheilk*, 188: 416–417.
61. Klein R M, and Glassman L (1985): Neurofibromatosis of the choroid. *Am J Ophthalmol*, 99: 367–368.
62. Kobrin J L, Blodi F C, and Weingeist T A (1979): Ocular and orbital manifestations of neurofibromatosis. *Survey Ophthalmol*, 24: 45–51.
63. Koch G (1972): Genetic aspects of the phakomatoses. in *Handbook of Clinical Neurology*, P J Vinken, and G W Bruyn, vol. 14. The phakomatoses, North Holland Publishing C°, Amsterdam, 488–561.
64. Krohel G B, Rosenberg P M, Wright J E, and Smith R S (1985): Localized orbital neurofibromatosis. *Am J Ophthalmol*, 100: 458–464.
65. Kurosawa A and Kurosawa H (1982): Ovoid bodies in choroidal neurofibromatosis. *Arch Ophthalmol*, 100: 1939–1941.
66. La Piana F G (1977): Sectorial retinal pigmentation in neurofibromatosis. *Ann Ophthalmol* 9: 413–422.
67. Lewis R A, and Riccardi V M (1981): Von Recklinghausen neurofibromatosis. Incidence of iris hamartomas. *Ophthalmology*, 88: 348–354.
68. Lewis R A, Gerson L P, Axelson K A Riccardi V M, and Whitford R P (1984): Von Recklinghausen neurofibromatosis. II. Incidence of optic gliomata. *Ophthalmology*, 91: 929–935.
69. Lisch K (1937): Ueber Beteiligung der Augen, insbezondere das Vorkommen von Irisknötchen bei der Neurofibromatose (Recklinghausen). *Ztschr Augenheilk*, 93: 137–143.
70. Lloyd L A (1974): Gliomas of the optic nerve and chiasm in childhood. *Trans Am ophthalmol Soc*, 71: 488–535.
71. Mans (1927): Neurofibromatose des Auges. *Klin Mbl Augenheilk*, 79: 548.
72. Manschot W A (1954): Primary tumours of the optic nerve in von Recklinghausen's disease. *Br J Ophthalmol*, 38: 285–289.
73. Martyn L J and Knox D L (1972): Glial hamartoma of the retina in generalized neurofibromatoses. Von Recklinghausen's disease. *Br J Ophthalmol*, 56: 487–491.
74. Meeker L H (1936): Plexiform neuroma of the choroid in a non-buphthalmic eye. *Arch Ophthalmol*, 16: 152.
75. Miller N R (1975): Optic nerve glioma and cerebellar astrocytoma in a patient with von Recklinghausen's neurofibromatosis. *Am J Ophthalmol*, 79: 582–588.
76. Miller N R (1988): Neurofibromatosis. in *Clinical Neuro-ophthalmology*, Walsh and Hoyt, 4th edition, vol. 3. 1747–1765.
77. Musger A (1972): Dermatological aspects of the phakomatoses. in *Handbook of clinical Neurology*, P J Vinken and G W Bruyn, vol. 14, The phakomatoses, North Holland Publishing C°, Amsterdam, 562–618.

78. Nitsch M (1929): Neurofibromatose des Auges. *Ztschr Augenheilk*, 69: 117–143.
79. Nordmann J, and Brini A (1970): Von Recklinghausen's disease and melanoma of the uvea. *Br J Ophthalmol*, 54: 641–648.
80. Paufique L, Etienne R, and Charleux J (1956): Exophtalmie pulsatile par malformation orbitaire dans la neurofibromatose de von Recklinghausen. *Bull Soc Fr Ophtalmol*, 69: 203–214.
81. Perry H D, and Font R L (1982): Iris nodules in von Recklinghausen's neurofibromatosis. Electron microscopic confirmation of their melanocytic origin. *Arch Ophthalmol*, 100: 1635–1640.
82. Pieck C F M (1936): Ein Fall von Neurinoma Retinae. *Von Graefe's Arch Ophthalmol*, 135: 451–461.
83. Politi F, Sachs R, and Barishak R (1978): Neurofibromatosis and congenital glaucoma. A case report. *Ophthalmologica*, 176: 155–159.
84. Pollet-de Lille and Pollet J (1953): Deux cas de thrombose de la veine ophtalmique chez deux jumelles atteintes de maladie de Recklinghausen. *Bull Soc Fr Ophtalmol*, 53: 286–288.
85. Riley F C, and Campbell R J (1979): Double phakomatosis. *Arch Ophthalmol*, 97: 518–520.
86. Robson S, Blackwood W, and Cookson H A (1941): Case of von Recklinghausen's disease with diffuse neurofibromatosis of choroid. *Br J Ophthalmol*, 25: 431–442.
87. Rush J A, Younge B R, Campbell R J, and MacCarty C S (1982): Optic glioma: long-term follow-up of 85 histopathologically verified cases. *Ophthalmology*, 89: 1213–1219.
88. Saran N, and Winter F C (1967): Bilateral gliomas of the optic disc associated with neurofibromatosis. *Am J Ophthalmol*, 64: 607–612.
89. Savino P J, Glaser J S, and Luxenberg M N (1977): Pulsating enophthalmos and choroidal hamartomas: two rare stigmata of neurofibromatosis. *Br J Ophthalmol*, 61: 483–488.
90. Schmoger E (1956): Myopia and von Recklinghausen's neurofibromatosis. *Von Graefe's Arch Ophthalmol*, 157: 260–277.
91. Shapland C D, and Greenfield J G (1935): A case of neurofibromatosis with meningeal tumour involving the left optic nerve. *Trans Ophthalmol Soc U.K.*, 55: 257–279.
92. Sheehan B (1952): Optic atrophy with altitudinal hemianopia in neurofibromatosis. *Br J Ophthalmol*, 36: 506–510.
93. Shokeir M H K (1970): Von Hippel-Lindau syndrome: a report on three kindreds. *J Med Genet*, 7: 155–157.
94. Spencer W H, and Borit A (1967): Diffuse hyperplasia of the optic nerve in von Recklinghausen's disease. *Am J Ophthalmol*, 64: 638–642.
95. Stallard H B (1938): A case of intra-ocular neuroma (von Recklinghausen's disease) of the left optic nerve head. *Br J Ophthalmol*, 22: 11–18.
96. Stern J, Jakobiec F A, and Housepian E M (1980): The architecture of optic nerve gliomas with and without neurofibromatosis. *Arch Ophthalmol*, 98: 505–511.
97. Stough J T (1937): Intraocular neurofibroma. Report of a case. *Arch Ophthalmol*, 18: 540–546.
98. Szekler R (1953): Ein Uvealsarkom bei einem Mitglied einer Familie mit Recklinghausenscher Krankheit. *Ophthalmologica*, 126: 248–251.
99. Thomas J V, Schwartz P L, and Gragoudas E S (1978): Von Hippel's disease in association with von Recklinghausen's neurofibromatosis. *Br J Ophthalmol*, 62: 604–608.
100. Tishler P V (1975): A family with coexistent von Recklinghausen's neurofibromatosis and von Hippel-Lindau's disease. Diseases possibly derived from a common gene. *Neurology*, 25: 840–844.
101. Trincao R, Cunha-Vaz J G, and Pires J M (1973): Astrocytic hamartoma of the optic disc in localized ocular neurofibromatosis (von Recklinghausen's disease). *Ophthalmologica*, 167: 465–469.
102. Trueman R H, and Rubin I E (1953): Tumor of the optic disc associated with neurofibromatosis. Presentation of a case. *Arch Ophthalmol*, 50: 469–474.

103. Turek E, Raistrick E R, and Hart C D (1977): Retinal tumours in neurofibromatosis. *Can J Ophthalmol*, 12: 68–70.

104. Turpin R, Saraux M, Caille B, Grignon J, and Chome J (1963): La forme oculo-faciale bilatérale de la neurofibromatose faciale. *Ann Ocul*, 776–789.

105. Ufermann K (1972): Doppelseitige Augenbeteiligung bei der Neurofibromatose von Recklinghausen. *Klin Mbl Augenheilk*, 161: 305–308.

106. Ulbright T M, Fulling K H, and Helveston E M (1984): Astrocytic tumors of the retina. Differentiation of sporadic tumors from phakomatosis-associated tumors. *Arch Pathol Lab Med*, 108: 160–163.

107. Unger K (1947): Neurofibromatosis iridis (Recklinghausen's disease). *Arch Ophthalmol*, 38: 654–659.

108. Van Der Hoeve J (1923): Eye diseases in tuberose sclerosis of the brain and in von Recklinghausen's disease. *Trans Ophthalmol Soc U.K.*, 43: 534–541.

109. Van Der Hoeve J (1932): Eye symptoms in phakomatoses. *Trans Ophthalmol Soc U.K.*, 52: 380–401.

110. Von Papolczy F (1932): Ueber ein aus einem hinteren Ciliarnerven entspringendes intra-retrobulbäres Neurinom. *Von Graefe's Arch Ophthalmol*, 128: 325–335.

111. Von Recklinghausen F D (1882): Ueber die multiplen Fibrome der Haut und ihre Beziehung zu den multiplen Neuromen. *Ed Hirschwald*, Berlin.

112. Waardenburg P J (1963): Genetics and ophthalmology. Vol. 2, Neuro-ophthalmology, *Ed. Van Gorcum*, Assen, 1340–1356.

113. Weleber R G, and Zonana J (1983): Iris hamartoma (Lisch nodules) in a case of segmental neurofibromatosis. *Am J Ophthalmol*, 96: 740–743.

114. Wheeler J M (1937): Plexiform neurofibromatosis (von Recklinghausen's disease) involving the choroid, ciliary body and other structures. *Am J Ophthalmol*, 20: 368–375.

115. White J P, and Loewenstein A (1946): Pigmented primary tumour of optic disc (contribution to knowledge of phakomata of eye). *Br J Ophthalmol*, 80: 253–260.

116. Wiener A (1925): A case of neurofibromatosis with buphthalmos. *Arch Ophthalmol*, 54: 481–488.

117. Wiznia R A, Freedman J K, Mancini A D, and Shields J A (1987): Malignant melanoma of the choroid in neurofibromatosis. *Am J Ophthalmol*, 86: 684–687.

118. Wolff P G (1947): Von Recklinghausen's disease. *Am J Ophthalmol*, 30: 1028.

119. Wolter J R (1965): Nerve fibrils in ovoid bodies with neurofibromatosis of the choroid. *Arch Ophthalmol*, 73: 696–699.

120. Wolter J R, and Butler R G (1963): Pigment spots of the iris and ectropion uveae. With glaucoma in neurofibromatosis. *Am J Ophthalmol*, 56: 964–973.

121. Wolter J R, Gonzales-Sirit R, and Mankin W J (1962): Neurofibromatosis of the choroid. *Am J Ophthalmol*, 54: 217–225.

122. Zakka K A, Summerer R W, Yee R D, Foos R Y, and Kim J (1979): Optociliary veins in a primary optic nerve sheath meningioma. *Am J Ophthalmol*, 87: 91–95.

123. Zamella F E, and Kirchhof B (1986): Computertomografische Befunde bei Orbitaveränderungen ins Rahmes der kindlichen Neurofibromatosis. *Klin Mbl Augenheilk*, 188: 57–59.

124. Zaret C R, Choromokos E A, and Meisler D M (1980): Cilio-optic vein associated with phakomatosis. *Ophthalmology*, 87: 330–336.

7   Tuberous sclerosis

According to Morgan and Walfort [90] Rayer in 1835 reported for the first time a case with facial cutaneous lesions, characteristic of what would later be described by Bourneville [18] as 'tuberous sclerosis'. Although von Recklinghausen [144] is credited with the first pathological description of the disease in an infant with multiple cardiac rhabdomyomas and cerebral sclerosis, Bourneville identified in a young child a syndrome consisting of mental retardation, epilepsy and cerebral lesions. The child eventually died and was found to have tumors of the brain and of the kidneys. Because of the similarity of the brain lesions with potatoes (tubers), Bourneville called his syndrome 'tuberous sclerosis'. Vogt in 1908 [141] defined the classical triad of sebaceous adenoma of the face, mental deficiency and epilepsy.

As mentionned in the previous chapter, Bielschowsky [10] was the first to associate tuberous sclerosis with neurofibromatosis. Van der Hoeve in 1921 [137] described for the first time retinal lesions in Bourneville's disease, which he called 'phakomas'. He introduced the term 'phakomatosis' to characterize both diseases [139].

I. Incidence and heredity

Tuberous sclerosis has been observed in all races [66] and both sexes are equally represented [145]. The reported incidence in the general population varies between 1 in 15,000 [40] and 1 in 100,000 [93]. However the incidence in institutes for epileptic and retarded children is much higher. It is estimated as 1 to 5 in 1,000. Pampligione and Pugh [101] carried out a survey of fifty-four patients with infantile spasms investigated at the Hospital for Sick Children in London in the years 1972 and 1973. Fourteen patients (26%) had three or more features undoubtedly diagnostic of tuberous sclerosis, while a further 10 cases (16%) had less obvious but similar features. Hoyt [59] examined 44 consecutive patients with infantile spasms, aged from 6 weeks to 28 months. In eight cases one or more retinal hamartomas were identified and in all eight patients a diagnosis of tuberous sclerosis was confirmed by genetic history, dermatologic examination and/or demonstration of subependymal calcification by CT-scanning of the brain.

Berg (1913) reported on the occurrence of tuberous sclerosis in three generations of a same family. Since this paper numerous reports have been published on the autosomal dominant pattern of heredity of this disease [4, 5, 15, 21, 38, 39, 66, 86, 87, 93, 98, 145]. The marked inter- and intrafamilial differences in expression and the lack of penetrance may account for the relatively high incidence of sporadic cases, but also the fact that a large number of tuberous sclerosis patients do not reproduce because of mental retardation or premature death [4]. It may also be assumed that most sporadic cases are the result of a mutation [35].

Based on the observation of tuberous sclerosis in two sibs whose parents were normal, an autosomal recessive form of inheritance or gonadal mosaicism has been suggested [75, 149].

Fryer et al. [40] carried out a linkage analysis in nineteen families with tuberous sclerosis, using 26 polymorphic markers. They demonstrated linkage between tuberous sclerosis and the ABO blood group locus. The tuberous sclerosis gene was mapped to the distal long arm of chromosome 9.

II. Diagnostic criteria

The diagnosis of tuberous sclerosis was initially based on the classic triad of epilepsy, mental retardation and adenoma sebaceum. Later intracerebral calcifications and ocular symptoms were included [38]. However these different manifestations of the disease are not always met in the same individual and for diagnostic purposes the criteria introduced by Gomez are generally accepted [48].

a. Primary criteria
The diagnosis of tuberous sclerosis can be made if only one of the following manifestations is present:
1. specific dermatologic lesions: facial angiofibroma (adenoma sebaceum), ungual fibroma or fibrous plaque on the forehead;
2. cortical tubers or subependymal hamartomas diagnosed either pathologically or by neuro-imaging (CT-scan or NMR);
3. multiple retinal hamartomas.

b. Secondary criteria
Two of the following secondary criteria allow a tentative diagnosis of tuberous sclerosis:
1. infantile spasms
2. hypopigmented macules (mountain ash leaf spots)
3. shagreen patch
4. single retinal hamartoma
5. renal angiomyolipomata or cysts
6. cardiac rhabdomyoma
7. a first degree relative with a primary diagnosis of tuberous sclerosis

III. Non-ocular manifestations of tuberous sclerosis

1. Cutaneous manifestations

Adenoma sebaceum (Figs. 7–1, 7–2)
Since Pringle's description in 1890 [106] this is the sign most frequently associated with tuberous sclerosis. It is present in 80 to 90% of the patients and usually appears between the ages of two to five years, sometimes however not until puberty [61]. Adenoma sebaceum is however a misnomer as on histopathology the lesion is primarily an angiofibroma while the sebaceous glands are only passively involved [94]. The lesions consist of flat or dome-shaped papules usually 1 to 2 mm and rarely larger than 5 mm in diameter. Some are yellowisch, others pink or red and covered with tele-angiectases [91]. The lesions are symmetrically distributed in the nasolabial folds, on the cheeks and chin. They can also be seen on the nose, whereas the upperlip is usually spared except immediately under the nose. They tend to progress until adult life and remain then stationary.

Leukoderma or hypopigmented macules (Fig. 7–3)
Hypopigmented macules are usually present at birth or appear early in the postnatal period. They probably represent the earliest detectable cutaneous lesion of tuberous sclerosis. The lesions may vary in form but they are often

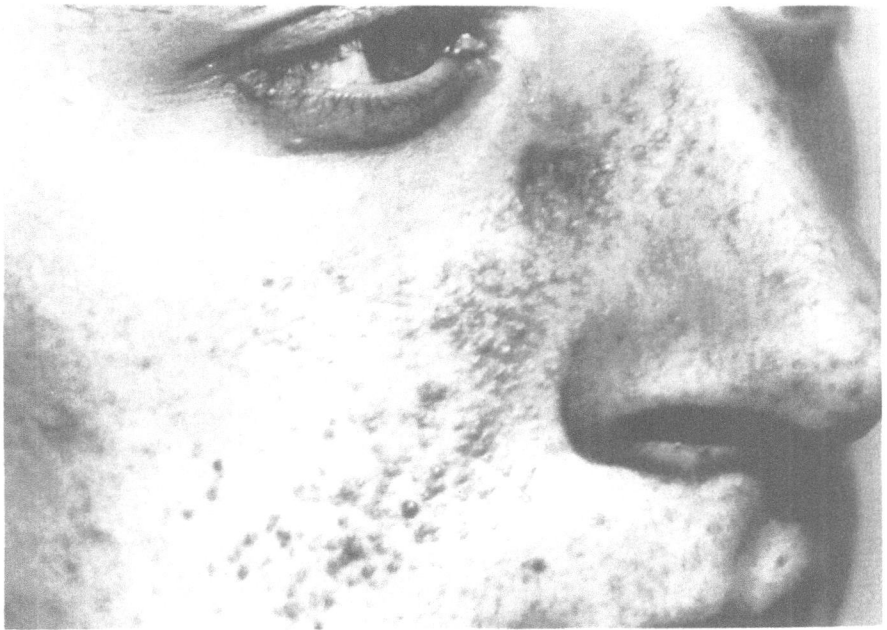

Figure 7–1. Adenoma sebaceum (case of Prof. A. Kint, Ghent).

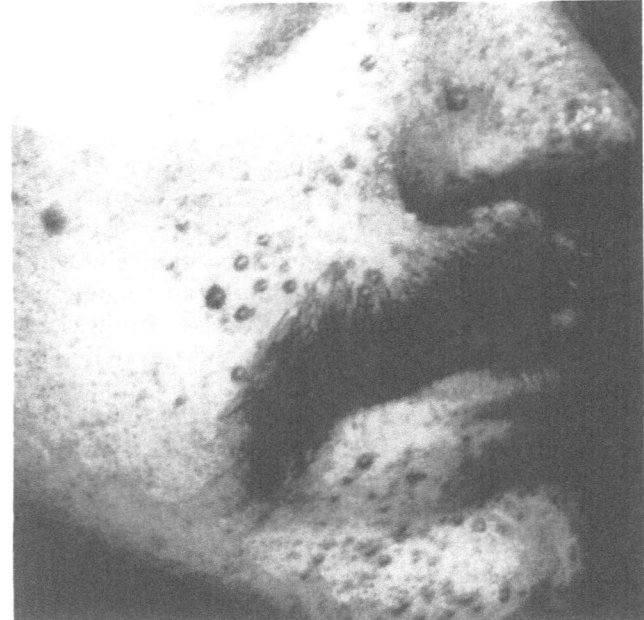

Figure 7–2.   Adenoma sebaceum (case of Prof. A. Kint, Ghent).

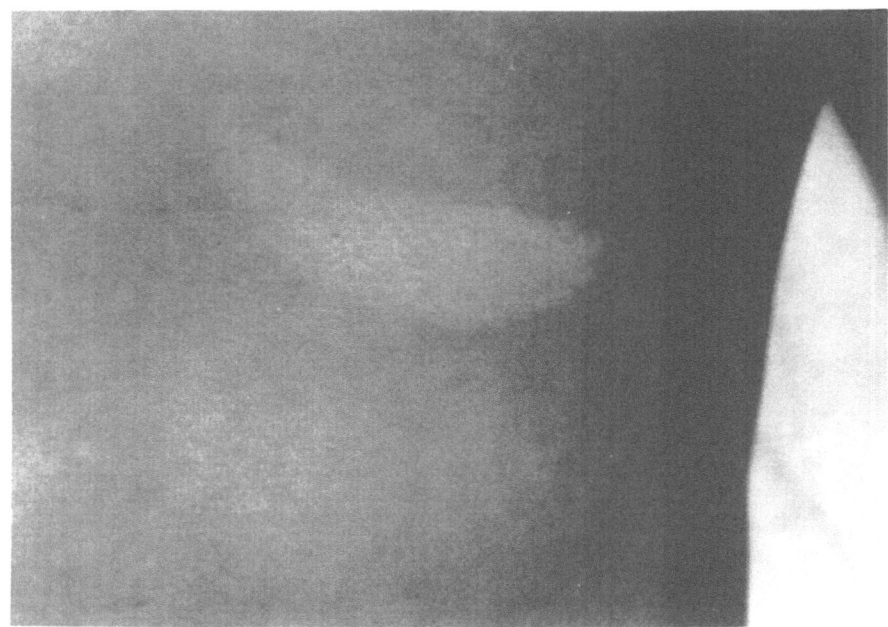

Figure 7–3.   Mountain ash leaf spot (case of Prof. A. Kint, Ghent).

oval at one end and tapered at the other end. Their appearance has therefore been compared to the leaf of the mountain ash tree (mountain ash leaf spots) [89]. Such lesions have often been considered as vitiligo [47] but in contrast to vitiligo, in ash leaf spots the melanocytes are present in normal number although the size of the melanocytes and their melanin content appear smaller [61]. They may be detected earlier with the help of Wood's ultraviolet light. Ash leaf spots are found in up to 78% of tuberous sclerosis patients [89, 100]. 'Café-au-lait' spots may also occur in tuberous sclerosis and are seen in 26% of the patients [61]. Tuberous sclerosis patients usually have only one or two 'café-au-lait' spots [88].

Ungual fibromas or Koenen tumors (Fig. 7–4)
These pathognomonic lesions of tuberous sclerosis usually appear at puberty [91]. They are thus of little use in the early diagnosis of the disease [61]. (Sub)ungual fibromas emerge from the groove of one or several nails of the fingers and especially of the toes.

Shagreen patches ('peau de chagrin')
Shagreen patches are raised plaques varying in size from a few millimeters to 1 to 2 centimeters. They are especially found on the eyelids, the face, the lumbar region or the trunk [148]. They are areas of fibromatous infiltration.

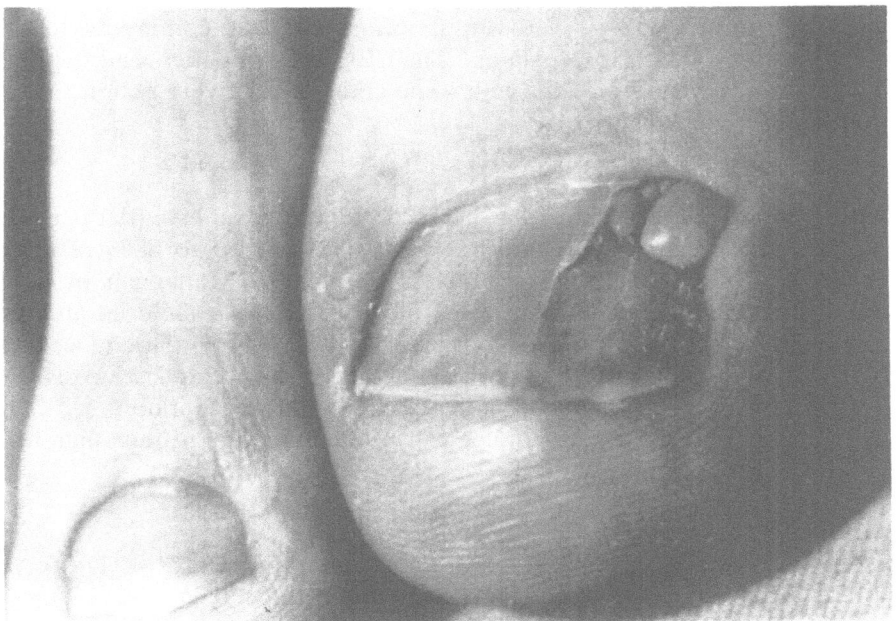

Figure 7–4.   Ungual fibroma (case of Prof. A. Kint, Ghent).

Shagreen patches usually appear at about the same time as the adenoma sebaceum [91]. Their frequency varies between 11 and 24% [89, 101].

Other cutaneous lesions
A white forelock [91] and poliosis of the eyelid [29] may be associated or not with mountain ash leaf spots and probably have the same diagnostic significance. Multiple fibromas of various sizes may be found on mucous membranes, especially on the gums [91]. Pedunculated fibromas on the trunk, neck, axillae or groins are usually seen in older patients and are not pathognomonic of tuberous sclerosis [91].

2. Neurological manifestations

Epilepsy
Seizures may be the first and are the most frequent manifestation of tuberous sclerosis [30, 51, 72]. They usually begin as infantile spasms [59, 89]. Infantile spasms or Salaam convulsions consist of repetitive massive spasms involving the muscles of the neck, of the trunk and of the limbs, either in extension or in flexion. Each spasm lasts more or less a second. They occur in bows of 10 to 50 or more attacks. They are mostly seen between the ages of 6 to 18 months and are accompanied by psychomotor retardation and gross EEG abnormalities [101]. Later in life the spasms may disappear and they are replaced by 'grand mal' seizures [88, 148]. Infantile spasms occur in up to 93% of the children who later will develop a tuberous sclerosis complex [72]. A grossly abnormal EEG is commonly found in epileptic tuberous sclerosis patients. The EEG abnormalities tend to progress towards multifocal alterations with some areas of relatively better preserved rhythmic activities [101].

Mental retardation
Although mental retardation has been considered as an essential part of the tuberous sclerosis complex and has been found in up to 88% of affected children [101], it probably occurs less frequently. Monaghan et al. [89] found mental retardation in 49 of 62 tuberous sclerosis children and Lagos and Gomez [72] in 43 of 71 patients. Six of the eighteen patients examined by Nevin and Pearce [93] had normal intelligence. Tuberous sclerosis is thus not necessarily associated with epilepsy or mental retardation [45, 52, 105], even in the presence of radiologically demonstrable intracranial lesions [132].

Intracranial lesions
There are two main cerebral lesions in tuberous sclerosis. The cortical tubers after which the disease was named and the subependymal giant-cell astrocytoma. In addition diffuse fibrillary gliosis may occur [88].

The sclerotic areas of the cortex first attracted the attention of Bourne-ville. Because of their appearance he called these lesions 'tubers' and the disease 'tuberous sclerosis' ('sclérose tubéreuse des circonvolutions céré-brales') [18]. Sclerotic tubers are yellow-white or pale in appearance and have a firm consistency, contrasting with the surrounding normal brain [30]. They may compress the convolutions in the vicinity and produce pressure atrophy. Histopathologically these tubers are composed of very large cells resembling swollen astrocytes [88].

Calcified hamartomas often involve the lateral and third ventricles and sometimes also the posterior fossa. They contain large astrocytic cells [36]. They are histologically benign but may enlarge slowly with time. If situated near the foramen of Monro or the aqueduct of Sylvius they produce intracranial hypertension with papiledema and even blindness due to secondary optic atrophy [88]. These tumors may be detected on skull radiography as calcified masses or 'brain stones'. The frequency of finding such lesions on plain skull röntgenograms in patients with tuberous sclerosis varies between 35 to 60% [72, 89, 100]. Computed tomographic findings suggest that these hamartomas are more common than generally thought [150] and CT-scan is considered as a vital test in the investigation of gene carriers of tuberous sclerosis [35]. Fryer et al. [41] however could not detect CT-scan abnormalities in parents of children with tuberous sclerosis, unless there was evidence of the disease on skin examination.

Whereas the periventricular calcified lesions are better visualized with Computer Cranial Tomography, the cortical tubers are more frequently demonstrated with Magnetic Resonance Imaging (MRI). The number of cortical lesions as found on MRI also correlates with the degree of seizure control and the severity of the disease [115].

3. Visceral manifestations

Von Recklinghausen's original case concerned a girl with cardiac rhabdo-myomas [144]. Rhabdomyomas of the heart may be single or multiple and bulge into the cardiac lumen [36].

The kidneys are frequently affected. The hamartomas of the kidneys are described as angiomyolipomas [36].

Lesions may be present in the skull, the vertebral column and pelvic bone [99], as well as cystic lesions in metacarpals, metatarsals and phalanges of hands and feet [30].

The lung lesions usually consist of cysts which may provoke emphysema, pulmonary insufficiency, spontaneous pneumothorax or chronic right heart failure [30, 88].

Other organs can also present hamartomatous lesions: the gastro-intestinal tract, the urinary bladder, the thyroid, the ovaries, the liver, the adrenal glands [30, 88, 99].

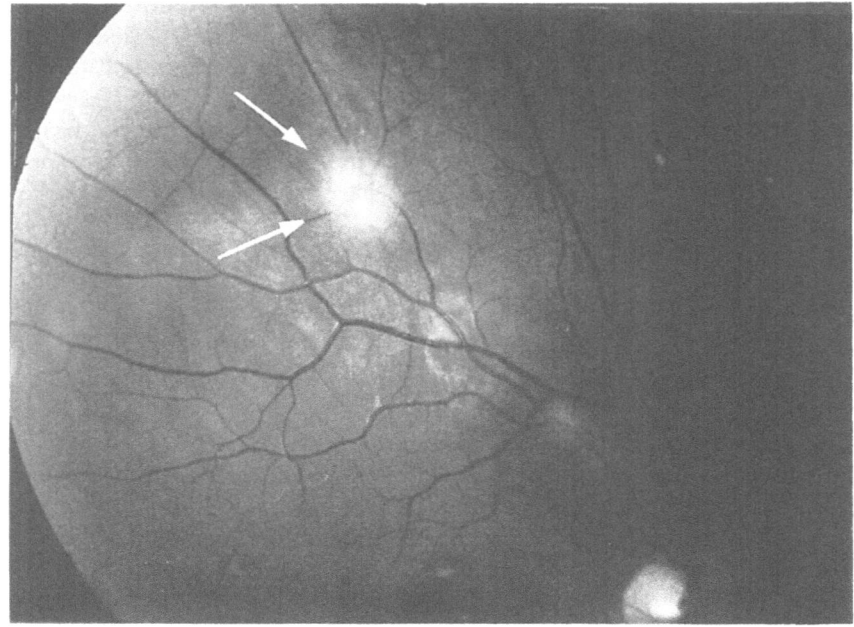

Figure 7–5.   Small translucent hamartoma (see arrows) overlying the superotemporal artery in a child with tuberous sclerosis. (Courtesy of Prof. Raspiller, Nancy)

IV. Ocular manifestations of tuberous sclerosis

1. Clinical aspect

Retinal and optic disc hamartomas

The most characteristic fundus lesion in tuberous sclerosis is a hamartoma in the posterior pole. It was originally called a phakoma by van der Hoeve [137]. Since Nitsch [95] as first stressed the importance of this lesion in the diagnosis of tuberous sclerosis, numerous cases have been described. Hamartomas may be situated in the retina [2–4, 8, 11, 13, 14, 20, 21, 36, 43–45, 51, 52, 55, 56, 58, 62, 67, 68, 74, 80, 82, 86–88, 96, 98, 99, 102, 105, 111, 112, 121, 137–140, 145, 147, 152, 153] or on the optic disc [15, 31, 44, 46, 82, 86, 88, 98, 111, 113, 132, 143, 148].

Retinal tumors may be found even in very young children: 3 months, 1 and 2 years in the cases of Rintelen and Wessing [113], 3.5 and 11 months in the cases of Yassur et al. [151], 6 and 9 months in those of McLean [80]. They may precede other manifestations of tuberous sclerosis [22, 80]. The reported incidence of fundus tumors varies. Nyboer et al. [96] examined 116 tuberous sclerosis patients and found retinal hamartomas in 56 of them. Shelton [129] noted the presence of retinal tumors in the 7 patients he examined. In three of them both eyes were affected. In earlier reports the

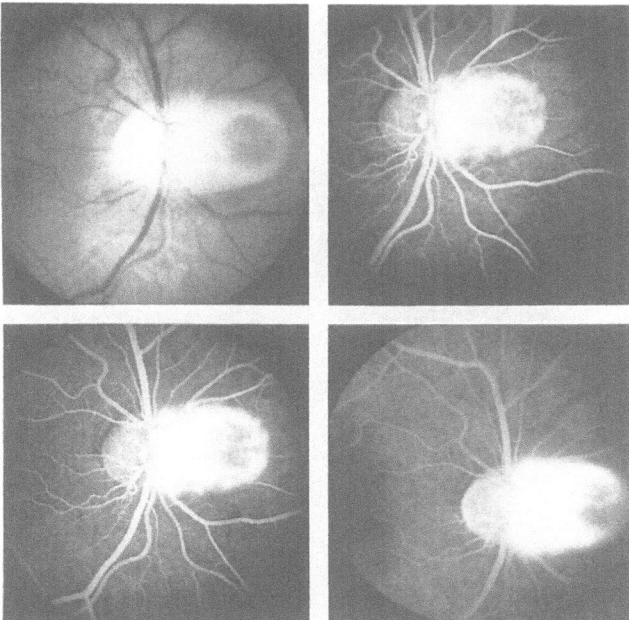

Figure 7–6. Juxtapapillary hamartoma in a child with tuberous sclerosis (same eye as Fig. 7–5). Note the vascularity of the tumor as seen on fluorescein angiography. Intense late staining of the lesion. (Courtesy of Prof. Raspiller, Nancy)

incidence is however much lower, varying between 3 to 4% [23] and 20% [67]. These conflicting figures are probably best explained by the difficulty of a careful fundus examination in mentally handicapped children.

There are two basic varieties of retinal tumors in tuberous sclerosis [59, 96, 125]. The most commonly observed are small round to oval, relatively small, soft or smooth appearing lesions. Their limits are often less well defined (Fig. 7–5). These hamartomas are usually found in the posterior pole but not in the macular region [125]. The lesions are frequently located superficially to retinal vessels and as they are translucent, they may easily be overlooked, especially if an indirect ophthalmoscope is used. Such lesions may be single or multiple, affect one or both eyes [96].

The second type is the more classical but relatively less frequent tumor [96, 125], which has been compared to a white mulberry [13] or to salmon eggs. This tumor is multinodular and protrudes into the vitreous. It is often found in the vicinity of the optic disc, partially covering it (Fig. 7–6). Disc hamartomas may resemble giant hyaline bodies or disc drusen. Their size varies between 0.5 to 4 disc diameters and their elevation may be up to 7 diopters [96]. Clear cystic spaces may be seen in the tumor [4, 44, 140].

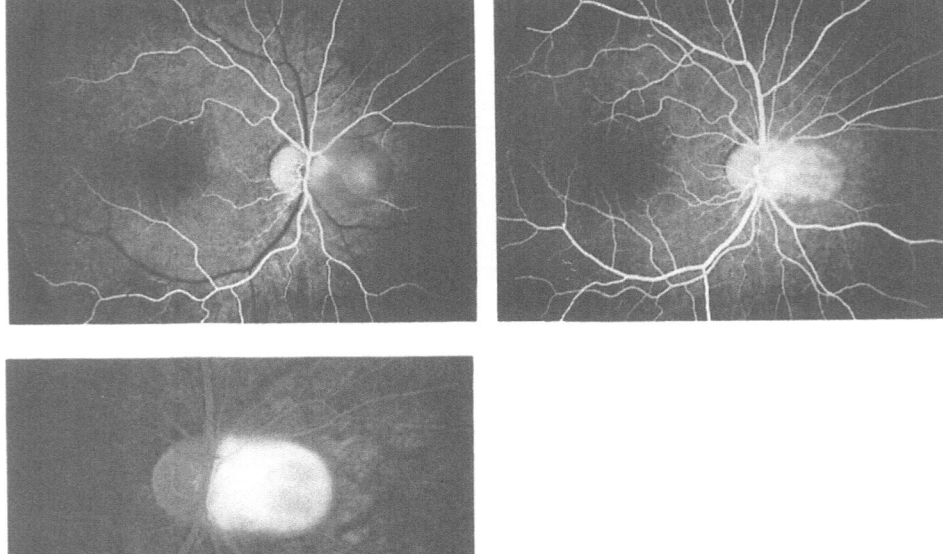

Figure 7–7.   Same lesion as Fig. 7–6. Unchanged aspect one year later. (Courtesy of Prof. Raspiller, Nancy)

Although most tumors are seen in the posterior pole, some have been found at the ora serrata [114] or at the ciliary body [2]. The two types of tumors may coexist in the same fundus and the question is still not settled if the two types are different stages of development of the same lesion [96].

Drusen of the optic disc are a feature of tuberous sclerosis [108] (Fig. 7–8) and some may even contain a mass of metaplastic bone [155]. According to Reese [108] they occur more frequently in the 'formes frustes' of the disease as one of its many clinical variants. They represent glial hamartomas of the optic disc [36, 154] and are situated anteriorly to the lamina cribrosa [154]. They should not be confused with the ordinary drusen of the optic disc or with a true glioma [36]. Hogan and Zimmerman [56] and Robertson [116] have discussed the similarities and differences between drusen of the optic nerve head and the ocular lesions in tuberous sclerosis. Although similar in clinical appearance, the giant drusen of the optic nerve head – seen as an incidental finding in the general population – differ from those seen in tuberous sclerosis and represent a degenerative process with deposition of hyaline material of unknown origin [92]. The contention of Reese that they represent a 'forme fruste' of tuberous sclerosis is no longer generally accepted [4, 44, 56].

Flat fundus lesions of tuberous sclerosis may be mistaken for medullated

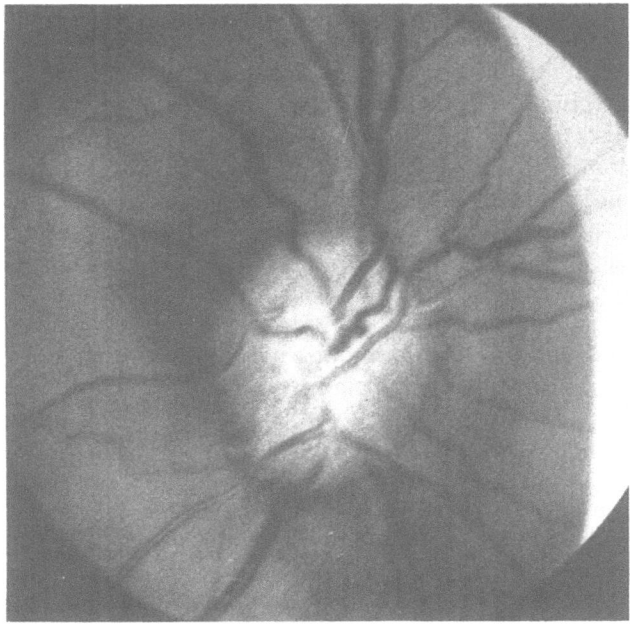

Figure 7–8.   Drusen of the optic disc in a child with tuberous sclerosis.

nerve fibers [51], larger tumors for retinoblastoma [62], amelanotic melanoma [17] or even a tuberculoma [63].

In small lesions fluorescein angiography may fail to reveal abnormal
staining [1], whereas large mulberry-like tumors usually show varying degrees
of vascularization resulting in intense staining [4, .6, 31, 44, 107, 110, 126]
(Fig. 7–6). Fluoroangiography may be helpful in differentiating young and
active retinal lesions from old hyalinized ones [51]. It may also be possible
to demonstrate the lesion with echography and with CT-scan [24].

The evolution of these tumors is variable. New lesions may appear during
follow-up [51]. Some of these tumors have little or no growth potential and
have remained essentially unchanged for periods of up to 20 years [132,
142]. Rettinger and Wessing [113] even observed the spontaneous regression
of a disc tumor. At first examination the child was 3 months old and
presented a tumor with an elevation of 6 diopters on the left optic disc. Half
a year later a small peripheral tumor was detected in the same eye. At the
age of 3 years the disc tumor had regressed to the half of its original size.

Cystic tumors may burst and the cyst may empty itself in the vitreous and
later refill [140]. Also small particles may get loose and float into the
vitreous [140]. Preretinal and vitreous hemorrhages are possible complications [6, 22, 58, 68, 140]. Progressive enlargement can sometimes be
observed [43, 68]. Optic disc tumors have been seen to extend through the

lamina cribrosa into the optic nerve [37]. In some cases the tumor undergoes a chronic necrotic process [22, 150] resulting in rubeosis iridis. A number of eyes have been enucleated for secondary glaucoma [42, 62, 63].

Although retinal or optic disc hamartomas are most commonly associated with tuberous sclerosis, they have been also noticed in von Recklinghausen's neurofibromatosis [12, 36, 84, 136]. Such tumors can also be found without any other indication of a systemic disease as an isolated tumor of the eye [20, 27, 37, 42, 63, 79, 110, 118]. The association of astrocytic hamartoma with retinitis pigmentosa has been reported [7, 25, 104, 116] (Fig. 7–9). The prevalence of astrocytic hamartomas of the optic nerve head in retinitis pigmentosa is estimated at 1.4% [25]. Awan [7], who observed a patient with Usher's syndrome and a mulberry-like lesion near the disc, considers the tumor as a reactive hyperplasia of the glial cells of the retina.

Retinal pigment epithelial lesions
Depigmented areas are occasionally observed in the fundus of tuberous sclerosis patients. They may be associated with hamartomas [3, 21]. Welge-Lussen and Latta [147] examined a young child with tuberous sclerosis and noted amongst other ocular anomalies (megalocornea and iriscoloboma) the presence of a white area at the temporal side of the left optic disc, which they at first considered as a colobomatous lesion. Three years later a 2 diopters elevated nodular tumor was noted in place of the depigmented area and in addition two flat tumors were also seen.

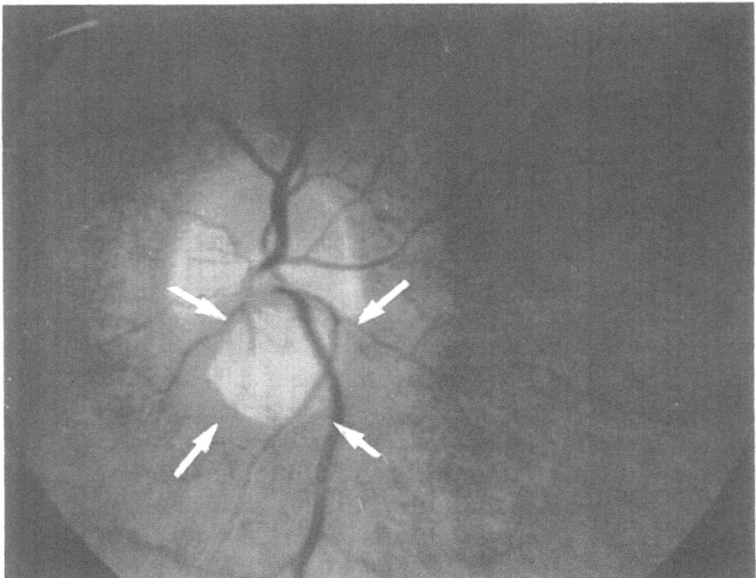

Figure 7–9.   Small Hamartoma on the optic disc of a patient with retinitis pigmentosa (arrows).

Depigmented punched-out lesions resembling those seen in presumed ocular histoplasmosis syndrome have been described in the midperiphery, some of them surrounded by pigment proliferation [96, 123, 128]. Luchesse and Goldberg [76] observed sector hypopigmentation of the iris and the fundus in a 12 year old girl with tuberous sclerosis and compared this to the changes seen in Waardenburg syndrome. They suggest that these changes are the consequence of faulty migration of cells derived from the neural crest.

Optic disc edema and optic atrophy
Papiledema and subsequent optic atrophy are the result of intracranial hypertension, usually related to the presence of giant cell astrocytomas in the vicinity of the foramen of Monro or the aqueduct of Sylvius [5, 19, 35, 67, 74, 88, 96, 112, 121, 127].

Other ocular manifestations
Sectorial iris depigmentation has been observed in a number of patients with tuberous sclerosis [76] and is considered as an early sign of the disease comparable to the mountain ash leaf spot [69]. On fluorescein angiography no atrophy nor increased vascularity was evident. The true incidence of depigmented iris spots in tuberous sclerosis is still unknown [50].

Colobomas of the iris, choroid or lens have been seen in association with other signs of tuberous sclerosis [39, 89, 114, 135, 147, 148]. Other associations are probably fortuitous such as megalocornea [147], band keratitis [5, 134], posterior embryotoxon, persistence of hyaloid remnants and cataract [135].

Conjunctival and eyelid tumors have been reported [78] as well as eyelid depigmentation [29].

Not surprisingly a number of patients will develop neuroophthalmological signs related to the cerebral involvement: eye muscle paralysis, nystagmus, hemianopia [19].

2. Histopathology

Glial tumors of the retina and optic disc are generally classified as hamartomas. As we already mentioned, although they are most frequently seen in association with tuberous sclerosis, they may be found also in von Recklinghausen's neurofibromatosis. Histologically and ophthalmoscopically the retinal hamartomas in tuberous sclerosis are indistinguishable from those seen in neurofibromatosis [36, 96]. In rare instances these tumors have been described unassociated with tuberous sclerosis or neurofibromatosis. They were called astrocytomas [14, 17, 20, 26, 37, 42, 67, 79, 107, 110], glioma [103, 118] or oligodendroglioma [16, 60]. Whether such tumors should be considered as hamartomas in the absence of other underlying or associated developmental anomalies is doubtful [14].

Histological descriptions of tumors of retina and optic disc in tuberous sclerosis were reported in a large number of cases [8, 9, 20, 22, 32–34, 36, 43, 54, 55, 58, 64, 65, 68, 71, 80, 81, 86, 108, 109, 117, 124, 138, 139, 146, 151, 155], as well as more extensive studies on the subject [4, 6, 88, 117]. The tumors have histologically been described as astrocytoma [20, 56, 150], astrocytic hamartoma [6, 22, 36, 38, 68, 92, 97], angio-astrocytic hamartoma [8], glial hamartoma [130, 154], glial blastoma [77], neurospongioblastoma or glioneurocytoma [117] and glioneuroma or glioneuromatous hamartoma [43].

According to Barsky and Wolter [8] the angioblastic basis of the tumor may provide the anatomic correlation between tuberous sclerosis and the other phakomatoses. It was also emphasized that neurofibromatosis and tuberous sclerosis affect primarily neuro-ectodermal structures with secondary angiomatous reaction of the mesoderm, while angiomatosis retinae and Sturge-Weber disease are primarily mesodermal with secondary reaction of the ectoderm [73, 77].

The retinal tumors occupy the inner retinal layers [20, 80, 96], involving the nerve fiber and ganglion cell layer [4, 6, 32–34, 36, 55, 56, 65, 71, 77, 81, 83, 86, 92, 122, 124, 155]. Less frequently the tumor invades all retinal layers [6, 43, 71, 77, 80, 83, 86, 124, 146] or even shows an exophytic growth pattern [64, 150]. The limitans interna may remain intact [20, 56], be displaced by the enlarging tumor [55] or ruptured by a tumor projecting into the vitreous cavity [55, 83, 124].

Optic disc tumors may similarly arise from the superficial layers [4, 22, 96], involve all layers [4] or even extend through the cribriform plate [37].

The different aspects suggest that the minute flat and localized tumors possibly develop into the larger multinodular lesions [83].

The tumors appear cytologically benign [56] without active mitosis [4] and do not generally infiltrate other structures [56], extend outside the eye or metastatize [56, 130]. Intraretinal metastases can however occur when buds of tumor detach, float in the vitreous and settle on the retina, producing a new growth [55, 83, 138, 139].

In some instances the tumor grows to large dimensions resulting in reactive inflammation [24, 43, 55], rubeosis iridis [22, 151], secondary glaucoma [22, 43, 151] and even in invasion of choroid, sclera, cornea and optic disc [64]. This may lead to enucleation of the blind painful eye [22]. The growth may also be the consequence of the enlargement of cystic spaces, increased ossification or concretion formation, necrosis and organization within the tumor [22]. It is also possible that aging of the lesion may cause hyalinization and obliteration of the blood vessels [8].

Microscopically all types of disc and retinal tumors have certain basic similarities [4, 80, 83] (Fig. 7–10, 7–11). They are composed of proliferating cells [4, 83, 124], separated by a coarse and non-fibrillated [154] or finer and fibrillated matrix [56, 155] or felt-like network [96] formed by the cell processes [154]. Although the cell type may frequently be difficult to classify [83], they have been identified as glial cells [65, 83, 86, 155], astroblasts [49,

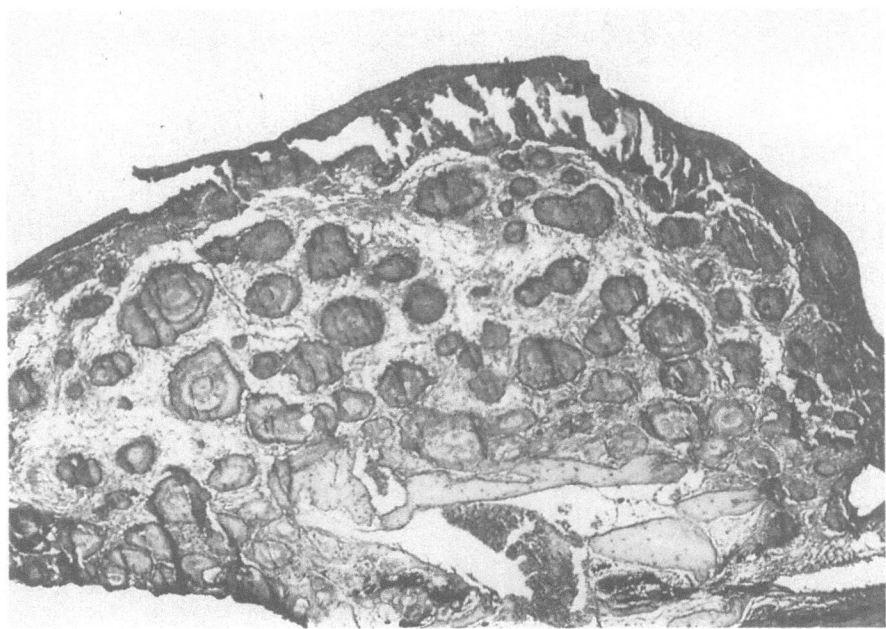

Figure 7–10. Retinal phakoma in tuberous sclerosis. Mulberry-shaped lesion on ophthalmo-scopy. Spherical calcified structures, commonly composed of concentric layers and separated by loosely arranged cells. Areas of ossification. (Courtesy of Prof. A Brini, Strasbourg, case 124, xix)

132, 155], astrocytes [4, 8, 22, 36, 43, 44, 55, 56, 68, 80, 92, 96, 98, 129, 130, 151], undifferentiated neurocytes [73, 138, 139] or spongioblasts [32, 73, 77, 86, 122]. Among the astrocytes further differentiation is made in proto-plasmic astrocytes [97], fibrous astrocytes [56, 97, 150] and gemistocytic astrocytes [130].

The cells are generally pleomorphic [4, 32, 43, 44, 64, 71, 97, 122, 138, 139]. They may be large and round or oval [4, 43, 44, 55, 77, 80, 130, 138, 139], plump [22], polygonal [97] or atypical [137, 138] with abundant cytoplasm [4, 22, 43] and poorly defined boundaries giving sometimes the appearance of a syncytium [4, 22, 81, 83, 138, 139]. Other cells are elongated [4, 20, 44, 56, 77, 81, 83, 97, 151, 155] or spindle-shaped [22, 55, 68] with elongated, interlacing fibre-like processes forming a network [32, 71, 98, 122, 138, 139] or taking sometimes a fascicular arrangement [77]. Some macrophage-like foamy cells may also be found [97].

According to the general configuration of the cells, the nuclei may be small [44, 56, 68, 98, 130, 151] or large [4, 22, 80, 138, 139], with prominent [4, 22, 43, 138, 139] or multiple nucleoli [138, 139]. Intracytoplasmatic fibers or filaments were demonstrated [4, 22, 55, 68, 83, 97, 98] although special staining techniques are often required to demonstrate these structures. [4,

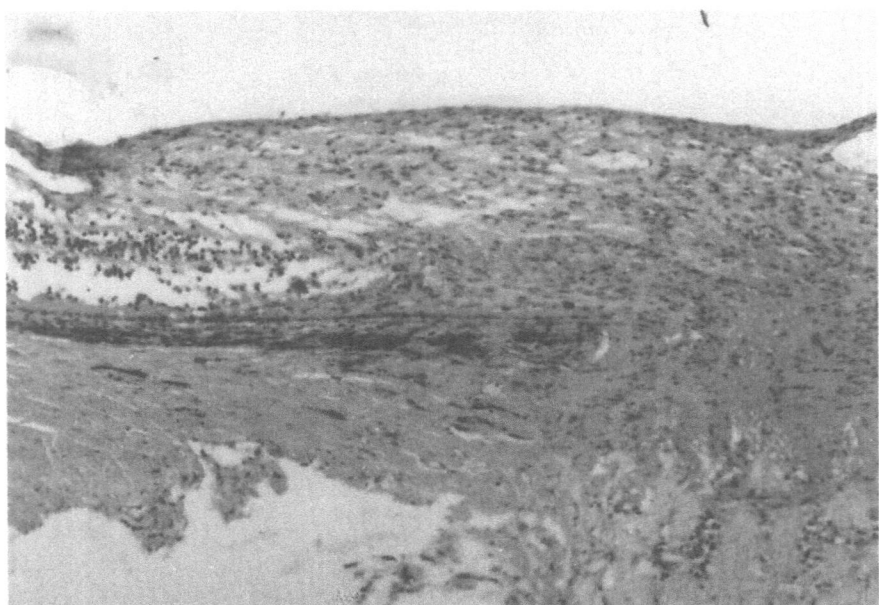

Figure 7–11.   Tuberous sclerosis. Papiledema on ophthalmoscopy. Proliferation of spindle-shaped cells at the edge of the optic disc. (Courtesy of Prof. A. Brini, Strasbourg, case 124, xix)

97]. Nerve fibers originating in the nerve fiber layer [151] have also been described in the tumor [138, 139].

During the evolution the tumor may undergo regressive or degenerative changes such as cystic degeneration [4, 22, 44, 55, 77, 81, 83, 96, 124, 138, 139] with the spaces occasionally filled with blood and serum [4, 44, 138, 139], necrosis [22, 64, 151], calcification [4, 20, 44, 77, 81, 83, 96, 124, 130, 138, 139, 151, 154, 155], ossification [4, 22, 64, 83, 155], hyalinization [55, 124] and presence of lamellated bodies or drusen [22, 43, 77, 96]. These regressive changes may be due to deficient vascularization [55] and the smaller, usually more peripheral, nodules generally do not present the calcification, cystic degeneration or ganglioform cells seen in the larger tumors [6, 42]. Other possible concomitant alterations include atrophy, fibrosis or ossification of the underlying choroid [4], diffuse retinal gliosis [98, 151] changes in the retinal pigment epithelium [4, 154], retinal detachment [6, 130, 151] and vitreous hemorrhage [22, 68]. These alterations are however not found in early lesions and probably represent secondary changes [4].

The vascularization of the tumor has been estimated in different ways. For some the vascularization is scant and poorly developed [55, 83, 107, 108] with even an apparent avascularity of the flat peripheral tumors [67]. For others the tumor is richly vascularized [20] with numerous vascular channels [68, 80, 96] or relatively large vessels forming the skeleton of the tumor [151]. Ocular lesions in tuberous sclerosis may thus contain a significant angiomatous element also with microaneurysms and intervascular fibrous strands [8]. Some authors have even suggested that these tumors are due to an irregular development of vessels with resulting hypoxia and that the degenerative changes are the consequence of the vascular anomalies [57].

V. Associations

A few patients have been reported who presented signs of Bourneville's disease and of another phakomatosis. Cutaneous angiomas were found in patients with tuberous sclerosis [70, 152, 153]. Schwartz et al. [126] reported the association of an exophytic retinal angioma with an epipapillary astrocytic hamartoma in a 62 year old patient, known to have tuberous sclerosis. However, the question arises if these were two separate tumors, especially as no histological proof exists. Loewenstein and Steel [73] found what they considered as a typical choroidal angioma in a young boy who presented multiple tumors in the other eye.

The simultaneous occurrence of a choroidal melanoma with a retinal hamartoma in the same eye has to be considered as a by chance association [42].

References

1. Ahmad A (1978): Fluorescein angiography in tuberous sclerosis. *Ann Ophthalmol*, 10: 453–455.
2. Andreani D (1960): Su di un caso di malattia di Bourneville con compromissione del corpo ciliare. *Boll Oculist*, 39: 319–327.
3. Anker H and Kveim A (1938): Drei Fälle von tuberöser Hirnsklerose mit van der Hoeve's 'phakoma retinae'. *Acta Ophthalmol*, 16: 454–466.
4. Archer D B and Nevin N C (1977): The phakomatoses. II. Tuberous sclerosis pp. 1219–1248 in: Krill (ed.). *Hereditary Retinal and Choroidal Diseases*, Vol. II, Harper and Row Publ.
5. Ardouin M, Feuvrier Y M and Urvoy M (1960): Sclérose tubéreuse de Borneville avec manifestation oculaire peu habituelle: oedème papillaire et kératite en bandelette. *Rev. Oto-Neuro-Ophtalmol*, 32: 499.
6. Atkinson A, Sanders M D and Wong V (1973): Vitreous haemorrhage in tuberous sclerosis. Report of two cases. *Br J Ophthalmol*, 57: 773–779.
7. Awan K J (1976): Presumed glial retinal hamartomas in Usher's syndrome. *Can J Ophthalmol*, 11: 256–267.
8. Barsky D and Wolter J R (1971): The retinal lesion of tuberous sclerosis: an angioglioma-tous hamartoma? *J Ped Ophthalmol*, 8: 261–265.
9. Bau-Prussakowa J (1933): Ueber einen Fall von tuberöser Hirnsklerose mit Netzhaut-veränderungen und benignes Verlauf. *Z Ges Neurol Psychiatr*, 145: 275–282.

10. Bielschowsky M (1914): Ueber tuberöser Sklerose und ihre Beziehungen zur Reckling-hausensche Krankheit. *Z Ges Neurol Psychiatr*, 26: 133–155.
11. Blanck C (1966): Sclérose tubéreuse de Bourneville. *Arch Ophtalmol*, 26: 29–32.
12. Bloch F J (1948): Retinal tumor associated with Neurofibromatosis (von Recklinghausen's disease). Report of a case. *Arch Ophthalmol*, 40: 433–437.
13. Bloch F J and Grove B A (1938): Tuberous sclerosis with retinal tumor. *Arch Ophthalmol*, 19: 34–38.
14. Boles W M, Naugle T C and Samson C L M (1958): Glioma of the optic nerve. Report of a case arising from the optic disc. *Arch Ophthalmol*, 59: 229–231.
15. Boles-Carenini B (1957): Sulle manifestazione oculari della sclerosi di Bourneville e la loco associazione con sintomi extraoculari. *Boll Oculist*, 36: 337–367.
16. Boniuk M and Bishop D W (1969): Oligodendroglioma of the retina. *Surv Ophthalmol*, 13: 284–289.
17. Boniuk M and Hawkins W R (1971): Transscleral migration of pigment following cryo-therapy of intraocular glioma. *Trans Am Acad Ophthalmol Otolaryngol*, 75: 60–69.
18. Bourneville D (1880): Contribution à l'étude de l'idiotie. Sclérose tubéreuse des circon-volutions cérébrales: idiotie et épilepsie hémiplégique. *Arch Neurol*, 1: 81–91.
19. Busch K Th and Busch G (1962): Neuro-ophthalmologische und neuropathologische Befunde bei der tuberösen Sklerose (Morb. Bourneville). *Klin Mbl Augenheilk*, 141: 388–401.
20. Cleasby G W, Fung W E and Shekter W B (1967): Astrocytoma of the retina. *Am J Ophthalmol*, 64: 633–637.
21. Constantine E F (1943): Tuberous sclerosis. *Arch Ophthalmol*, 30: 494–498.
22. Coppeto J R, Lubin J R and Albert D M (1982): Astrocytic hamartoma in tuberous sclerosis mimicking necrotizing retinochoroiditis. *J Ped Ophthalmol Strabismus*, 19/6: 306–313.
23. Critchley M and Earl C J C (1932): Tuberous sclerosis and allied condition. *Brain*, 55: 311–346.
24. Daily M J, Smith J L and Dickens W (1976): Giant drusen (astrocytic hamartoma) of the optic nerve, seen with computerized axial tomography. *Am J Ophthalmol*, 81: 100–101.
25. De Bustros S, Miller M R, Finkelstein D and Massop R (1983): Bilateral astrocytic hamartomas of the optic nerve heads in retinitis pigmentosa. *Retina*, 3: 21–23.
26. Dejean Ch (1934): Le vrai gliome de la rétine. Astrocytome de la rétine adulte. *Arch Ophtalmol (Paris)*, 51: 257–276.
27. Dekking H M (1951): Presentation of cases: tuberous sclerosis of the retina. *Ophthal-mologica*, 122: 386–387.
28. Dickey L B (1949): Tuberous sclerosis or epiloic. *Stanf Med Bull*, 7: 74.
29. Di Tizio A (1963): Manifestazioni oculari atipiche in 4 casi di sclerosi tuberosa di Bourneville. *Boll Oculist*, 42: 32–52.
30. Domegami G, Crattarola F R, and Wildi E (1972): Tuberous sclerosis, pp. 340–389. in P J Vink and G W Bruyn (ed.) *Handbook of Clinical Neurology*, Vol. 14, The phakomatoses, North Holland Publishing Co, Amsterdam.
31. Farnarier G, Roumagnou J and Mulfinger N (1975): Considérations sur le réseau capillaire radiaire de la papille [à propos d'une étude angiographique de sclérose tubéreuse de Bourneville). *Ann Oculist*, 208/3: 207–216.
32. Feriz H (1930): Ein Beitrag zur Histopathologie der tuberösen Sklerose. *Virchow's Archiv*, 278: 690.
33. Fleischer B (1935): Ueber klinischen und anatomischen Befunde bei tuberöser Hirnskle-rose. *Ztschr Augenheilk*, 88: 158–159.
34. Fleisher B (1935): Ueber klinischen und anatomische Befunde bei tuberöser Hirnsklerose. *Klin Mbl Augenheilk*, 95: 397.
35. Flinter F A and Neville B G R (1986): Examining the parents of children with tuberous sclerosis. *Lancet*, 2: 1167.

36. Font R L and Ferry A P (1972): The phakomatoses. *Int Ophthalmol Clin*, 12: 1–50.
37. Foos R Y, Straatsma B R and Allen R A (1965): Astrocytoma of the optic nerve head. *Arch Ophthalmol*, 74: 319–326.
38. Francois J (1972): Ocular aspects of the phakomatoses. in P J Vink and G W Buryn, *Handbook of Clinical Neurology*, vol. 14, The Phakomatoses, North Holland Publishing C°, Amsterdam, 619–667.
39. Francois J and Deweer J P (1952): Sclérose tubéreuse cérébrale de Bourneville. *Ophthalmologica*, 124: 321–339.
40. Fryer A E, Chalmers A, Connor J M, Fraser I, Povey S, Yazes A D, Yates J R W and Osborne J P (1987): Evidence that the gene for tuberous sclerosis is on chromosome 9. *Lancet*, 1: 659–660.
41. Fryer A E, Chalmers A H and Osborne J P (1986): Examining the parents of children with tuberous sclerosis. *Lancet*, 2: 1467.
42. Ganley J P and Streeten B W (1971): Glial nodules of the inner retina. *Am J Ophthalmol*, 71: 1099–1103.
43. Garron L K and Spencer W H (1964): Retinal glioneuroma associated with tuberous sclerosis. *Trans Am Acad Ophthalmol Otolaryngol*, 68: 1018–1021.
44. Gass J D M (1987): Stereoscopic atlas of macular diseases. Diagnosis and treatment. Third Edition, the C V Mosby C°, St Louis, 626–633.
45. Gifford S R (1940): Phakoma retinae and adenoma sebaceum. *Arch Ophthalmol*, 24: 967–971.
46. Glicklich E A, Schultz A and Benjamin J E (1944): Tuberous sclerosis associated with tumor of the optic disc (phacoma). *Arch Ophthalmol*, 32: 60–62.
47. Gold A G and Freeman J M (1965): Depigmented nevi: the earliest sign of tuberous sclerosis. *Pediatrics*, 35: 1005.
48. Gomez M R (1979): Tuberous sclerosis. New York, Raven Press.
49. Grinker R R (1932): Tumors of the retina. in Penfield W (ed.), Cytology and Cellular Pathology of the Nervous System, Paul B Hoeber Inc., New York, vol. 3, 1058.
50. Gutman I, Dunn D, Behrens M, Gold A P, Odel J and Olarte M R (1982): Hypopigmented iris spot: an early sign of tuberous sclerosis. *Ophthalmology*, 89: 1155–1159.
51. Harley R D and Grover W D (1970): Tuberous sclerosis. Description and report of 12 cases. *Ann. Ophthalmol*, 1: 477–481.
52. Hayden P M (1954): Tuberous sclerosis. *Am. J. Ophthalmol*, 38: 573–574.
53. Heilmann K (1970): Tuberöse Sklerose. *Klin. Mbl. Augenheilk*, 156: 71–76.
54. Hirose K and Nagae R (1940): Au sujet des altérations du fond de l'oeil et de l'examen histologique de l'oeil dans la sclérose tubéreuse (maladie de Bourneville). *Ann. Oculist.*, 177: 1–16.
55. Hofman H (1959): Tuberöse Hirnsklerose. Von Graefe's *Arch. Ophthalmol*, 161: 122–143.
56. Hogan H J and Zimmerman L E (1962): Ophthalmic Pathology. An atlas and textbook. 2nd edition, W B Saunders C°, Philadelphia, London, 525–530.
57. Horniker E (1932): Klinischer und Histologischer Beitrag zur Kenntnis der tuberösen Sklerose. *Ber. Dtsche Ophthalmol. Ges.*, 49: 357–362.
58. Horniker E and Salom G (1932): Alterazioni oculari nella sclerosi tuberosa (contributo clinico ed istopathologico). *Boll. Oculist*, 11: 497–539.
59. Hoyt C S (1979): The ocular findings in infantile spasms. *Ophthalmology*, 86: 1794–1800.
60. Huggert A and Hultquist T (1947): True glioma of the retina. A case of probable oligodendroglioma. *Ophthalmologica*, 113: 193–202.
61. Hurwitz S and Braverman M (1970): White spots in tuberous sclerosis. *J Pediatr*, 77: 587–594.
62. Jakobiec F A, Brodie S E, Haik B and Iwamoto T (1983): Giant cell astrocytoma of the retina: a tumor of possible Mueller cell origin. *Ophthalmology*, 90: 1565–1576.
63. Jordano J, Galera H, Toro M and Carreras B (1974): Astrocytoma of the retina. Report of a case. *Br. J. Ophthalmol*, 58: 555–559.

64. Kimura H, Setogawa T, Tamai A et al. (1974): Histology of retinal tumor with Bourne-ville Pringle's disease. *Folia Ophthalmol. Jap.*, 25: 643–645.
65. Kinder R S L (1972): The ocular pathology of tuberous sclerosis. *J. Ped. Ophthalmol*, 9: 106–107.
66. Kogh G (1972): Genetic aspects of the phakomatoses. in P J Vinken and G W Bruyn, *Handbook of Clinical Neurology*, vol. 14, The phakomatoses, North Holland Publishing C°, Amsterdam, 488–561.
67. Koch F L G and Walsh M N (1939): Syndrome of tuberous sclerosis. Report of a case. *Arch. Ophthalmol*, 21: 465–475.
68. Kroll A J, Ricker D P, Robb R M and Albert D M: Vitreous hemorrhage complicating retinal astrocytic hamartoma.
69. Kranias G and Romano P T (1977): Depigmentated iris sector in tuberous sclerosis. *Am. J. Ophthalmol*, 83: 758–759.
70. Krug E F and Echlin F A (1944): Tuberous sclerosis. Report of a case. *Arch. Ophthalmol*, 31: 68–73.
71. Kuchenmeister E (1934): Ueber einem Fall von Pringlescher Krankheit mit Veränderungen am Augenhintergrund und an den Schleimhauten von Blase und Mastdarm. *Dermat. Wchnschrift*, 99: 1333–1337.
72. Lagos J C and Gomez M R (1967): Tuberous sclerosis: reappraisal of a clinical entity. Mayo Clin. Proc., 42: 26–49.
73. Loewenstein A and Steel J (1941): Retinal tuberous sclerosis (Bourneville's disease). *Am. J. Ophthalmol*, 24: 731–741.
74. Lowe R J (1938): Intra-ocular Phakomata — A report of three cases. *Br. J. Ophthalmol*, 32: 847–853.
75. Lowry R B, Dunn H G and Paris R P (1979): Inheritance of tuberous sclerosis. *Lancet*, 1: 216.
76. Luchesse M J and Goldberg M F (1981): Iris and fundus pigmentary changes in tuberous sclerosis. *J. Ped. Ophthalmol. Strabismus*, 18: 45–46.
77. Lund O E (1960): Histologische und morphogenetische Untersuchungen an Auge und Hirn bei Phakomatosen. *Von Graefe's Arch. Ophthalmol*, 162: 369–399.
78. Luo T H (1940): Conjunctival lesions in tuberous sclerosis. *Am. J. Ophthalmol*, 23: 1029–1034.
79. McLean J M (1937): Astrocytoma (true glioma) of the retina. Report of a case. *Arch. Ophthalmol*, 18: 255–262.
80. McLean J M (1956): Glial tumors of the retina. In relation to tuberous sclerosis. *Am. J. Ophthalmol*, 41: 428–432.
81. Martin A J (1968): The Tuberous Sclerosis Complex. *Scot. Med. J.*, 13: 295–296.
82. Martin J P and Savin L H (1941): A case of tuberous sclerosis with 'phakomata'. *Br. J. Ophthalmol*, 25: 305–313.
83. Martyn L (1971): Tuberous sclerosis of Bourneville. in Retinal diseases in Children, W. Tasman ed., Harper and Row Publ., New York, 98–103.
84. Martyn L J and Knox D L (1972): Glial hamartoma of the retina a generalized neuro-fibromatosis. Von Recklinghausen's disease. *Br. J. Ophthalmol*, 56: 487–491.
85. Messinger H C (1936): Tuberous sclerosis with tumor of the optic nerve. *Am. J. Ophthalmol*, 19: 516–517.
86. Messinger H C and Clarke B E (1937): Retinal tumors in tuberous sclerosis: review of the literature and report of a case, with special attention to microscopic structure. *Arch. Ophthalmol*, 18: 1–11.
87. Miles P W and Dixon J M (1949): Tuberous sclerosis in three siblings. *Arch. Ophthalmol*, 41: 473–480.
88. Miller R M (1988): The phakomatoses. in Walsh and Hoyt's *Clinical Neuro-Ophthalmology*, 4th edition, Williams and Wilkins, Baltimore, Chapter 54, 1747–1827.
89. Monaghan H P, Krapchik B R, McGregor L and Fitz C R (1981): Tuberous sclerosis

complex in children. *Am. J. Dis. Child.*, 135: 912–917.

90. Morgan J E and Wolfort F (1979): The early history of tuberous sclerosis. *Arch. Dermatol*, 115: 1317–1319.

91. Musger A (1972): Dermatological aspects of the phakomatoses. in P J Vinken and G W Bruyn, *Handbook of Clinical Neurology*, vol. 14, The phakomatoses, North Holland Publishing C°, Amsterdam, 562–618.

92. Naumann G O H and Apple D J (1986): Pathology of the eye. Springer Verlag, New York, 929.

93. Nevin M C and Pearce W C (1968): Diagnostic and genetical aspects of tuberous sclerosis. *J. Med. Genet*, 5: 273–280.

94. Nickel W R and Reed W B (1968): Tuberous sclerosis. *Arch. Dermatol*, 85: 209.

95. Nitsch M (1927): Augenhintergrundsbefund bei tuberöser Hirnsklerose. *Ztschr. Augenheilk*, 62: 73–75.

96. Nyboer J H, Robertson D M and Gomez M R (1976): Retinal lesions in tuberous sclerosis. *Arch. Ophthalmol*, 94: 1277–1280.

97. Ohta T, Matsuo N, Egi K and Tanaka T (1980): Histopathological studies of retinal tumor in tuberous sclerosis. *Folio Ophthalmol. Jap.*, 31/7: 1095–1102.

98. Orzalesi N and Grignolo F M (1977): Tuberous sclerosis without mental deficiency or epilepsy. The abortive Bourneville disease. *Ophthalmologica*, 175/5: 241–249.

99. Pagenstecher W J (1955): Tuberous sclerosis. Historical review and report of two cases. *Am. J. Ophthalmol*, 39: 663–676.

100. Pampiglione G and Moyahan E J (1976): The tuberous sclerosis syndrome: clinical and EEG studies in 100 children. *J. Neurol. Neurosurg. Psychiatr.*, 39: 666–673.

101. Pampiglione G and Pugh E (1975): Infantile spasms and subsequent appearance of tuberous sclerosis syndrome. Lancet, 2: 1046.

102. Pascheff C (1940): Vergleichende Studiën ueber die 'Phakome' des Auges und seiner Adnexe. *Klin. Mbl. Augenheilk*, 104: 595–609.

103. Paufique L, Audibert J and Lauret C (1960): Gliome de la rétine. J. Méd. Lyon, 41: 1555.

104. Pillai S, Limaye S R and Saimovici L B (1983): Optic disc hamartoma associated with retinitis pigmentosa. Retina, 3: 24–26.

105. Prompitak A, Maberley A L and Shea H (1973): An abortive case of tuberous sclerosis without mental deficiency or epilepsy in an adult. *Am. J. Ophthalmol*, 76/2: 255–259.

106. Pringle J J (1890): A case of congenital adenoma sebaceum. *Br. J. Dermatol*, 2: 1.

107. Ramsay R C, Kinyoun J L, Hill C W, Aturaliya U P and Knobloch W H (1979): Retinal astrocytoma. *Am. J. Ophthalmol*, 88: 32–36.

108. Reese A B (1940): Relation of drusen of the optic nerve to tuberous sclerosis. *Arch. Ophthalmol*, 24: 187–205.

109. Reese A B (1963): Tumors of the eye. 2nd edition, Harper and Row, 173–177.

110. Reeser F H, Aaberg Th. M and Van Horn D L (1978): Astrocytic hamartoma of the retina not associated with tuberous sclerosis. *Am. J. Ophthalmol*, 86: 688–698.

111. Remler O (1949): Augen- und Allgemeinveränderungen bei tuberöser Sklerose. Ber. D O G Heidelberg, 55: 368–370.

112. Remler O and Pieck K (1950): Ueber ophthalmologische Veränderungen bei der tuberösen Sklerose. *Klin. Mbl. Augenheilk*, 116: 522–536.

113. Rettinger E and Wessing A (1967): Seltene Hautveränderungen bei Morbus Bourneville. Ber. D O G Heildelberg, 68: 228–234.

114. Rintelen F (1935): Fundusveränderungen bei tuberöser Hirnsklerose. *Ztschr. Augenheilk*, 88: 15–19.

115. Roach E S, Williams D P and Laster D W (1987): Magnetic resonance imaging in tuberous sclerosis. *Arch. Neurol.*, 44: 301–303.

116. Robertson D M (1972): Hamartoma of the optic disc with retinitis pigmentosa. *Am. J. Ophthalmol*, 74: 526–531.

117. Rodriguez B, Medoc J and Turturiello O (1953): Sclérose tubéreuse (maladie de Bourne-

ville). Esclerosis tuberosa. Enfirmedad de Bourneville. Importancia del llamado 'Adenoma sebacco de Pringle'. *An. Fac. Med., Montevideo*, 37: 195–220, 1952. *Arch. Ophthalmol*, 13: 206.

118. Rosa D (1961): Contributo allo studio dei cosi detti 'gliomi della retina'. Descrizione di un caso in un uomo di 59 anni. Boll. Oculist., 40: 492–505.

119. Ross A T and Dickerson W W (1943): Tuberous sclerosis. *Arch. Neurol. Psychiatr.*, 50: 233–257.

120. Rougier M J (1963): Syndrome fruste de la sclérose tubéreuse de Bourneville. *Bull. Soc. Ophtalmol. Fr.*, 63: 288–290.

121. Schmidt M (1939): Vorweisungen zur Krankheitsgruppe der Phakomatosen. *Klin. Mbl. Augenheilk*, 102: 286–287.

122. Schob F (1925): Beitrag zur Kenntnis der Netzhauttumoren bei tuberöser Sklerose. *Ztschr. Ges. Neurol. Psychiatr.*, 95: 731.

123. Schwab F (1956): Die Augenhintergrundveränderungen bei tuberöser Hirnsklerose. *Klin. Mbl. Augenheilk*, 128: 257–297.

124. Schwab F (1960): Einiges zur Histologie der tuberösen Hirnsklerose. *Wien. Med. Wochr.*, 110: 228–231.

125. Schwab F (1966): Die Tumoren der Netzhaut und der Aderhaut mit Ausnahme des Retinoblastoms und des bösartigen Melanoms der Aderhaut. Ophthalmologica, 151: 231–259.

126. Schwartz P L, Beards J A, Maris P J G (1980): Tuberous sclerosis associated with a retinal angioma. *Am. J. Ophthalmol*, 90: 485–488.

127. Seidel E (1938): Ueber eine sehr seltene Netzhauterkrankung als Teilerscheinung einer Allgemeinerkrankung auf ererbten Grundlage. *Von Graefe's Arch. Ophthalmol*, 139: 520–525.

128. Shelton R W (1975): The incidence of ocular lesions in tuberous sclerosis. *Ann. Ophthalmol*, 7: 771–774.

129. Shields J A (1983): Intra-ocular tumors. The C V Mosby C°, St. Louis, 650–656.

130. Spencer W H: Ophthalmic Pathology. An atlas and textbook. 3rd edition, W B Saunders, Philadelphia, London, Toronto.

131. Storchheim F and Taube E L (1936): Fundus findings in tuberous sclerosis. *Am. J. Ophthalmol*, 19: 508–509.

132. Szopa R (1949): Demonstration eines Falles von Papillengeschwulst. *Ber. D O G Heidelberg*, 55: 346–349.

133. Tarlau M and McGrath H (1940): Pathological changes in the fundus oculi in tuberous sclerosis. *J. Nerv. Ment. Dis.*, 92: 22.

134. Thomas C, Cordier J and Algan B (1948): Kératite en bandelette et sclérose tubéreuse de Bourneville. *Bull. Soc. Ophtalmol. Fr.*, 48: 465–467.

135. Tridon P, Marchand P and Coffe P (1977): Sclérose tubéreuse de Bourneville et malformations oculaires. *Rev. Oto-Neuro-Ophtalmol*, 49: 43–46.

136. Turek E, Raistrick E R and Hart C D (1977): Retinal tumours in neurofibromatosis. *Can. J. Ophthalmol*, 12/1: 68–70.

137. Van der Hoeve J (1921): Augengeschwülste bei der tuberösen Hirnsklerose (Bourneville). *Von Graefe's Arch. Ophthalmol*, 105: 880–898.

138. Van der Hoeve J (1923): Augengeschwülste bei der tuberösen Hirnsklerose (Bourneville). *von Graefe's Arch. Ophthalmol*, 111: 1–16.

139. Van der Hoeve T (1923): Eye diseases in tuberous sclerosis of the brain and in Recklinghausen's disease. *Trans. Ophthalmol. Soc. U.K.*, 43: 534–541.

140. Van der Hoeve J (1932): Eye symptoms in phakomatoses. *Trans. Ophthalmol. Soc. U.K.*, 52: 380–401.

141. Vogt H (1908): Zur Diagnostik der Tuberöse Sklerose. Z. Erforsch. Behandl. jugend f. Schwachsinns, 2: 1–12.

142. Vogt A (1934): Seltener Maulbeertumor der Retina bei tuberöser Hirnsklerose, 9 Jahre verfolgt. *Ztschr. Augenheilk*, 84: 18.
143. Von Herrenschwand (1929): Ueber Augenhintergrundsveränderungen bei tuberöser Hirnsklerose. *Klin. Mbl. Augenheilk*, 83: 732–736.
144. Von Recklinghausen F (1863): Ein Herz von einem Neugeborenen welches mehrere theils nach ausser theils nach der Hohler prominierende Tumoren (Myomen) trug. *Verhandl. Gesellsch. Geburtsh*, 15.
145. Waardenburg P J (1963): *Genetics and ophthalmology*. Vol. 2, Neuro-Ophthalmology, Ed. Van Gorcum, Assen, 1334–1339.
146. Wagner F (1957): Das Bild der tuberösen Hirnsklerose. Mit histologischen Befunde des Auges und der inneren Organe. *Klin. Mbl. Augenheilk*, 180: 577–584.
147. Welge-Lussen L and Latta E (1976): Tuberöse Sklerose mit Megalokornea und Iriskolobom. *Klin. Mbl. Augenheilk*, 168: 557–563.
148. Williams R and Taylor D (1986): Tuberous sclerosis. *Surv. Ophthalmol*, 30: 143–154.
149. Wilson J and Carter C O (1978): Genetics of tuberous sclerosis. *Lancet*, 1: 340.
150. Winter J (1982): Computed tomography in the diagnosis of intracranial tumors versus tubers in tuberous sclerosis. *Acta Radiol*, 23: 337–344.
151. Wolter J R and Mertus J M (1969): Exophytic retinal astrocytoma in tuberous sclerosis. Report of a case. *J. Ped. Ophthalmol*, 6: 186–191.
152. Yassur Y, Melamed S and Ben-Sira I. (1977): Retinal involvement in tuberous sclerosis. *J. Ped. Ophthalmol*, 14: 379–381.
153. Yassur Y, Melamed S and Ben-Sira I. (1978): Retinal involvement in tuberous sclerosis. *Metab. Ophthalmol*, 2: 385–386.
154. Yanoff M and Fine B S (1975): Ocular Pathology. A text and atlas. *Harper and Row Publ.*, 35–36.
155. Zimmerman L E and Walsh F B (1956): Clinical pathologic conference. *Am. J. Ophthalmol*, 42: 737–747.
156. Zolli C, Rodrigues M M and Shannon G M (1976): Unusual eyelid involvement in tuberous sclerosis. *J. Ped. Ophthalmol*, 13: 156–158.

8   Congenital Retinal telangiectasis

In 1883 Story and Benson [122] observed a peculiar fundus lesion in the right eye of a 20 year old man. They described the lesions as follows:

> Three bright well-defined cherry-like globular protrusions of one of the walls of the artery running above the macula were observed . . . a cylindrical dilatation on the trunk of the artery, which so suddenly and evenly became enlarged as to have quite the appearance of an intussusception. There was also much white fibrous thickening along the arteries, so that in place the blood column could hardly be seen. On the small vein near the artery was observed a three headed swelling and a little further on a single swelling of the same vein. The remainder of the fundus was carefully searched for any similar appearance but none were visible. There were in many places prominent masses of fibrous tissue in the retina, in some of which blood vessels ran.

The patient was further followed and three years later Story [121] reported an increase in number of the aneurysms. This is probably the first clinical description of congenital retinal telangiectasis, a disease which is mainly linked to the names of Coats and of Leber. Even before Coats published his original paper in 1908, other similar cases were described either clinically or histopathologically [28, 38, 39, 59, 78, 97, 107, 115].

Coats [22] in his original paper described three types of retinal diseases characterized by massive exudation:
– group 1: external exudative retinopathy
– group 2: external hemorrhagic retinopathy and
– group 3: with arteriovenous communication.
This was based on the pathological examination of cases from the literature and of six personal cases. The same author in 1912 [24] considered that the similarities between the two first groups were greater than their differences and he put the two first groups together. Meanwhile, von Hippel [134] had identified retinal angiomatosis as a separate entity and Coats recognized that his third group was in fact von Hippel's disease.

Coats already clearly defined the clinical and pathological characteristics of his disease: predominant occurrence in young male patients, unilaterality, progressive evolution with new hemorrhages and exudates leading to retinal detachment, ocular hypotony or secondary glaucoma.

In 1912, the same year Coats published his second paper on the subject, Leber [83] described what he called 'miliary aneurysms'. He collected eleven cases previously described in the literature [28, 38, 39, 59, 78, 97, 102, 107, 115, 122] and added two personal observations. He presumed that miliary aneurysms were a genuine manifestation of Coats' disease and was followed in this view by many authors [48–51, 65, 73, 89, 92, 106, 110, 117, 120, 129, 131, 132, 137]. Others however contested a direct relationship between the two conditions [25, 95, 112, 139].

The literature on the subject became extremely confused and the term 'Coats' disease' was used as a waste basket for a number of diseases with massive retinal and subretinal exudation. Some even did not consider Coats' disease as a specific entity but rather as a reaction to varying causes of illness [128]. Instead of Coats' disease the terms of 'Coats' syndrome' [32] and 'Coats' lesion' were used, which only added to the confusion.

Reese [110] critically reviewed the problem and introduced the denomination of retinal telangiectasis to characterize the typical lesion of Coats-Leber's disease. Unfortunately, some of his cases appear to be examples of cavernous hemangiomas of the retina.

Manschot and De Bruyn [90] consider that the diagnosis of Coats' disease should be restricted to cases of exudative retinopathy resulting from congenital retinal vascular anomalies. Adult Coats' disease [63] and Coats-like lesions associated to retinitis pigmentosa are not the same entity even if they share some characteristics with congenital telangiectasis or Leber-Coats' disease. These specific forms of acquired retinal vascular anomalies will be discussed respectively in chapter 10 and 11. With the introduction of fluorescein angiography a more detailed analysis of retinal vascular changes was made possible. Next to the relatively more common form of peripheral retinal telangiectasis, localized juxtafoveolar telangiectasis was described [52, 69]. We will consider this form separately in chapter 9.

I. Pathogenesis

Diverse pathogenic processes have been considered. According to Coats [22–24] the process is initiated by capillary hemorrhages due to abnormal blood constituents or to primary changes in the smaller vessels. For Leber [84] the lesions are inflammatory in nature and the hemorrhages are only of secondary importance. An inflammatory origin was also considered by Ogata et al. [101]. Manschot and De Bruyn [90] stressed that intraretinal hemorrhages are not obligatory for the pathogenesis of this condition. Berg [10] proposed an embolic origin after an infectious disease. Sattler [114] also considered the disease as a toxic-embolic process leading to severe alteration with secondary hemorrhage. Orzalesi [103] believed it to be a primary proliferative and degenerative disease of the retinal pigment epithelium, with the retinal vascular abnormalities playing an important role in aggravating the secondary inflammatory process.

For Wolff [142] the disease is generally the consequence of an exudative choroiditis while Hada [60] stated that ischemia plays an essential role. This could be due to congenital anomalies, circulatory disturbances and inflammation, while an allergic constitution could also play a role. Finally Young and Harris [146] suggested that fatty exudates passing from the vitreous through the retina into the subretinal space might explain the clinical aspect.

Actually the general view is that Leber-Coats' disease is primarily due to congenital alterations of the retinal vessels [2, 14, 36, 45, 48–51, 66, 82, 105, 119, 133]. The evidence of the congenital origin of these vascular anomalies is supported by the fact that the disease may occur at an advanced stage early in life and also that they may be associated with incomplete retinal and vitreous differentiation [33]. The breakdown of the blood-retinal barrier at the level of these abnormal vessels [2, 87, 99, 133] is the cause of secondary exudative phenomena, which may sometimes remain static or provoke a degeneration of neuronal tissue and even progress to total retinal detachment.

In conclusion Leber's and Coats' diseases are to be considered as a same clinical entity, whereby Coat's disease indicates a more progressed stage of the disease with massive intra- and subretinal exudates which may lead to total retinal detachment. Follow-up examination of cases originally diagnosed as Leber's disease showed the possible progression to the typical Coats' picture [57, 120, 129]. The term 'Leber-Coats' disease' should be reserved to cases of exudative retinopathy due to the presence of congenital retinal telangiectasis.

II. Incidence

Congenital retinal telangiectasis is a relatively uncommon disease, although some large series of cases have been reported [18, 35, 42, 65, 96, 113, 120, 125, 138]. The disease predominantly affects young males in a proportion of more than 70%. This was already noted by Coats [24] and confirmed by many authors [42, 96, 120, 125, 144].

The disease usually affects only one eye. Although some authors [141] reported an increased involvement of the left eye, others could not find preference for the right or the left eye [18]. Bilaterality occurs in less than 10%. Morales [96] found no bilateral cases in his series of 51 patients. Coats [24] had two bilateral cases in 46 patients, Egerer [18] 3 in 31 cases, Fox [42] 1 in 28 cases, Woods and Duke [144] 3 in 18 patients and Spitznas et al. [120] 10 in 112 patients. It is well worth noting that bilateral cases appear to be relatively more common in female patients [13, 20, 29, 87, 144] or in association with other anomalies [130]. The incidence of bilateral cases may be underestimated as the lesions in the least affected eye may be so discrete [135] that they can be sometimes missed.

The age at diagnosis varies. Leber-Coats' disease was detected before the age of one year in a number of cases [42, 79, 96, 110, 144]. Probably the youngest patient in the literature was described by Judisch and Apple [72].

They diagnosed Coats' disease in an 8 weeks old infant. Their diagnosis was later confirmed histologically. The majority of cases are detected before the age of 20 years, the mean age at presentation being 10 years [42, 126]. The disease is rarely found between the age of 21 and 40 years, but a second peak is noted between 41 and 60 years [120, 138]. This second peak probably represents cases of so-called adult Coats which share common clinical and histopathological characteristics with the congenital cases, but are to be considered as a separate entity (see chapter 11).

III. Heredity

There is no indication that Leber-Coats' disease is an inherited disorder. Pajtas [104] described the occurrence of pseudoglioma in four males in three generations of the same family and considered this as possible sex-linked Coats' disease. However the paucity of the clinical informations and the absence of histology cast some doubts concerning the diagnosis. Also the association with epilepsy in two of the affected members is more suggestive for a phakomatosis.

Renard et al. [111] observed a typical congenital telangiectasis in a 15 year old boy. The grandmother was diabetic and presented capillary dilatation and collaterals in the posterior pole, associated with peripheral aneurysmal dilatations, whereas her sister had a probable retinal branch vein occlusion. Although the authors suggested a possible familial occurrence, the vascular lesions in the grandmother and in the grandaunt are most likely acquired in origin. The familial cases of retinal telangiectasia with hypogammaglobulinemia described by Frenkel and Russe [46] are in fact examples of cavernous hemangiomas of the retina.

Familial cases of bilateral retinal telangiectasis have however been described in association with muscular dystrophy [40, 58, 118] and in association with hair and nail defects and intracranial calcifications [130].

IV. Clinical aspects

1. Presenting symptoms

The presenting symptoms are very variable and depend on the extent and severity of the retinal vascular involvement. The younger the age of the patient at diagnosis, the more likely the parents may have noticed an abnormal pupillary reflex or squint. In older children or in young adults the most common reason for consultation is blurred or decreased vision. Typical congenital telangiectasis is sometimes found during routine examination in otherwise asymptomatic eyes.

2. Ophthalmoscopy

The two major ophthalmoscopic signs are telangiectasis and exudates. Telangiectasis most probably precedes the exudates as cases with typical vascular anomalies but with minimal exudative reaction are known [83, 109, 137]. The lesions are predominantly localized in the superotemporal periphery [35, 132] and are characterized by numerous saccular and fusiform dilatations surrounded by hard white to yellowish exudates. The affected area is usually slightly elevated. The capillaries are primarily affected [119] but the retinal arterioles and veins can be involved predominantly [62]. The large aneurysms have a typical lightbulb aspect (Figs. 8–1, 8–2). The smaller vessels are tortuous, dilated or beaded. They are sometimes sheathed and form interarterial or arteriovenous anastomoses [6, 11, 35, 62]. Retinal neovascularization may be present [62], probably as a consequence of peripheral capillary occlusion. Even when the telangiectatic area is limited, the exudative response may be quite impressive. Exudates are commonly found at the limit of the affected area. The macular area may be spared in

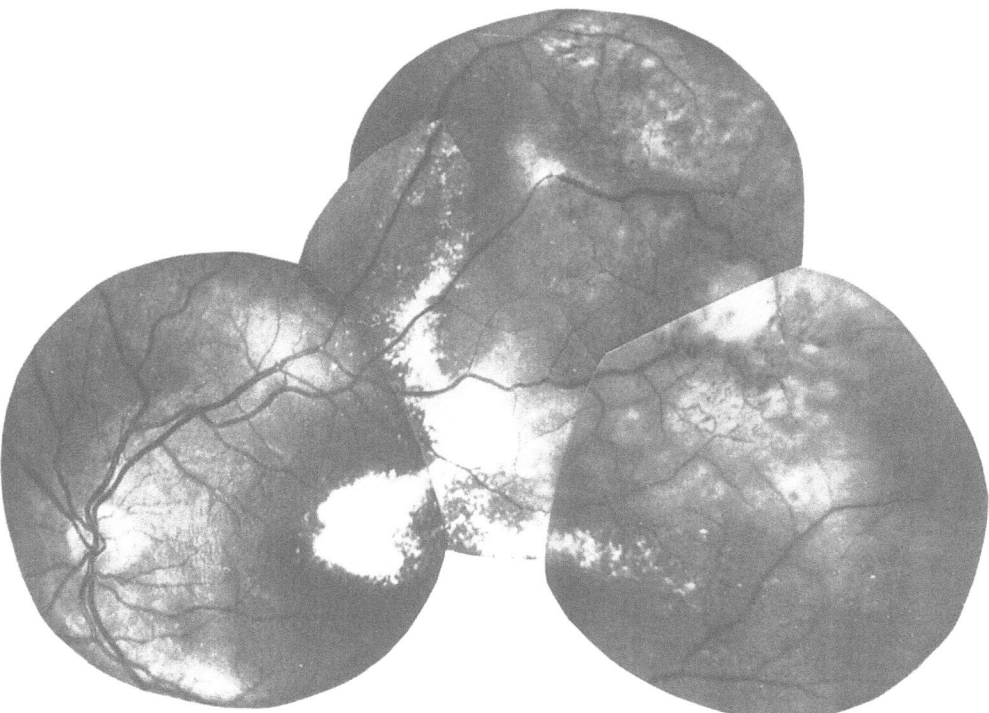

Figure 8–1.   Retinal telangiectasis with light bulbs, coarsening of the capillary bed and shunt vessels. Photomontage in red-free light.

some cases. However exudates may extend to the fovea. They may form a macular star or progress to form a macular plaque (Fig. 8–3). Cystoid macular edema and preretinal fibrosis (Fig. 8–7) are sometimes seen but are considered as relatively uncommon manifestations [48]. Although hemorrhages may occur, they usually are not very marked. Pseudotumoral lesions, more common in older patients with telangiectatic changes, may exceptionally be found also in younger patients with Coats' disease (Fig. 8–5).

3. Fluorescein angiography

Fluorescein angiography better outlines the peripheral vascular changes (Figs. 8–2, 8–4, 8–6). It indicates that the light-bulbs are not limited to terminal arterioles but may affect capillaries and veins. The circulation in the affected area is usually slow (Fig. 8–6). There is a coarsening of the

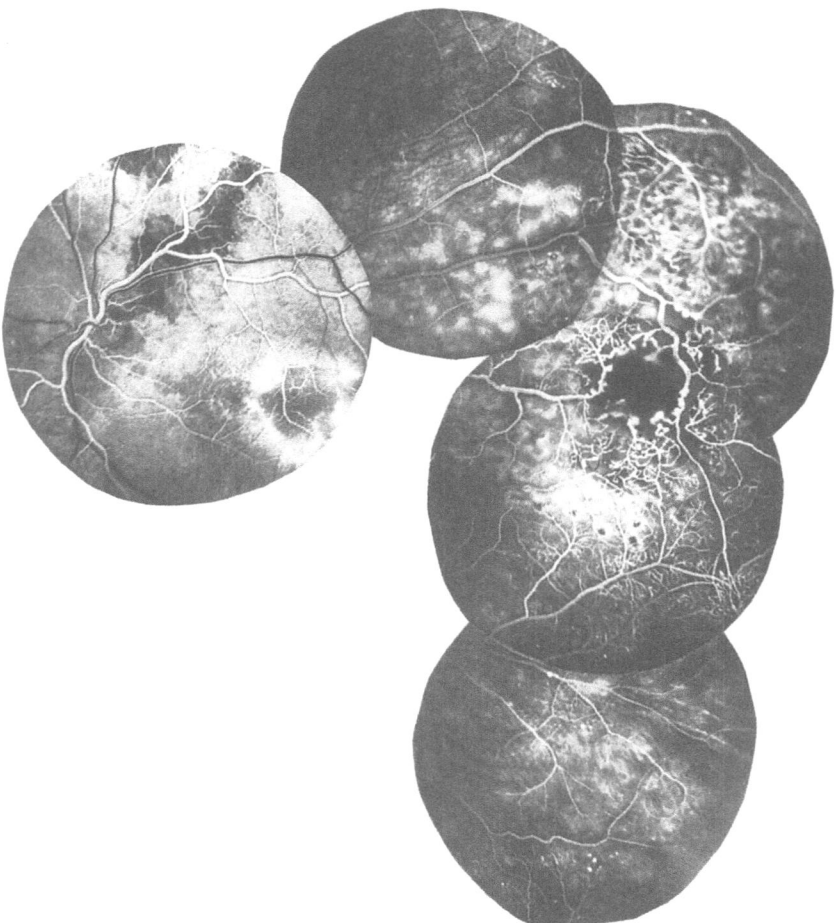

Figure 8–2.   Same eye as Fig. 8–1. Photomontage of the fluoroangiography.

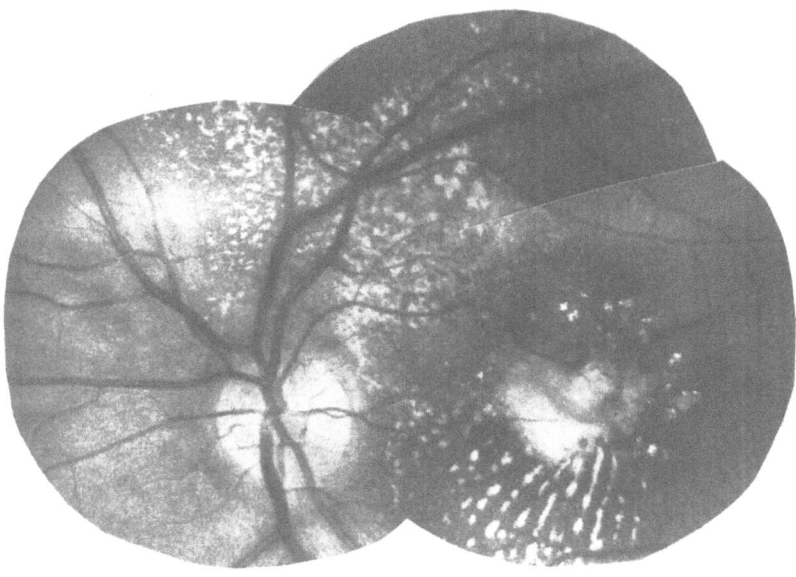

Figure 8–3.   Macular scar and lipoid exudates in a 10 year old boy with peripheral telangiectasis.

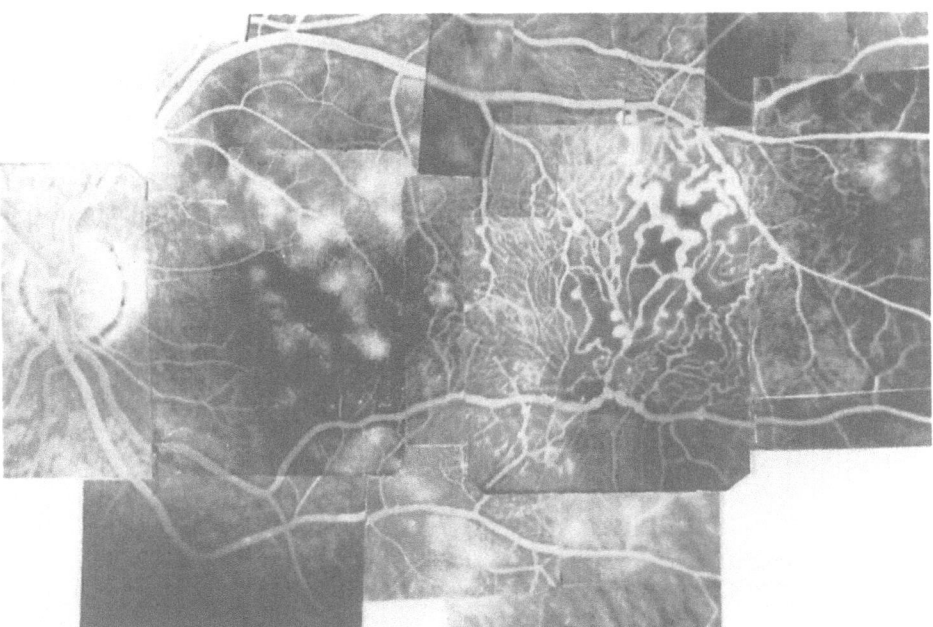

Figure 8–4.   Photomontage of the fluoroangiography in a case of Leber-Coats' disease. Note the telangiectasis temporal to the macula, the coarsening of the capillary bed and the leakage from the perifoveal capillaries.

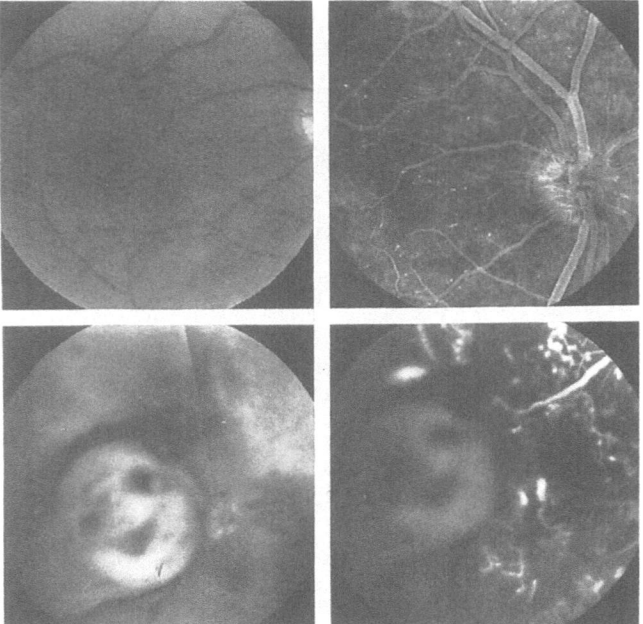

Figure 8–5.   Leber-Coats' disease in a 22 year old man. Cystoid macular edema and pseudotumoral lesion surrounded by telangiectasis in the inferotemporal periphery.

capillary bed. Capillary occlusion and even arteriolar occlusions are commonly found in the affected area and more peripherally large non-perfusion areas may be seen, usually bordered by shunt vessels. In these non-perfusion areas pigmentary changes sometimes occur (Fig. 8–6). Leakage of dye is variable and is not limited to the area of telangiectatic vessels. It can also be seen in the perifoveal region (Fig. 8–4).

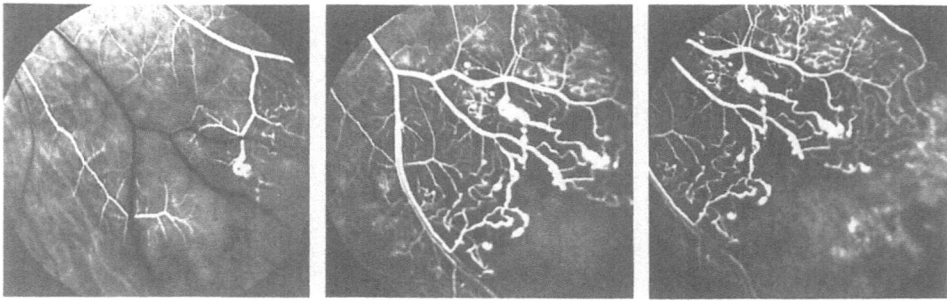

Figure 8–6.   Fluorescein angiography in a case of Leber-Coats' disease: retarded retinal circulation, coarsening of the capillaries, aneurysms on the arterioles and in the capillaries, shunt vessels and peripheral non-perfusion area with pigmentary changes.

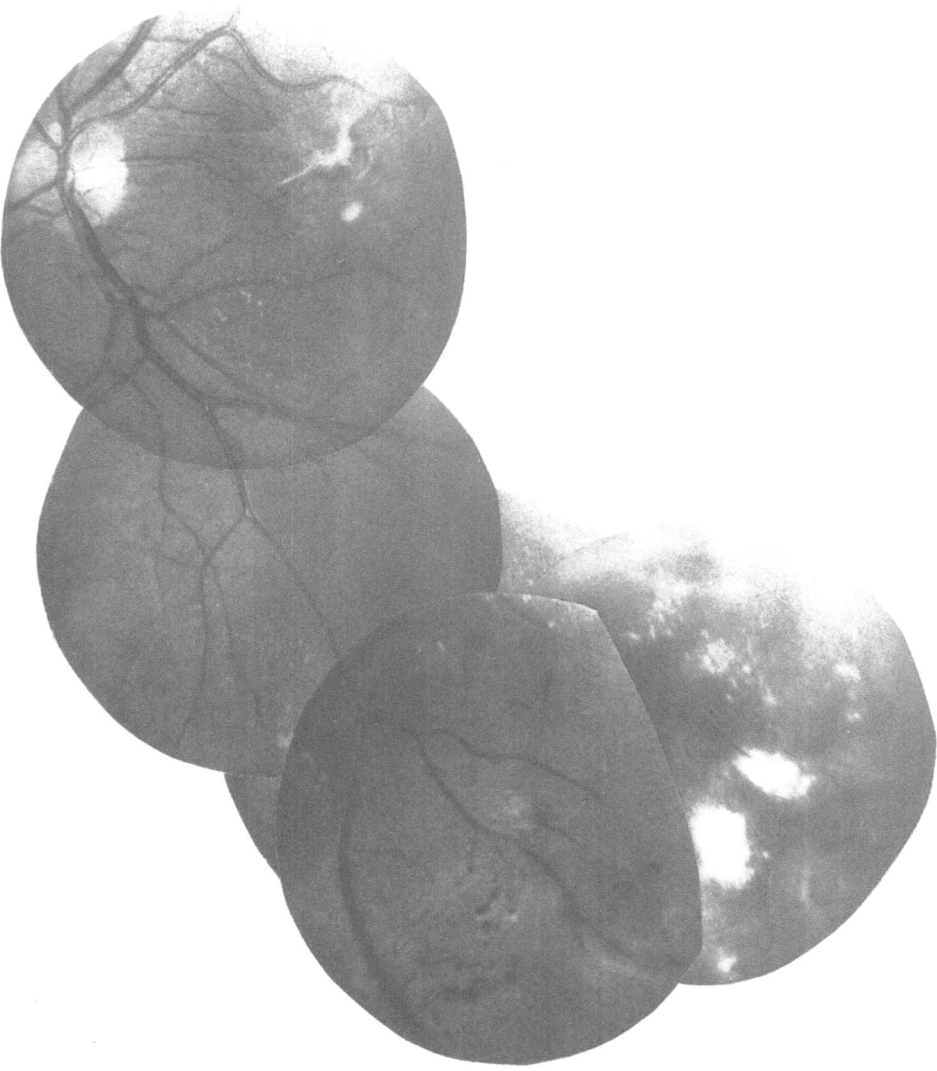

Figure 8–7.   Same eye as Fig. 8–6. Photomontage in red-free light. Preretinal fibrosis and macular scar. Typical light bulbs in the temporal periphery. Only few lipoid exudates are seen in the posterior pole.

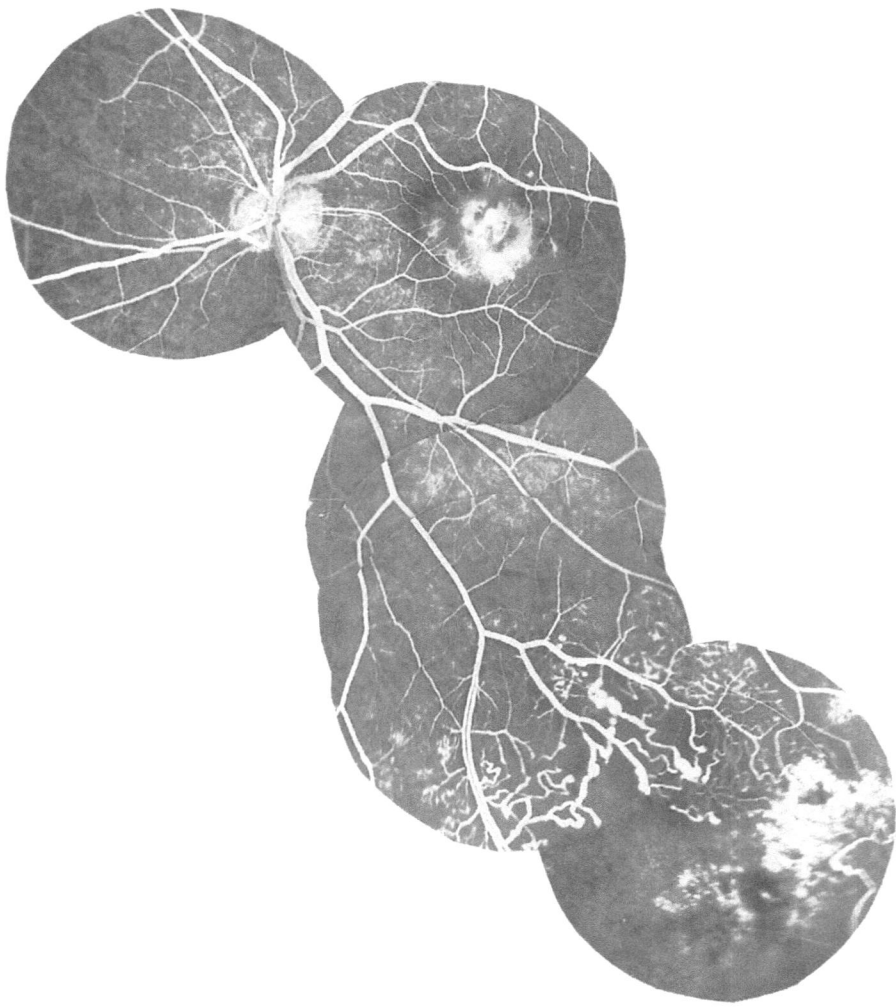

Figure 8–8.   Same eye as Fig. 8–6. Photomontage of the fluoroangiography. The macular scar is better outlined as well as the vascular changes in the temporal periphery. The retinal vessels between the posterior pole and the temporal periphery have a normal aspect.

4. *Natural history*

The evolution is variable. Morales [96] in a study of 22 untreated cases found that slightly less than 50% remain unchanged for a prolonged period of time. The other cases will gradually develop increased intra- and sub-retinal exudation (Figs 8–1, 8–3, 8–9, 8–10, 8–11), leading to loss of macular function and to exudative retinal detachment. The eye may ulti-mately be lost by total retinal detachment, neovascular glaucoma, total cataract or bulbus atrophy.

Even if the course is not so dramatic, central vision may be permanently impaired by secondary neuro-retinal degeneration due to persisting lipoid exudates in the macula, or exceptionally by retinal hole formation due to chronic cystoid macular edema [9]. Even after regression of the macular exudates a pigmentary scar may remain (Figs. 8–7, 8–8).

Judisch and Apple [72] observed a severe orbital cellulitis in a baby with known advanced Coats' disease. The inflammatory signs promptly regressed after enucleation. This was considered as an inflammatory reaction, due to the release of toxic intraocular breakdown products.

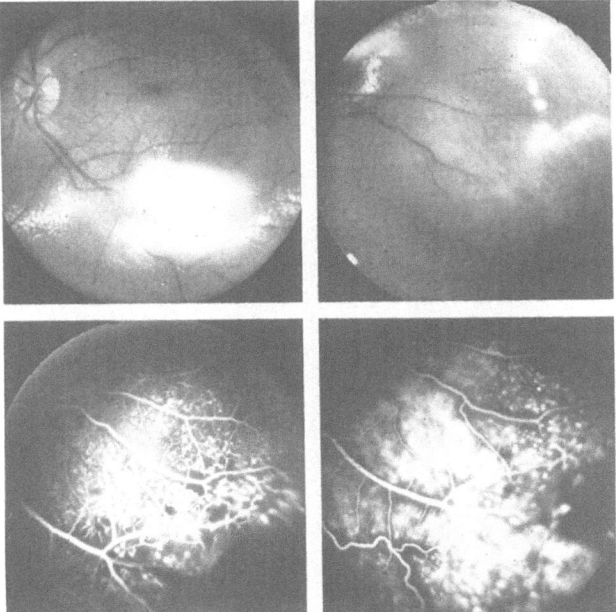

Figure 8–9. Localized exudative retinal detachment, lipoid exudates and preretinal fibrosis in a patient with Coats' disease.

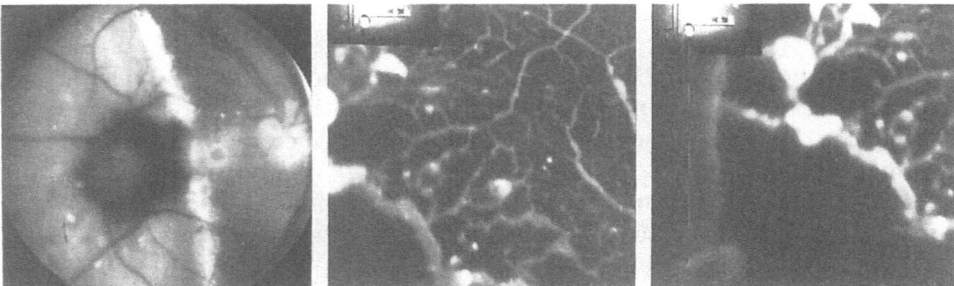

Figure 8–10.   Massive lipoid exudative reaction involving the temporal part of the macular region. Typical telangiectasis in the temporal periphery.

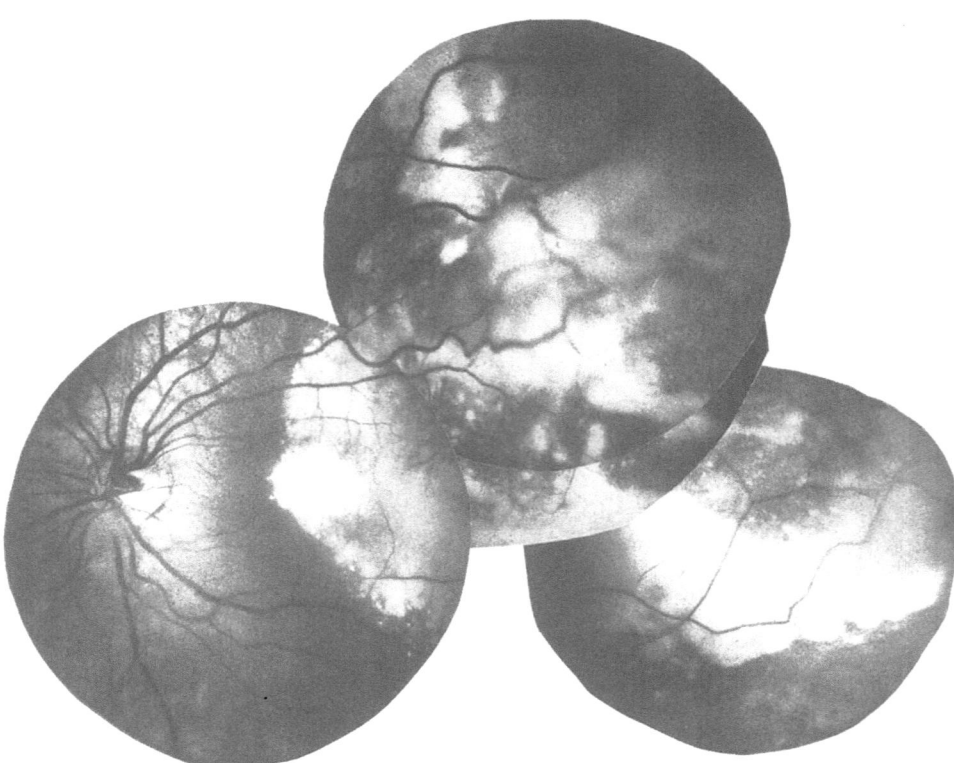

Figure 8–11.   Extensive retinal detachment with massive exudation in a case of Coats' disease.

Spontaneous regression is relatively rare. Already in 1929 Zinsser [147] observed a progressive resorption of lipoid exudates in the macular region of one of the patients originally described by Coats. A chorioretinal macular scar with cilio-retinal anastomosis was left. The telangiectasis was still present in the temporal periphery.

Deutsch et al. [27] documented the spontaneous regression of the retinal lesions in a patient. The case of spontaneous regression described by Offret et al. [100] is dubious as it is most probably a retinal arteriolar macroaneurysm which was treated by perivascular argonlaser photocoagulation.

Yet, the observation of extensive macular scars in patients with classical peripheral telangiectasis and only minimal lipoid exudates (Figs. 8–7, 8–8) is an indication that spontaneous resorption of macular exudates may occur. This is possibly related to occlusive phenomenons in the affected vessels with reduction of vascular leakage. In a young patient with peripheral telangiectasis associated with a limited retinal detachment in the inferotemporal periphery, we noted a marked horizontal pigmentary demarcation line crossing the posterior pole. A second pigmentary line was clearly visible on fluorescein angiography and extended from the first demarcation line temporal to the macula to the inferonasal periphery (Fig. 8–12). These demarcation lines suggest that the retinal detachment at a certain moment extended up to the posterior pole but that the retina spontaneously reattached at least partially.

According to the importance of the exudation Morales [96] classified his cases in 5 groups:
1. isolated local exudates;
2. massive elevated exudation;
3. partial detachment of the retina;
4. total retinal detachment;
5. secondary complication such as iridocyclitis, glaucoma or cataract.

A more or less similar classification was used by Spitznas et al. [120]:
1. vascular involvement of less than a total of one quadrant of the fundus and no large coherent lipoid deposits;
2. vascular involvement of less than a total of two quadrants of the fundus and/or large coherent lipoid deposits;
3. vascular involvement of more than a total of two quadrants of the fundus and/or partial exudative detachment of the retina;
4. total retinal detachment.

V. Associated conditions

Usually patients with congenital retinal telangiectasis are in good health. In particular serum lipid studies were normal in young patients with Coats' disease [31]. However association with dysbetalipoproteinemia [55] or dysproteinemia and hyperlipidemia [74] have been noted. As mentioned

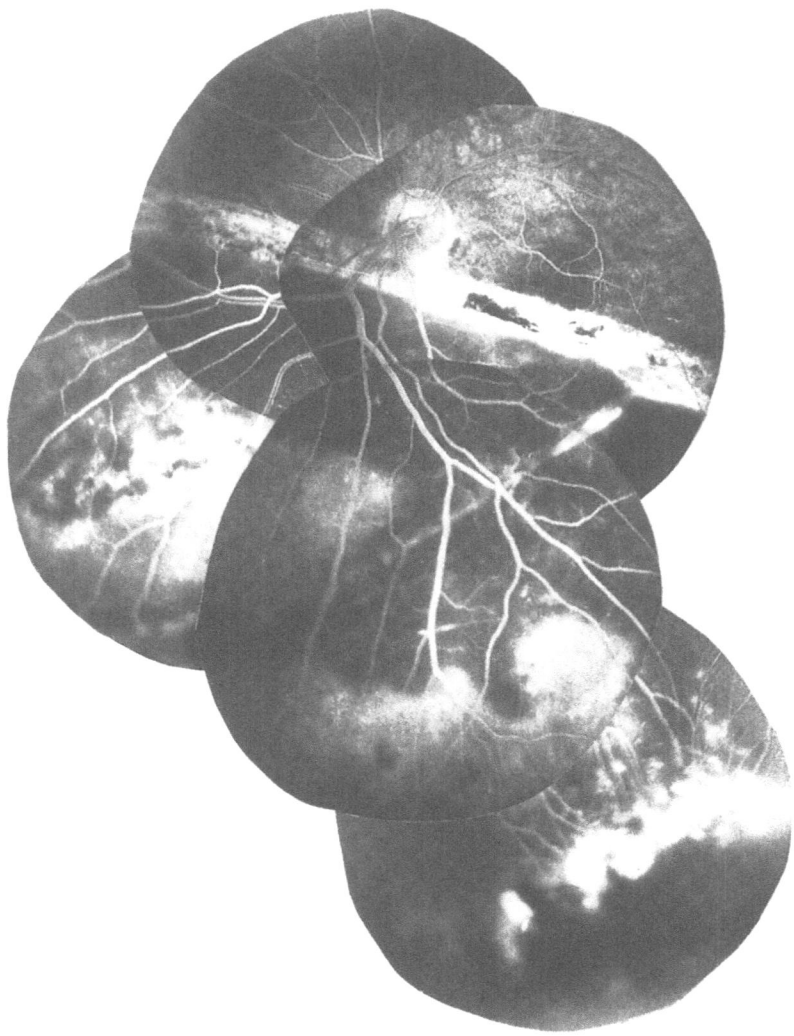

Figure 8–12.   Possible spontaneous regression of an exudative detachment in a case of Coats' disease. Double demarcation line: one horizontally through the posterior pole, the second extending from the first demarcation line towards the inferonasal periphery. Limited exudative detachment still present in the inferotemporal periphery.

previously, the patients of Frenkel and Russe [46] with hypogammaglobuli-nemia present retinal cavernous hemangiomas rather than Coats' disease. Such associations are possibly fortuitous as well as other associations with Coats' disease which have sometimes be noted: facial angioma [51], cavernous hemangioma of the retina [53], telangiectasis of the nasal mucosa [47], hypogonadism [5], Alport syndrome [76], ichtyosis hystrix [16], progressive facial hemiatrophy [51], morning glory optic disc anomaly [79] or Stargardt's disease [26].

Although congenital telangiectasis of cerebral vessels exist, no cases are known of the association of congenital cerebral and retinal telangiectasis [51]. However, Huet et al. [68] observed a cerebrovascular accident in a 39 year old man with Coats' disease and Bryson and Wolter [14] described a 20 year old man with typical retinal telangiectasis and central nervous system dysfunction (seizures, disciplinary problems at school and bizarre behaviour). A neuro-psychiatric examination was suggestive for an organic brain syndrome, probably vascular in nature. Arteriography was refused and no further information concerning the neurological problem was obtained.

Archer and Krill [4] observed a young man with retinal telangiectasis in the left eye, who developed progressive optic atrophy in the right eye. The progressive visual loss and an altitudinal visual field defect suggested more a vascular etiology of the optic atrophy than a demyelinating disorder.

Retinal telangiectasis may also be part of an inherited syndrome. The best known example is the association of retinal telangiectasis with facioscapulohumeral muscular dystrophy [40, 58, 118, 127, 145]. There is no correlation between the severity of the muscle disease and the extent of the

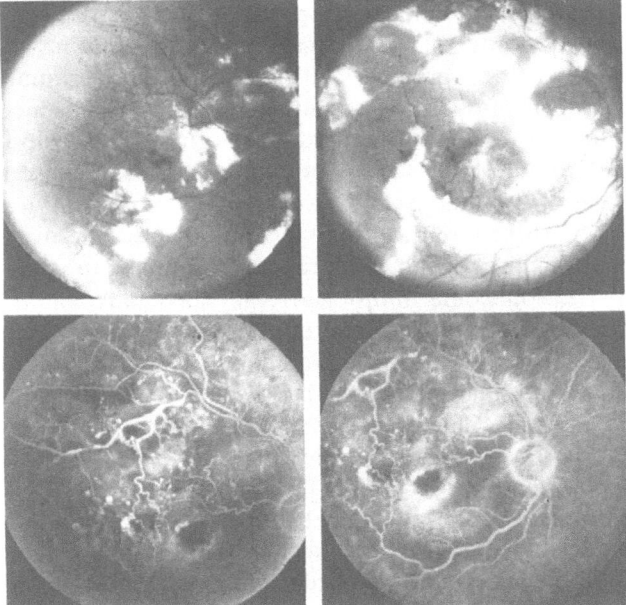

Figure 8–13.   Massive exudative respon:e after retinal branch vein occlusion (78 year old patient).

retinal vascular abnormality [35]. It is worthwhile to note that most cases in this syndrome present bilateral fundus disease which, as we have already seen, is highly unusual in Leber-Coats' disease.

Tolmie et al. [130] reported on two sisters with bilateral Coats' disease, intracranial calcification, sparse hair and dysplastic nails. The younger child also presented an angioma in one eye.

The association of Coats-like fundus lesions and retinitis pigmentosa will be discussed in details in chapter 10.

VI. Differential diagnosis

When reviewing the literature it is amazing to note the number of cases which were misdiagnosed as Coats' disease. These include cases of branch vein occlusion [106], acquired retinal macroaneurysms [9, 123], Eales' disease [106] and retinal cavernous hemangiomas [46, 110].

In young children presenting with a massive exudative retinal detachment the differential diagnosis will include other cases of leucocoria or total retinal detachment such as retinoblastoma, retinopathy of prematurity, familial exudative vitreoretinopathy, Toxocara canis infection and incontinentia pigmenti [49, 51, 126].

The most important differential diagnosis in this group is certainly retinoblastoma. Both diseases may show telangiectatic vessels and subretinal exudates. In retinoblastoma the superficial vessels are continuous with larger vessels extending into the tumor [51]. The finding of calcification, whether with ocular echography, skull radiography or cranial CT-scan, is a strong argument in favour of retinoblastoma. The absence however of calcification does not rule out the possibility of a retinoblastoma. As we will further see, treatment of massive exudation in Coats' disease may consist in cryocoagulation of the telangiectatic vessels and subretinal drainage. If such a procedure is performed in a retinoblastoma eye erroneously diagnosed as Coats' disease, this may result in extraocular tumor extension and mortality [61]. For this reason some authors [61, 80] have advocated to perform a controlled fine needle biopsy of subretinal fluid prior to surgery. If distinct large oval cells, round cells with pigment granules scattered through the cytoplasm or foamy macrophages with intracellular lipid droplets, are found a definite diagnosis of Coats' disease can be made. As cholesterol plaques, characteristic of Coats' disease, may dissolve during routine cytological staining procedures, Haik et al. [61] advocate the use of wet preparation cytodiagnosis, a procedure which is also faster.

In adult patients Coats' disease must be differentiated from branch vein occlusion [18, 116], carotid artery occlusion [17], acquired retinal arteriolar macroaneurysms (see chapter 12), retinal angiomas (see chapters 2 and 11), diabetic or hypertensive retinopathy and radiation retinopathy [48, 51, 126].

VII. Histopathology

The disease is histologically characterized by retinal vascular changes, PAS-positive exudates predominantly located in the outer retina and massive hemorrhagic or albuminous subretinal exudate with lipid macrophages and cholesterol clefts. When occurring simultaneously, these alterations are pathognomonic for Coats' disease [2, 72, 99].

Vascular alterations of retinal arterioles, venules and capillaries are observed in most cases, although some authors do not consider them as prerequisite criteria for the diagnosis [144]. They were described as thin-walled vessels [10, 22–24, 32, 33, 36, 66, 91, 114, 128, 134, 135, 143, 147] occurring especially in the inner layers [65], telangiectasis [2, 15, 19, 33, 36, 60, 66, 72, 90, 99, 110, 119] sometimes mainly located in the retinal periphery [20, 101], arteriovenous anastomoses or shunt [2, 72, 99] or aneurysms [60, 64, 72]. These aneurysms may present as microaneurysms [2, 75, 99, 119] or as larger aneurysms of a size between 50 and 350 microns. They may have large, sausage-like or beaded outpouchings and are sometimes situated on shuntvessels [33] (Figs. 8–14, 8–15, 8–16, 8–17). Vacuolization in the outer layers of the wall may lead to the formation of dissecting aneurysms [90]. Even an appearance of cavernous hemangioma [94] or neovascularization was reported [72]. The vessels may show obliterative

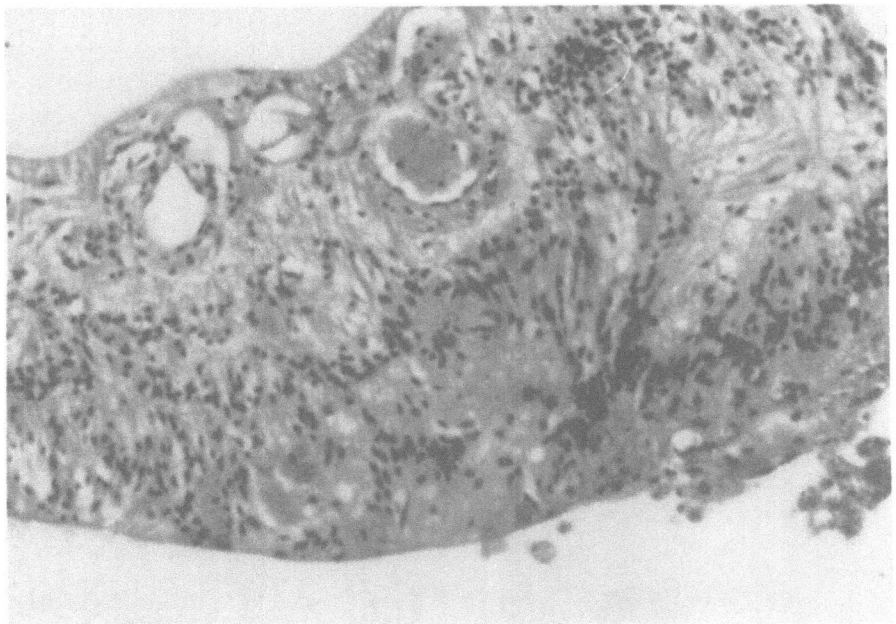

Figure 8–14. (Case 5100–82). Telangiectatic vessels in the inner layers of the severely disorganized retina.

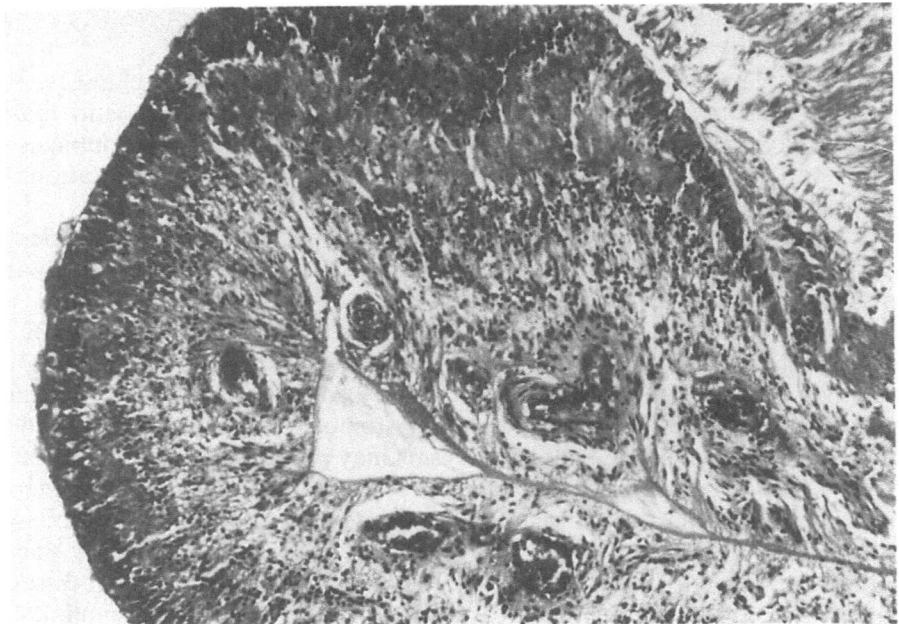

Figure 8–15.   (Case 1722–63). Disorganized and thickened retina. Telangiectatic vessels in the inner layers. Eosinophilic exudates in the outer layers.

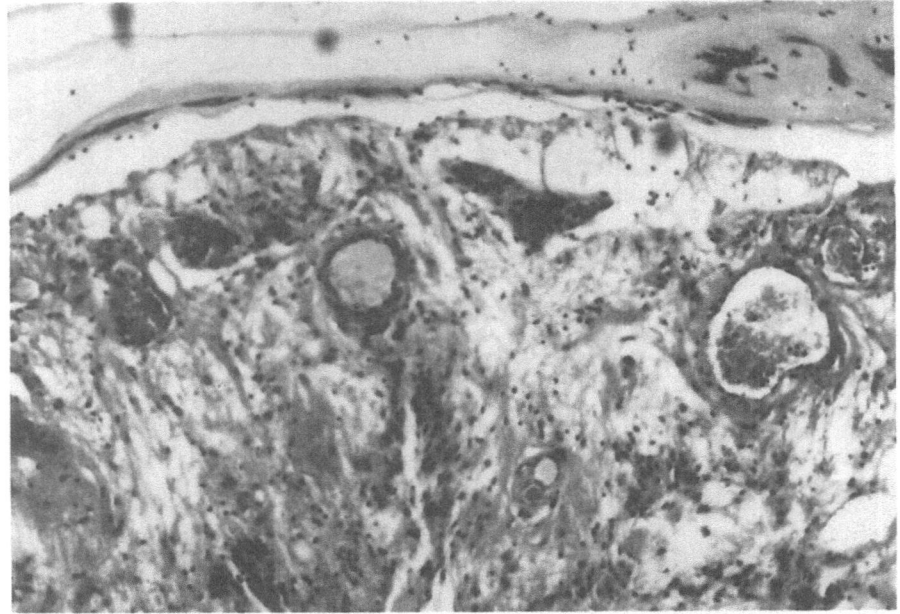

Figure 8–16.   (Case 4222–77). Disorganized and edematous retina. Thin-walled telangiectatic vessels in the inner layers. Preretinal membrane.

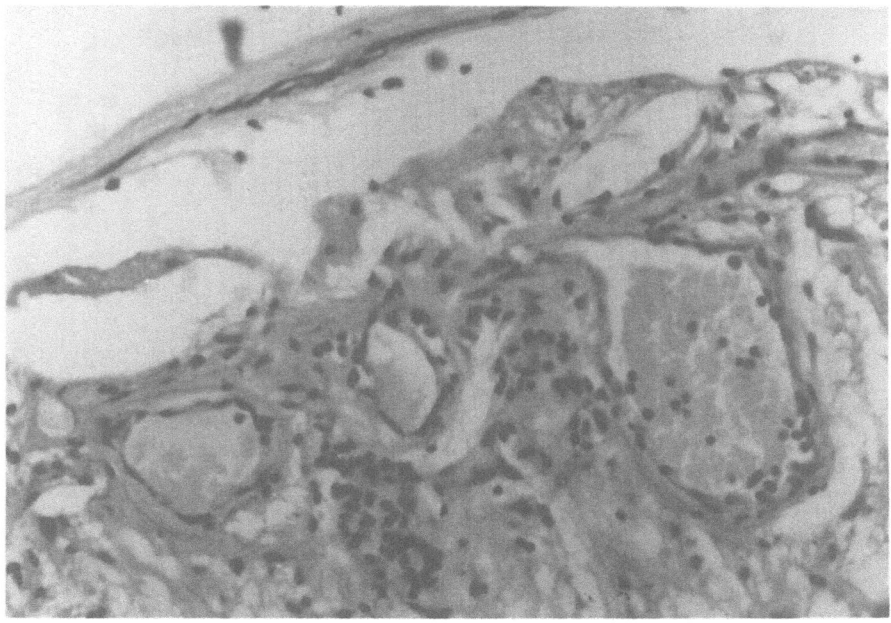

Figure 8–17.   (Case 4222–77). Thin-walled telangiectatic vessels in the inner retinal layers. Disorganized and edematous retina.

changes [2, 32, 94, 144], sclerosis [32], hyalinosis [2], sheathing [32] or perivasculitis [32, 56, 81, 110, 133, 144], suggesting a mild to low-grade inflammatory reaction [32, 81, 133]. Fibrin was found in and around the vessel walls as well as intimal and subintimal deposition of PAS-positive mucopolysaccharides [31, 110, 142]. Lipoidal cells may be present in the vessel wall [63, 86, 90, 133].

Proliferation [60, 75], loss [11, 133] or swelling [60, 90] of endothelial cells were found together with acellular strands [33]. Fenestration in the endoth lium was observed on electron microscopy [60, 86, 87]. The increased vessel permeability is evidenced by abundant endothelial pinocytic vesicles and micro-villi [60], the presence of enlarged intercellular spaces between the endothelial cells [86, 87] and the decrease or loss of endothelial tight junctions [2, 3]. Blood fluids and lipids can be deposited within the vessel wall (plasmatic vasculosis) and perivascular interstitial tissue [3, 86, 133]. This results in a thickening of the wall [2, 86, 90, 133] and intramural deposits consisting of a network of fibrils and homogeneous basement like material [2] similar to what is found in hypertensive or in diabetic retinopathy. Thickening [2, 11, 12, 75, 86, 133] and vacuolization [75] were also noted. This possibly leads to the occlusion of the vascular lumen [12].

Intraretinal hemorrhages, which are usually not prominent [66, 133], have been described [32, 66, 133] as well as edematous or albuminous exudate

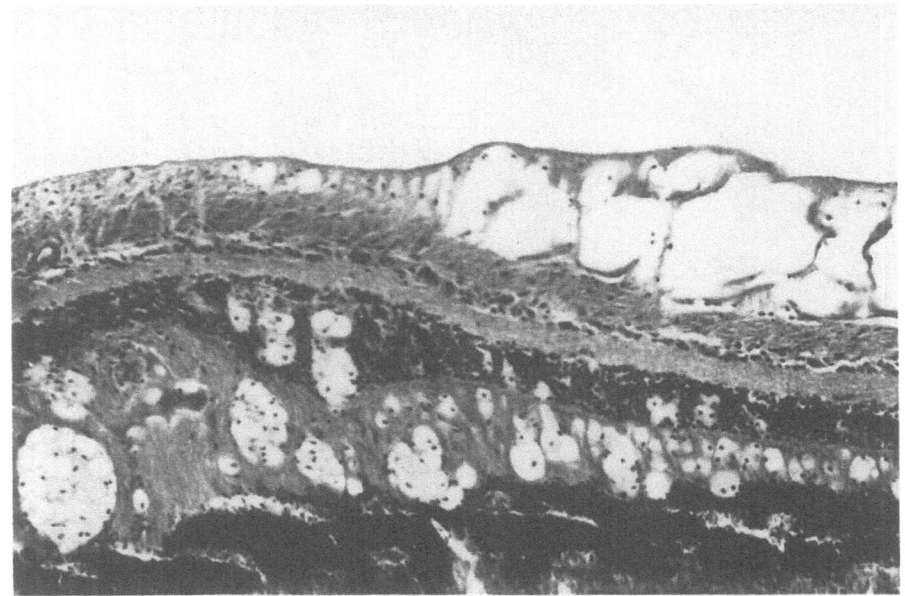

Figure 8–18.'   (Case 838–55). Thickened and disorganized retina. Cystic spaces in the nerve fiber layer. Clusters of lipoidal histiocytes in the outer layers.

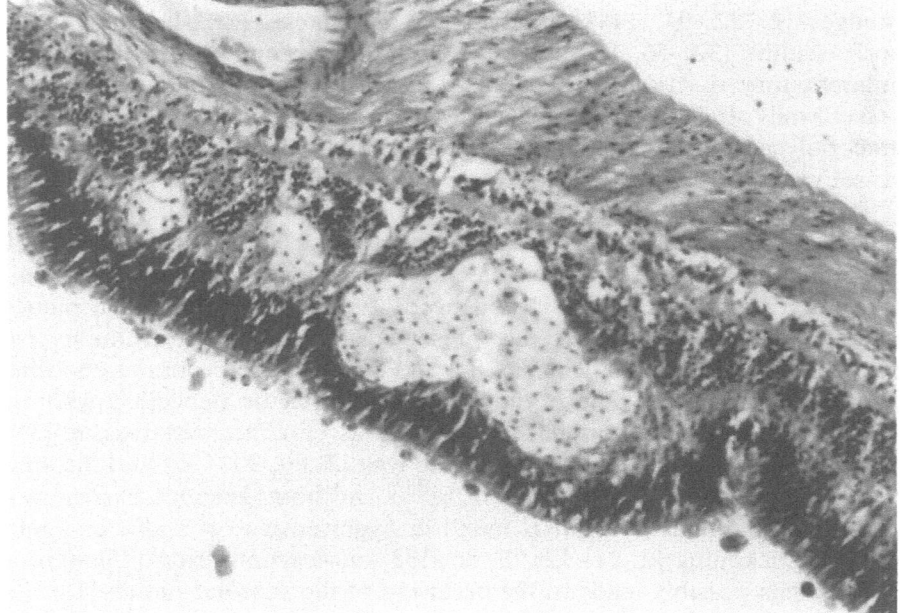

Figure 8–19.   (Case 5100–82). Thickened and disorganized retina. Gliosis. Clusters of lipoidal histiocytes in the outer layers.

with hyaloid eosin-staining foci [32, 110], fibrin [86], PAS-positive deposits [2, 72, 99, 136], lipid exudates with cholesterol clefts [2, 3, 72] and macrophages containing lipid, hemosiderin or cellular debris [2, 72, 86] (Figs. 8–18, 8–19). The exudation is mainly found in the outer retinal layers [32, 66, 99, 144]. This finding may even be considered as a histologic criterion [144], although all retinal layers may about equally be affected [81]. Cellular elements degenerate and are spread apart by the exudate [15, 99] and may even provide an aspect of retinoschisis [133].

Other retinal alterations include gliosis [10, 56, 64, 75, 93, 110, 114, 133], the presence in early cases of macrophages on the inner surface of the retina [81], dysplastic rosettes or true infoldings in the outer retinal layers [54].

The retina can be partially or totally detached by subretinal exudates or connective tissue. The exudate is sometimes albuminous or serous [32, 66], hemorrhagic [32, 66] or PAS-positive [2, 99]. It contains lipid macrophages, cholesterol clefts, epitheloid or giant cells [32, 44] and fatty deposits [133]. The origin of these exudates was considered to be the choroid [1, 142], the pigment epithelium [77], the retina [32] or the leaking vessels [37, 60]. In the exudate numerous ghost or foamy cells are found. These cells are macrophages or histiocytes [32, 36, 56, 57, 66, 70, 72, 81, 90, 92, 99, 133] which contain cholesterol [70], lipid droplets, cell debris or retinal pigment granules [56, 66, 119, 124] (Figs. 8–20, 8–21, 8–22). On electron microscopy phagosomes with lamellar inclusion bodies, a well developed rough endoplasmic

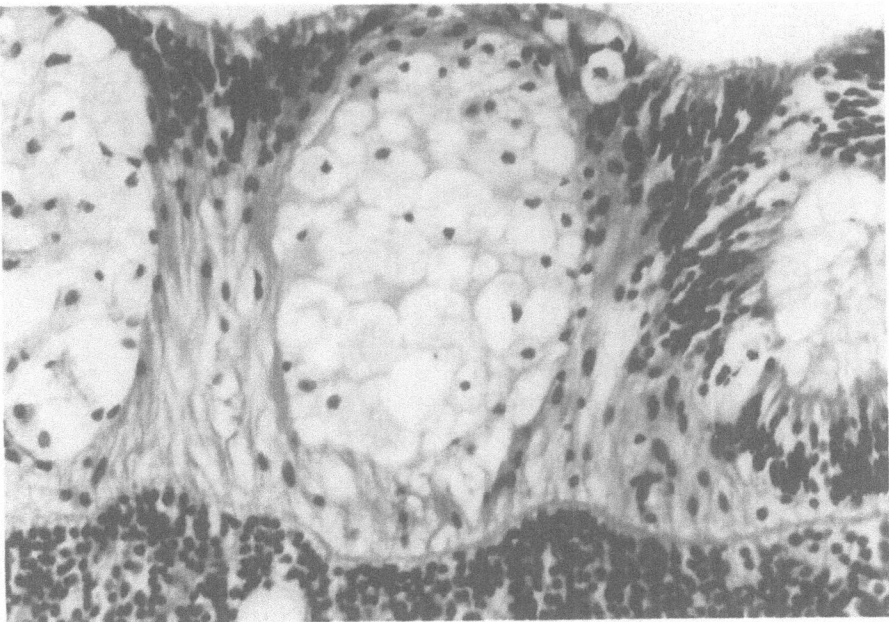

Figure 8–20.   (Case 5100–82). Clusters of lipoidal histiocytes.

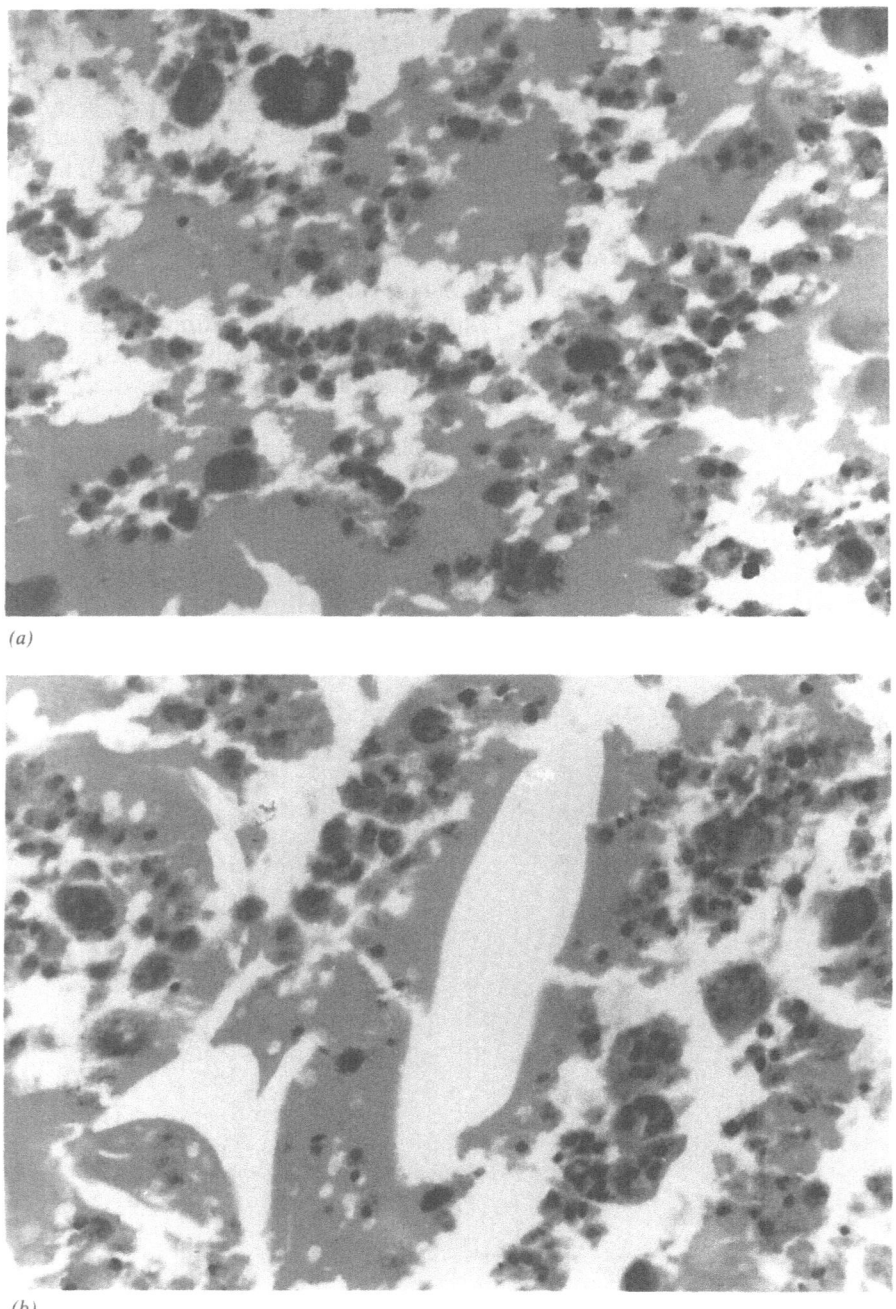

(a)

(b)

Figure 8–21.   (Case 1319–59). Subretinal eosinophilic exudate with ghost cells containing pigment granules, cholesterol clefts and some giant cells.

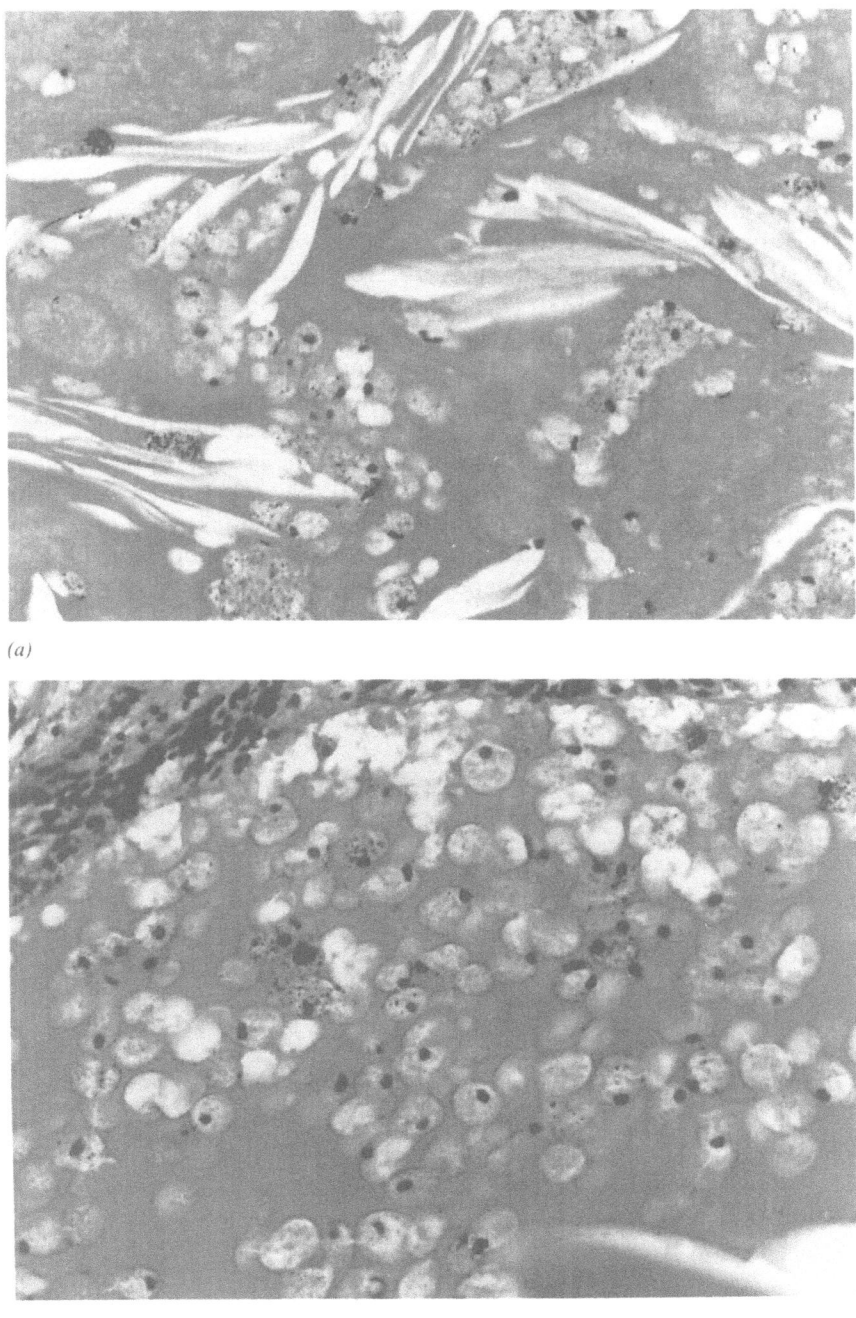

(a)

(b)

Figure 8–22. (Case 1722–63). Subretinal exudate with foamy cells (bladder cells, ghost cells) containing pigment granules and cholesterol clefts.

reticulum and scanty smooth endoplasmic reticulum were found [124]. The ghost cells generally accumulate in the vicinity of the retinal pigment epithelium and the detached retina, or float in the subretinal space [124]. They have been considered to derive from the retinal pigment epithelium [44, 60, 64, 81, 84, 90, 103, 114, 124] as the epithelial cells may detach, proliferate and assume phagocytic activities [32, 86, 90, 119, 133]. According to other authors there is no evidence of phagocytic activity in proliferated retinal pigment epithelial cells or in the diseased retina [70]. Degenerated leukocytes [22–24], monocytes [60, 70, 101], microglia [32], macrophages from the blood stream [133], the adventitia of blood vessels [36] or the local proliferation of resting retinal macrophages [133] have also been considered as possible sources of foamy cells. According to some authors the ghost cells originate in the retina and migrate into the subretinal space [70, 90], while for others the cells may originate from the choroid as well [119].

In the later stages of the disease the exudate is replaced by connective tissue which can be found in the choroid [10, 22–24], subretinally or in the retina itself (Figs. 8–23, 8–24). This connective tissue may be present under the macula, even when the vascular changes are located in the periphery [133]. The variations in size, shape and complexity of the connective tissue, from loose and cellular to dense, reflect the different stages of its development [70]. It presents itself as thick subretinal fibrosis [70] (Fig. 8–25), a

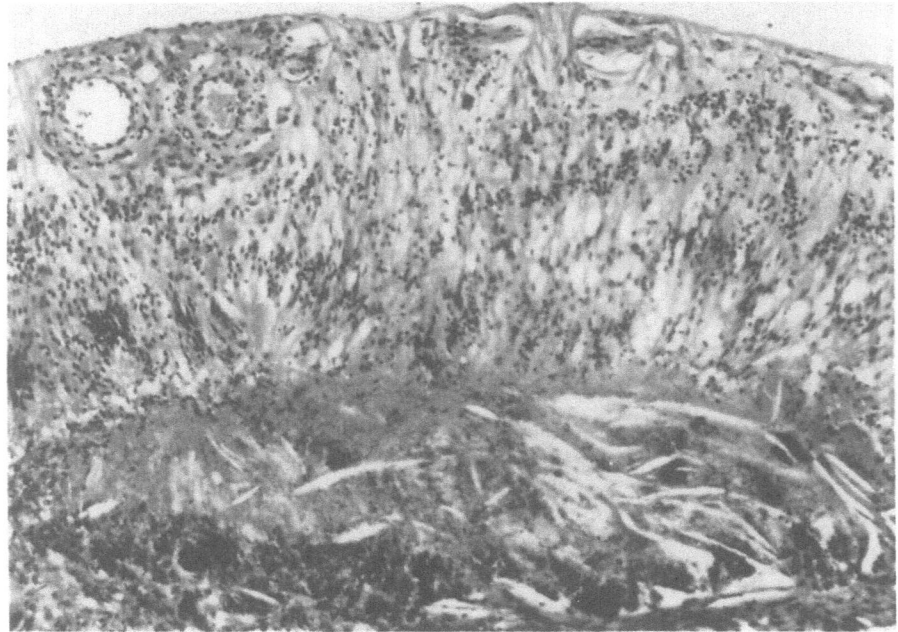

Figure 8–23.   (Case 5100–82). Thickened, disorganized and edematous retina. Subretinal organized exudate with cholesterol clefts.

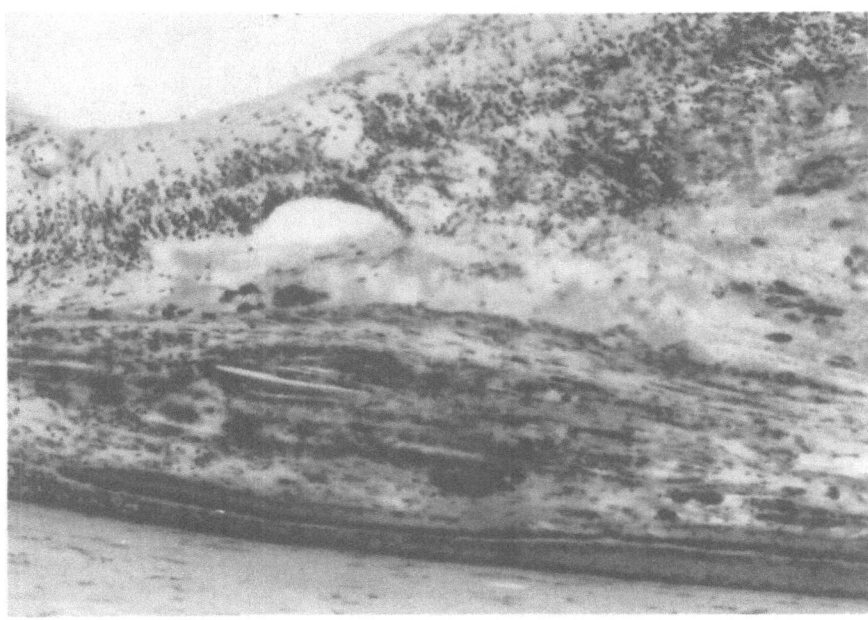

Figure 8-24. (Case 1553-61). Disorganized retina. Subretinal organized hemorrhagic exudates. Subretinal fibrous tissue with laminated hyperplastic retinal pigment epithelium. Small cholesterol clefts.

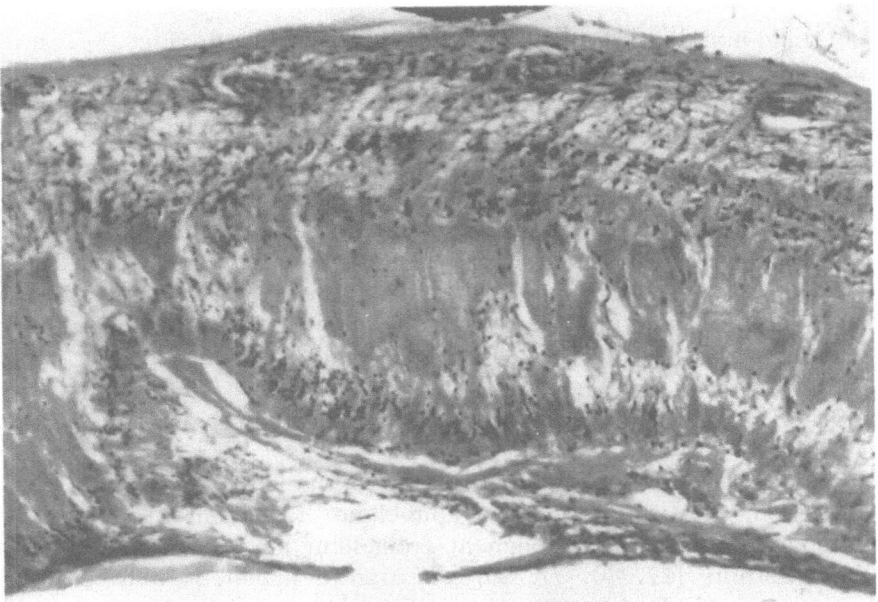

Figure 8-25. (Case 1722-63). Thickened and disorganized retina. Outer layers markedly engorged with exudates. Subretinal fibroblastic tissue.

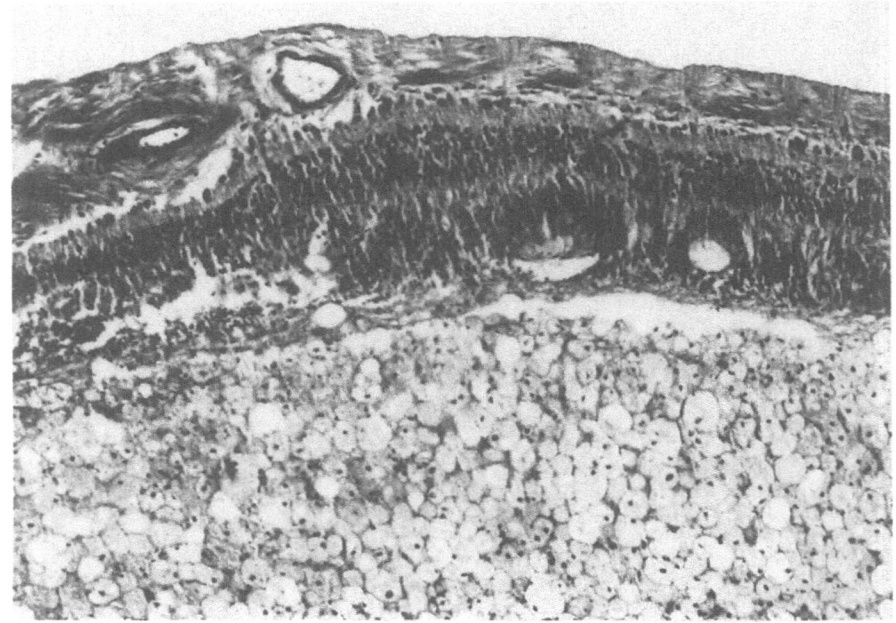

Figure 8–26.   (Case 838–55). Disorganized retina with subretinal foamy cells.

subretinal nodule with foamy cells and cholesterol clefts (Figs. 8–26), a thin subretinal fibroblastic layer along the detached retina [70, 90] or as finger-like projections from the retinal pigment epithelium [70]. All varieties have in common to be connected to the retinal pigment epithelium or to be surrounded by a sheet of epithelial cells [70]. Vessels coming from the choroid can be traced into the submacular disciform nodule [133].

Different opinions were advanced as to the origin of the fibrous tissue.

For Coats [22–24] retinal hemorrhages and subsequent retinal degenera-tion cause an influx or phagocytes and a proliferation of connective tissue, while in the opinion of Berg [10] it originates from the retinal pigment epithelium. For Sattler [114] the tissue comes from the anterior choroidal layers.

Lamb [81] incriminated the macrophages through their ability to become fibroblasts.

For Elwyn [36] it was formed by fibroblasts from mesodermal elements by metaplasia of retinal pigment epithelium. The proliferation and fibrous metaplasia of the retinal pigment epithelium have been incriminated by many authors [19, 70, 71, 90] and transitional steps between pigment epithelium and fibroblasts have been demonstrated [90, 133].

The cicatricial connective tissue may present cavities [32, 82] containing all kind of debris, remnants of hemorrhages, cholesterol or other crystals, pigment foam cells [32, 36, 71, 93, 101], hyaline, glial tissue [32, 93], cholesterol clefts [45, 54, 70, 72], foreign body giant cells [32, 45, 54, 63, 93, 101], calcareous particles [19, 32, 36] or ossification [7, 19, 22–24, 36, 45, 84, 98].

Special attention has been paid to the deposition of lipids in Coats' disease. Although highly characteristic, they are a measure of the severity or of the chronicity of the process, rather than a specific feature [133]. They are free cholesterol, cholesterol esters or unidentified crystalline associated with fatty acids [31]. In adult cases there seems to be a definite hyperlipemia, involving especially the cholesterol fraction. In juvenile cases, in which the trigger of a previous inflammatory process is missing, a tissue factor is necessary for the local deposition of cholesterol. It was suggested that this could be an acid mucopolysaccharide, which by combination with plasma lipoproteins formed new complexes which on hydrolysis could deposit the cholesterol [144].

The retinal pigment epithelium may show degenerative changes [1, 10, 64, 103] or proliferation [10, 32, 70, 103, 124], occurring sometimes in a perivascular pattern [63] or penetrating into the deep retinal and choroidal layers [93]. Transformation into fibroblasts has already been discussed. Some authors stated that the pigment epithelial cells probably always become macrophages before changing into fibroblasts [81]. Multinucleated giant cells as well as immature small retinal pigment epithelial cells were often encountered in non-proliferative areas of the retinal pigment epithelium [70].

The choroid may be normal [64, 114, 124, 125, 133], minimally affected [7, 34] or initially unchanged with inconstant secondary involvement [32]. Choroidal involvement can occur as a moderate to heavy inflammatory infiltration [34, 36, 45, 56, 90, 114, 144], especially at the site of chorioretinal adhesions [36, 114, 144], localized atrophy [144] or exudative changes in the vessels and in the suprachoroidal space [60].

Bruch's membrane may be intact [36, 133] or disrupted [4, 34]. Blood vessels can extend from the choroid to the base of the mounds or subretinally [7, 34, 45, 70] or even through the retina into the vitreous as reported in Coats-like response in retinitis pigmentosa [41].

The vitreous may show varying amounts of inflammatory cells [34], cholesterol deposits [15] or neovascularisation invading through gaps in the internal limiting membrane [19, 34].

Among other aspecific ocular changes we may mention cataract, rubeosis iridis and secondary glaucoma [19, 125] as well as inflammatory changes in the anterior segment [125, 144] and even orbital cellulitis in an advanced case of Coats' disease [72]. This orbital cellulitis was probably secondary to the release of toxic intraocular cellular breakdown products via the scleral emissaries.

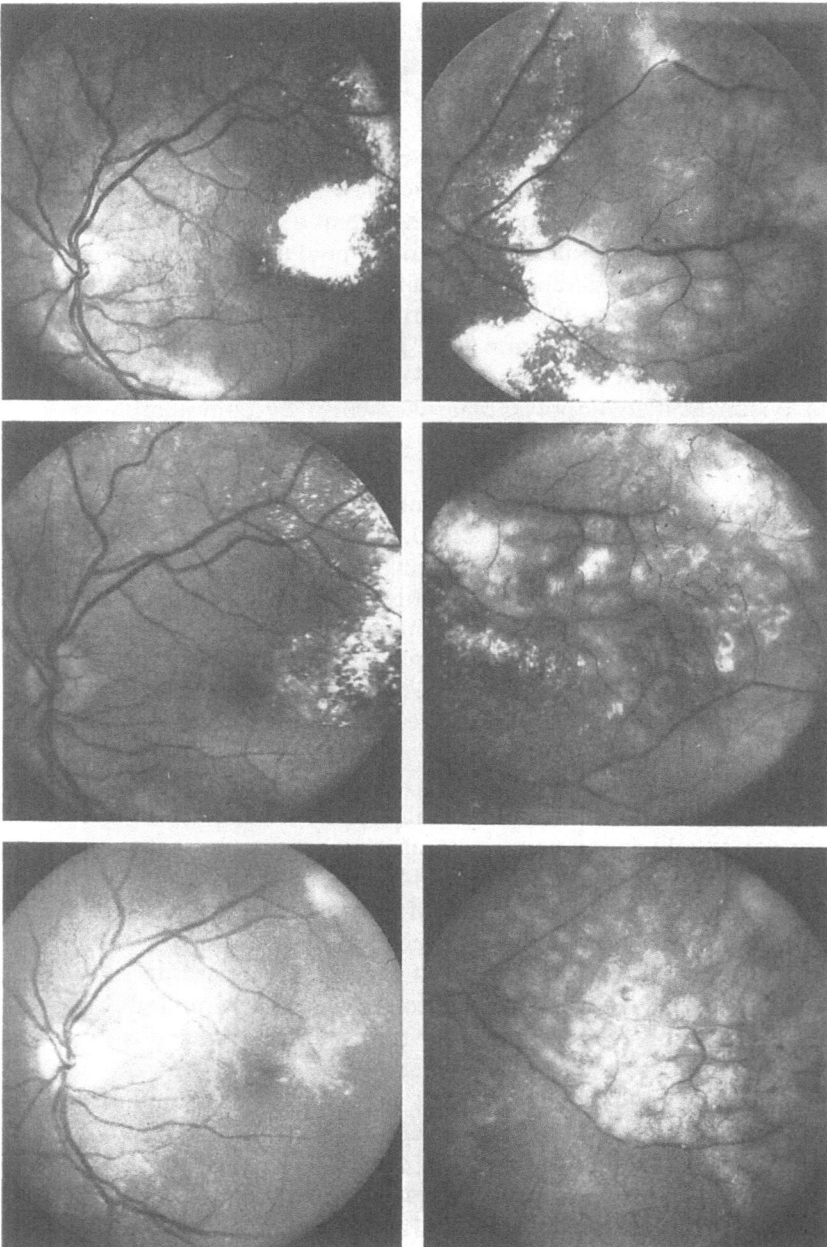

Figure 8–27.   Coats' disease in a 11-year old boy. Top: aspect two months after the first treatment. Middle: six months after treatment. Bottom: two years after treatment.

VIII. Treatment

Although some eyes with Leber-Coats' disease may stabilize or even show signs of regression, a majority of untreated cases will eventually loose vision either by secondary macular degeneration or by exudative retinal detachment and its complications.

The aim of the treatment is to improve or stabilize visual acuity and to prevent total retinal detachment, neovascular glaucoma and phthisis bulbi. In order to arrest the exudative reaction several methods of destroying telangiectatic vessels have been employed: diathermy, cryocoagulation or photocoagulation with the Xenon arc or with the Argon laser [11, 21, 35, 42, 48–51, 67, 85, 88, 112, 113, 125, 138, 141].

If the retina is still attached, the treatment of choice is photocoagulation. The treatment should be restricted to the area with telangiectatic vessels. Usually, several treatment sessions are needed [35, 125]. It has been our experience that Xenon photocoagulation is often more effective in treating such cases than the Argon laser. According to L'Espérance [85] the polychromacity of the Xenon arc, particularly in the infrared region, makes this more destructive and penetrating than Argon laser. If the lesions are associated with marked subretinal exudation and exudative retinal detachment, cryocoagulation is indicated. This can be done transconjunctivally or after release of subretinal fluid. In extensive retinal detachment, scleral buckling or encircling procedures may be necessary [11, 35, 125]. The prognosis is however relatively poor if more than two quadrants are involved.

Especially in young children, the treatment has to be aggressive [113, 125].

If the abnormal vessels are eliminated, exudates will progressively regress (Fig. 8–27). This starts within the first two months. However, the visual prognosis will depend on the extent of the lesions and the duration of involvement of the macular region. In longstanding cases, after total regression of the exudates in the macular region, a chorioretinal scar may sometimes be seen, which explains why vision has not improved despite a successful treatment.

After treatment 75% or more of the eyes will either improve or stabilize [113, 125, 138]. This figure has to be compared with the more than 50% deterioration in Morales' series of untreated cases [96].

Treatment complications are relatively rare; the most serious complication being the rupture of a large aneurysm [85]. This may provoke extensive retinal or even vitreous hemorrhages. Therefore, it is better to initially treat around large aneurysms. This sometimes is sufficient to produce their occlusion. If they do not disappear, mild coagulations of the aneurysms are indicated.

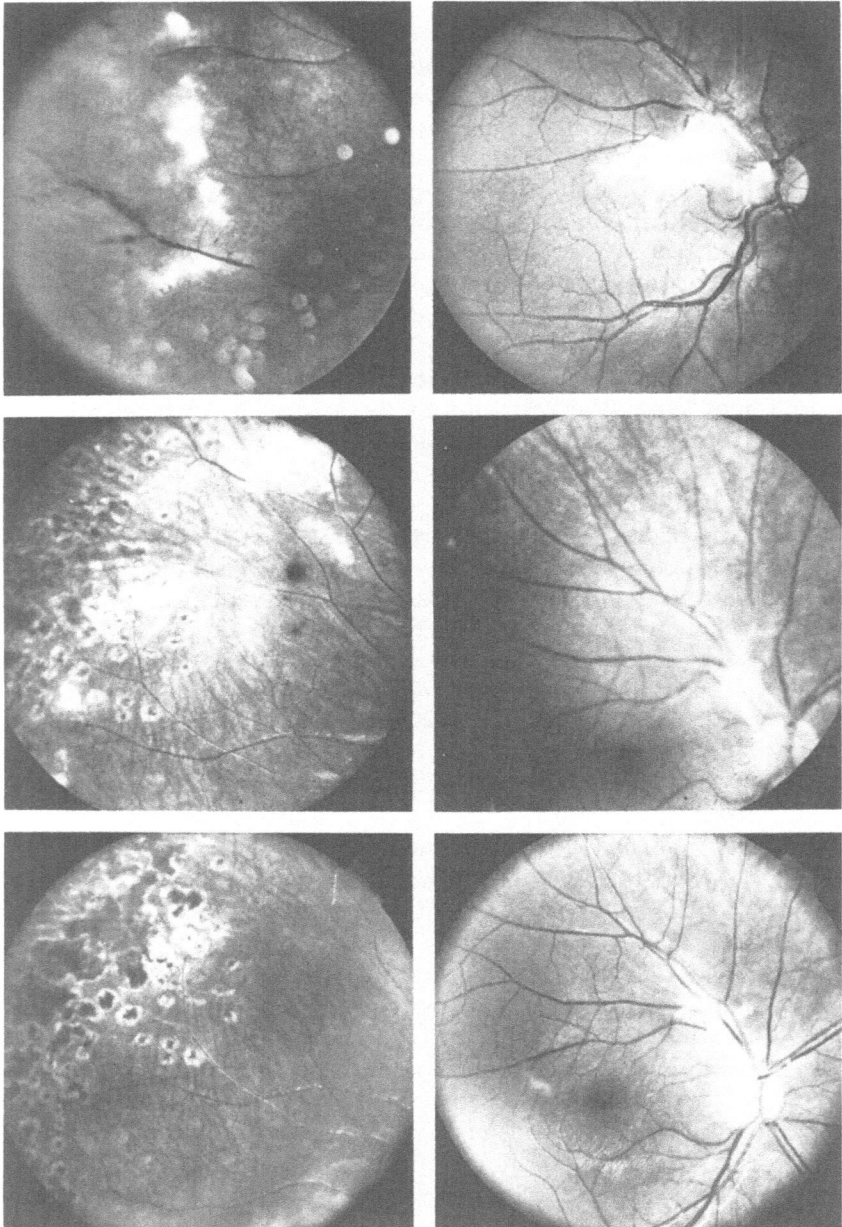

Figure 8–28.   Coats' disease with premacular fibrosis. Top: aspect before treatment. Middle: aspect two months after laser photocoagulation of the temporal lesions. Bottom: aspect three years after treatment. Note the peeling of the premacular fibrosis after treatment.

Another potential hazard is the increased retraction of pre-existing preretinal fibrosis. This complication is usually caused by too heavy burns. In one of our patients with pre-existing premacular fibrosis we observed an unusual favourable reaction (Fig. 8–28). The photocoagulation of the telangiectasis in the temporal periphery was followed by a progressive peeling of the preretinal membrane. This resulted in a vision improvement from 2/10 to 8/10.

After treatment the patients should be followed carefully as new lesions may appear [35, 112]. Recurrences may develop even five years after a successful treatment [35]. Further treatment is also necessary if telangiectatic vessels are still leaking and the exudates do not regress.

References

1. Alajmo B (1936): Retinite di Coats. Contributo clinico ed istopathologico. Considerazione patogenetiche. *Boll Oculist* 15: 405–416.
2. Apple D J, Gieser D K and Goldberg M F (1981): Pathologische Befunde bei einem Erwachsenen mit Morbus Coats. *Klin. Mbl. Augenheilk*, 79: 336–339.
3. Apple D J and Rabb M F (1978): *Clinicopathologic correlation of ocular diseases: a text and stereoscopic atlas*. the C V Mosby C°: St. Louis. pp. 382–385.
4. Archer D and Krill A E (1971): Leber's miliary aneurysms and optic atrophy. *Survey Ophthalmol*, 15: 384–400.
5. Artifoni E and Brancato R (1965): Su di un caso di retinopatia microaneurysmatica con degenerazione retinica di Leber, associata ad ipogonadismo primitivo. *Ann. Ophthalmol*, 91: 1303–1311.
6. Ashton N and Langley D (1951): Multiple aneurysms of the retina. *Br. J. Ophthalmol*, 35: 424–426.
7. Axenfield T (1915): Retinitis exsudativa externa mit Knochenbildung im Sehfähigen Auge. *Von Graefe's Arch. Ophthalmol*, 90: 452–470.
8. Babel J (1972): Angiomatoses et malformations rétiniennes. *Bull. Soc. Ophtalmol. Fr.*, 72: 65–74.
9. Bengisu M (1968): Maladie de Coats et trou maculaire. *Ann. Oculist*, 201: 158–162.
10. Berg F (1919): Beiträge zur pathologischen Anatomie des Retinitis exudativa. *Von Graefe's Arch. Ophthalmol*, 98: 211–242.
11. Bonnet M (1980): Le syndrome de Coats. *J. Fr. Ophtalmol*, 3: 57–66.
12. Brini A (1957): Maladie de Coats. Argument en faveur de la thèse vasculaire. *Bull. Soc. Ophtalmol. Fr.*, 57: 148–150.
13. Brunelle J C and Duval R (1971): Les angiopathies de Leber et de Coats. Réflexions à propos d'un cas d'angiomatose miliaire. *Bull. Soc. Ophtalmol. Fr.*, 71: 834–840.
14. Bryson J M and Wolter J R (1966): Leber's miliary aneurysms: with central nervous system dysfunction. *J. Pediatr. Ophthalmol*, 3: 26–27.
15. Bun J, Yamamoto M, Tatsugami H, and Itoh H (1980): A case of Coats' disease which was initially diagnosed as retinoblastoma with yellow nodules. *Folia Ophthalmol. Jap.*, 31: 1075–1081.
16. Burch J V, Leveille A S and Morse P H (1980): Ichthyosis hystrix (epidermal nevus syndrome) and Coats' disease. *Am. J. Ophthalmol*, 89: 25–30.

17. Campo R V and Reeser F H (1983): Retinal telangiectasia secondary to bilateral carotid artery occlusion. *Arch. Ophthalmol*, 101: 1211–1213.
18. Capier M J, Francois P and Madelain F (1974): Pseudo-angiopathie de Leber par thrombose veineuse. *Bull. Soc. Ophtalmol. Fr.*, 74: 813–815.
19. Chang M, McLean I W and Merritt J C (1984): Coats' disease: a study of 62 histologically confirmed cases. *J. Ped. Ophthalmol. Strabismus*, 21: 163–168.
20. Chic F, Langlois M and Madelain F (1985): La bilatéralité dans l'angiomatose de Leber-Coats. *Bull. Soc. Ophtalmol. Fr.*, 85: 53–54.
21. Chopdar A (1978): Retinal telangiectasis in adults: fluorescein angiographic findings and treatment by Argon laser. *Br. J. Ophthalmol*, 62: 243–250.
22. Coats G (1908): Forms of retinal disease with massive exudation. Royal London Ophthalmol. Hosp. Rep., 17: 440–525.
23. Coats G (1911): A case of exudative retinitis. *Ophthalmol. Rev.*, 30: 289–297.
24. Coats G (1912): Ueber Retinitis exsudativa (Retinitis haemorrhagica externa). *Von Graefe's Arch. Ophthalmol*, 81: 275–525.
25. Colyear B (1966): Retinal vascular lesions treated by photocoagulation. *Trans. Pac. Coast Oto-Ophthalmol. Soc.*, 52: 175.
26. Deutman A F (1976): Unexpected findings in hereditary macular dystrophy. *Doc. Ophthalmol. Proc. Series*, 7: 281–312.
27. Deutsch T A, Rabb M F and Jampol L M (1982): Spontaneous regression of retinal lesions in Coats' disease. *Can. J. Ophthalmol*, 17: 169–172.
28. Doyne R W (1896): Case of peculiar condition of retina, due to the formation of small aneurysms and large extravasation of blood, which has become decolourized. *Trans. Ophthalmol. Soc. U.K.*, 16: 94.
29. Dufour D, Francois P, Corbel M and Capier M J (1972): La micro-angiopathie de Leber. *Bull. Soc. Ophtalmol. Fr.*, 72: 277–279.
30. Duke J R (1963): The role of cholesterol in the pathogenesis of Coats' disease. *Trans. Am. Ophthalmol. Soc.*, 61: 492–544.
31. Duke J R and Woods A C (1963): Coats' disease. II. Studies on the identity of the lipids concerned and the probable role of mucopolysaccharides in its pathogenesis. *Br. J. Ophthalmol*, 47: 413–434.
32. Duke-Elder S and Dobree J H (1967): System of Ophthalmology. Vol. X, Diseases of the retina. *H. Kimpton, London*, 164–179.
33. Egbert P R, Chan C C and Winther F C (1977): Flat preparations of the retinal vessels in Coats' disease. *J. Ped. Ophthalmol*, 13: 336–339.
34. Egerer I., Rodrigues M M and Tasman W S (1975): Retinal dysplasia in Coats' disease. *Can. J. Ophthalmol*, 10: 79–85.
35. Egerer I, Tasman W and Tomer T L (1974): Coats' disease. *Arch. Ophthalmol*, 92: 109–112.
36. Elwyn H (1940): The place of Coats' disease among the diseases of the retina. *Arch. Ophthalmol*, 23: 507–521.
37. Farkas T G, Potts A M and Boone C (1973): Some pathologic and biochemical aspects of Coats' disease. *Am. J. Ophthalmol*, 75: 289–301.
38. Feilchenfeld H (1901): Eine ungewöhnliche Form von Erkrankung der Netzhautmitte. *Ztschr. Augenheilk*, 5: 115–126.
39. Fischer J H (1903): Aneurismal dilatation on diseased retinal arteries. *Trans. Ophthalmol. Soc. U.K.*, 23: 73–74.
40. Fitzsimons R B, Gurwin E B and Bird A C (1987): Retinal vascular abnormalities in facioscapulohumeral muscular dystrophy: a general association with genetic and therapeutic implication. *Brain*, 110: 631–648.
41. Fogle J A, Welch R B and Green W R (1978): Retinitis pigmentosa and exudative vasculopathy. *Arch. Ophthalmol*, 96: 696–702.
42. Fox K R (1980): Coats' disease. *Metab. Ped. Ophthalmol*, 4: 121–124.

43. Fracassi L (1956): Contributo allo studio della Malattia di Coats. *G. Ital. Oftalmol*, 9: 235–241.
44. Francois J, Rabaey M, Evens L and Devos E (1956): Etude histopathologique d'une rétinite de Coats probablement toxoplasmique. *Ophthalmologica*, 132: 1–12.
45. Frayer W C (1955): Coats' disease. A clinical and pathologic study. *Arch. Ophthalmol*, 54: 240–244.
46. Frenkel M and Russe H P (1967): Retinal telangiectasia associated with hypogammaglobulinemia. *Am. J. Ophthalmol*, 63: 215–220.
47. Gartner J and Draf W (1975): Leber's miliary aneurysm associated with telangiectasia of the nasal mucosa. *Am. J. Ophthalmol*, 79: 56–58.
48. Gass J D M (1968): A fluorescein angiographic study of macular dysfunction secondary of retinal vascular disease. V. Retinal telangiectasis. *Arch. Ophthalmol*, 80: 592–605.
49. Gass J D M (1974): Differential diagnosis of intraocular tumors: a stereoscopic presentation. *The C. V. Mosby C°, St. Louis*, 247–264.
50. Gass J D M (1977): Treatment of retinal vascular anomalies. *Trans. Am. Acad. Ophthalmol. Otolaryngol*, 83: 432–442.
51. Gass J D M (1987): *Stereoscopic atlas of macular diseases. Diagnosis and treatment*, 3rd ed. The C. V. Mosby C°: St. Louis, pp. 384–397.
52. Gass J D M and Oyakawa R T (1982): Idiopathic juxtafoveolar retinal telangiectasis. *Arch. Ophthalmol*, 100: 769–780.
53. Giuffre G (1985): Cavernous hemangioma of the retina and retinal telangiectasis. *Retina*, 5: 221–224.
54. Givner J (1954): Coats' disease (Retinitis exsudativa). A clinico-pathologic study. *Am. J. Ophthalmol*, 38: 852–854.
55. Godel V, Regenbogen L and Lazar M (1980): Leber's miliary aneurysm and dysbetalipoproteinemia. A case report. *Acta Ophthalmol*, 58: 825–830.
56. Green W R (1967): Bilateral Coats' disease. Massive gliosis of the retina. *Arch. Ophthalmol*, 77: 378–383.
57. Gronvall H (1961): Three year old boy with complete picture of Coats' exudative retinitis in the left eye and Leber's multiple miliary aneurysms with retinal degeneration in the right eye. *Acta Ophthalmol*, 39: 72–73.
58. Gurwin E B, Fitzsimons R B, Sehmi K S and Bird A C (1985): Retinal telangiectasis in facioscapulohumeral muscular dystrophy with deafness. *Arch. Ophthalmol*, 103: 1695–1700.
59. Gutzmann E (1907): Zwei Fälle einer sehr seltenen Netzhauterkrankung. *Ztschr. Augenheilk*, 17: 40–45.
60. Hada K (1973): Clinical and pathological studies on Coats' disease. I. Clinical and histopathological observations. *Acta Soc. Ophthalmol. Jap.*, 77: 438–459.
61. Haik B G, Koizumi J, Smith M E and Ellsworth R M (1985): Fresh preparation of subretinal fluid aspiration in Coats' disease. *Am. J. Ophthalmol*, 100: 327–329.
62. Harley R D (1983): *Pediatric Ophthalmology*, 2nd ed., W B Saunders C°: Philadelphia, pp. 612–614, 720–725.
63. Henkind P and Morgan G (1966): Peripheral retinal angioma with exudative retinopathy in adults (Coats' lesion). *Br. J. Ophthalmol*, 50: 2–11.
64. Hervouet F (1954): Travaux d'Anatomie pathologique oculaire. *1-ière Série, Ed. Masson, Paris*, 153–163.
65. Hiller H (1971): Morbus Coats — Miliaraneurysmenretinitis Leber. *Klin. Mbl. Augenheilk*, 158: 225–234.
66. Hogan M I and Zimmerman L E (1962): Ophthalmic Pathology. An atlas and textbook. W B Sauders C°: Philadelphia, 530–534.
67. Höpping W (1966): Erfahrungen mit der Lichtkoagulation bei Angiomatosis retinae, Miliaraneurysmenretinitis (Leber), Morbus Coats und ähnlichen Veränderungen. *Mod. Probl. Ophthalmol*, 4: 24–30.

68. Huet J F, Massin M and Leroux Les Jardins S (1979): Indications thérapeutiques dans la maladie de Leber. *Bull Soc. Ophtalmol. Fr.*, 79: 449–450.

69. Hutton W L, Snyder W B, Fuller D and Vaiser A (1978): Focal parafoveal retinal telangiectasis. *Arch. Ophthalmol*, 96: 1362–1367.

70. Ishikawa T (1976): Fine structure of subretinal fibrous tissue in Coats' disease. *Jap. J. Ophthalmol*, 20: 63–74.

71. Ishikawa T, Ikui H and Inomata H (1975): A case of Coats' disease. *Jap. J. Ophthalmol*, 29: 1243–1248.

72. Judisch ·G B and Apple D J (1980): Orbital cellulitis in an infant secundary to Coats' disease. *Arch. Ophthalmol*, 98: 2004–2006.

73. Junius P (1934): Zur Ätiologie der Retinitis exudativa Coats. *Klin. Mbl. Augenheilk*, 92: 748–763.

74. Kahan A, Kahan I L and Pirityi K (1964): Humorale Ursache der Miliaraneurysmen-Retinitis (Leber). *Klin. Mbl. Augenheilk*, 144: 361–370.

75. Kawata K, Ikui H and Ishikawa T (1975): A case of Coats' disease. *Jap. J. Clin. Ophthalmol*, 29: 1243–1248.

76. Kondra L, Gangemi F E and Pitta C G (1983): Alport's syndrome and retinal telangiectasis. *Am. J. Ophthalmol*, 15: 550–556.

77. Koyanagi Y (1935): Ueber die sekretorische Tätigkeit des retinalen Pigmentepithels bei Retinitis exsudativa (Coats). *Von Graefe's Arch. Ophthalmol*, 133: 173–184.

78. Krauss W and Bruckner A (1907): Zur Kenntniss der Tuberkulose des Augenhintergrundes. *Arch. Augenheilk*, 57: 157–173.

79. Kremer I, Cohen S, Bar Izhak R and Ben Sira I (1985): An unusual case of congenital unilateral Coats' disease associated with morning glory optic disc anomaly. *Br. J. Ophthalmol*, 69: 32–37.

80. Kremer I, Nissenkorn I and Ben Sira I (1989): Cytologic and biochemical examination of the subretinal fluid in diagnosis of Coats' disease. *Acta Ophthalmol*, 67: 342–346.

81. Lamb J D (1938): Exudative retinitis (anatomic findings in six early and two late cases). *Am. J. Ophthalmol*, 21: 618–641.

82. Laval J (1944): Coats' disease. *Am. J. Ophthalmol*, 27: 163–167.

83. Leber Th. (1912): Ueber eine durch Vorkommen multipler Miliaraneurysmen charakterisierte Form von Retinaldegeneration. *Von Grafe's Arch. Ophthalmol*, 81: 1–14.

84. Leber Th. (1916): Die Retinitis exsudativa (Coats), Retinitis und Chorioretinitis serofibrinosa degenerans, p. 1267 in Graefe O und Saemisch T (ed.), Handbuch der gesammten Augenheilkunde Vol. 7, pt 2 W Engelmann: Leipzig.

85. L'Esperance F A Jr (1989): Ophthalmic Lasers. Third Edition. The C V Mosby C°, St. Louis, 322–332.

86. Löffler K (1986): Histopathologischer und elektronenmikroskopischer Befund in einem Fall von Morbus Coats. XIV Jahrestreffen D O P, Essen.

87. McGettrick P M and Löffler K U (1987): Bilateral Coats disease in an infant. (A clinical, angiographic, light and electronmicroscopic study.) Eye, 1: 136–145.

88. McGrand J C (1970): Photocoagulation in Coats' disease. *Trans. Ophthalmol. Soc. U.K.*, 90: 47–56.

89. Maggi C (1963): Leber's retinal degeneration with miliary aneurysms. *Am. J. Ophthalmol*, 56: 901–907.

90. Manschot W A and de Bruyn W C (1967): Coats' disease: definition and pathogenesis. *Br. J. Ophthalmol*, 51: 145–157.

91. Marchesani O (1930): Zur Anatomie der Angiomatosis Retinae und Retinitis exsudativa. Arch. Augenheilk, 103: 643–656.

92. Marshall J and Michaelson I (1933): Exudative retinitis in childhood. *Trans. Ophthalmol. Soc. U.K.*, 53: 102–118.

93. Meythaler H (1970): Zur pathologischen Anatomie der Retinitis exsudativa externa. *Klin. Mbl. Augenheilk*, 156: 644–653.

94. Miyashita S and Nisyake Y (1921): The pathological anatomy of retinal degeneration with

multiple aneurysms. *Br. J. Ophthalmol*, 5: 448–453.

95. Mondon H, Lecoq P, Hamard H and Bregeat P (1971): A propos de quelques cas de maladie de Leber ou angiomatose rétinienne miliaire. *Bull. Soc. Ophtalmol Fr.*, 71: 22–25.

96. Morales A G (1965): Coats' disease. Natural history and results of treatment. *Am. J. Ophthalmol*, 60: 855–864.

97. Morton A S (1908): A peculiar form of retinal disease. *Trans. Ophthalmol. Soc. U.K.*, 28: 214–216.

98. Mylius K (1935): Klinisches und anatomisches zum Krankheisbilde der Retinitis Coats. *Klin. Mbl. Augenheilk*, 95: 257–258.

99. Naumann G O H (1980): Pathologie des Auges. Springer Verlag, Berlin, 646–647.

100. Offret H, Nou B, Morax S and Saraux H (1974): L'angiomatose rétinienne miliaire de Leber. A propos d'un cas guéri spontanément. Bull. Soc. Ophtalmol. Fr., 74: 1169–1174.

101. Ogata J, Oshima K and Kano M (1975): A case of Coats' disease with retinal detachment and glaucoma. *Folio Ophthalmol. Jap.*, 26: 1241–1247.

102. Oller (1897): Aneurysmata miliar. arterior. retin. oc. d. Atlas d. Ophthalmol, C. XVI.

103. Orzalesi F (1934): Retinite prolifero-degenerativa del foglietto esterno (Retinitis exsudativa externa—aemorragica externa—exsudativa serofibrinosa degenerativa). *Boll. Oculist*, 13: 833–874.

104. Pajtas J (1950): Cas de pseudogliome familial héréditaire dans 3 générations (Retinitis exsudativa Coats). *Ophthalmologica*, 120: 411–415.

105. Paufique L and Charleux J (1961): Angiomatose rétinienne de Leber. Traitement par photocoagulation. *Bull. Soc. Ophtalmol. Fr.*, 516: 479–480.

106. Paufique L, Ravault M P, Bonnet M and Istre M (1964): L'angiomatose miliaire rétinienne de Leber. *Ann. Oculist*, 197: 937–955.

107. Pergens E (1896): Aneurismatische Erweiterungen der Maculargefässe. *Klin. Mbl. Augenheilk*, 34: 170–173.

108. Pesch K J and Meyer-Schwickerath G (1967): Lichtkoagulation bei Morbus Coats und Retinitis Leber. *Klin. Mbl. Augenheilk*, 151: 846–853.

109. Pringle J A (1917): A case of multiple aneurysms of the retinal arteries. *Br. J. Ophthalmol*, 1: 87–92.

110. Reese A B (1956): Telangiectasis of the retina and Coats' disease. *Am. J. Ophthalmol*, 42: 1–8.

111. Renard G, Bernard J A, Pouliquen Y M, Bons G, Dureuil J and Lebuisson D K (1974): Forme familiale de l'angiomatose rétinienne miliaire de Leber. *Bull. Soc. Ophtalmol. Fr.*, 74: 1163–1167.

112. Ricci A (1963): La photocoagulation dans un cas de microanévrysme de Leber. *Ophthalmologica (Basel)*, 145: 427–430.

113. Ridley M E, Shields J A, Brown G C and Tasman W (1982): Coats' disease: evaluation of management. *Ophthalmology*, 89: 1381–1387.

114. Sattler H (1925): Ueber die pathologisch-anatomischen Veränderungen der Retinitis exsudativa (Coats). *Klin. Mbl. Augenheilk*, 74: 222–223.

115. Schieck (1900): Ueber choroiditis exudativa plastica. *Ber. Dtsche Ophthalmol. Ges.*, 28: 88–93.

116. Scimeca G, Magargal T E and Augsburger J J (1986): Chronic exudative ischemic superior temporal branch retinal vein obstruction simulating Coats' disease. *Ann. Ophthalmol*, 18: 118–120.

117. Seitz R (1968): Klinik und Pathologie der Netzhautgefässe. Miliaraneurysmenretinitis (Leber). *Enke Verlag. Stuttgart*, 369–380.

118. Small R G (1968): Coats' disease and muscular dystrophy. *Trans. Am. Acad. Ophthalmol. Otolaryngol*, 72: 225–231.

119. Spencer W H (1986): Ophthalmic pathology. An atlas and textbook. Third Edition. W B Saunders C°: Philadelphia, 624–634.

120. Spitznas M, Joussen F, Wessing A and Meyer-Schwickerath G (1975): Coats' disease. An

epidemiologic and fluorescein angiographic study. *Von Graefe's Arch. Klin. Exp. Ophthalmol*, 195: 241–250.

121. Story J B (1886): Aneurismal dilatations of retinal veins and arteries. Trans. Ophthalmol. Soc. U.K., 6: 336–338.
122. Story J B and Benson A H (1883): Aneurysms on retinal vessels in a peculiar case of retinitis *Trans. Ophthalmol. Soc. U.K.*, 3: 108–110.
123. Sugar H S (1958): Coats' disease: telangiectatic or multiple vascular origin? *Am. J. Ophthalmol*, 45: 508–517.
124. Takei Y (1976): Origin of the ghost cells in Coats' disease. *Invest. Ophthalmol*, 15: 677–681.
125. Tarkkanen A and Laatikainen L (1983): Coats' disease: clinical, angiographic, histopathological findings and clinical management. *Br. J. Ophthalmol*, 67: 766–776.
126. Tasman W (1971): Coats' disease. in Retinal Disease in Children, Ed. Harper and Row, New York, 59–69.
127. Taylor D A, Carroll J E, Smith M E, Johnson M O, Johnston G B and Brooke M H (1982): Facioscapulohumeral dystrophy associated with hearing loss and Coats' syndrome. *Ann. Neurol*, 12: 395–398.
128. Ten Doesschate G (1927): Ueber Retinitis exsudativa externa. *Klin. Mbl. Augenheilk*, 79: 505–509.
129. Theodossiadis G P, Bairaktaris-Kouris E and Kouris T (1979): Evolution of Leber's miliary aneurysms: a clinicopathological study. *J. Ped. Ophthalmol. Strabismus*, 16: 364–370.
130. Tolmie J L, Browne B H, McGettrick P M and Stephenson J B P (1988): A familial syndrome with Coats' reaction retinal angiomas, hair and nail defects and intracranial calcification. Eye, 2: 297–303.
131. Tornquist R (1966): Treatment of Coats' disease. *Acta Ophthalmol*, 144: 457–459.
132. Tour R L (1957): Miliary retinal aneurysms. *Am. J. Ophthalmol*, 43: 426–432.
133. Tripathi R and Ashton N (1971): Electron microscopical study of Coats disease. *Br. J Ophthalmol*, 55: 289–301.
134. Von Hippel E (1911): Die anatomische Grundlage der von mir beschriebenen 'sehr seltenen Erkrankung der Netzhaut'. *Von Graefe's Arch. Ophthalmol*, 79: 350–377.
135. Von Hippel E (1913): Anatomischer Befund bei einem Fälle von Retinitis exsudativa (Coats). *Von Graefe's Arch. Ophthalmol*, 86: 443–456.
136. Von Hippel E (1931): Angiomatosis Retinae und Retinitis exsudativa Coats. Pseudogliom durch Tuberkulose. *Arch. f. Ophthalmol*, 127: 27–45.
137. Wessing A (1968): Fluoreszenzangiographie der Retina. Lehrbuch und Atlas. Georg Thieme Verlag, Stuttgart, 133–137.
138. Wessing A and Spitznas M (1975): Morbus Coats und Lebersche Miliaraneurysmenretinitis. *Ber. Dtsche Ophthalmol. Ges.*, 74: 199–204.
139. Wise G N (1957): Retinal microaneurysms. *Arch. Ophthalmol*, 57: 151–156.
140. Wise G N and Horava A (1963): Coats' disease. *Am. J. Ophthalmol*, 56: 17–23.
141. Witmer R (1985): Die retinale Angiomatosen. *Klin. Mbl. Augenheilk*, 187: 434.
142. Wolff E (1949): La maladie de Coats. Rétinite hémorrhagique ou exsudative externe. *Bull. Soc. Ophthalmol. Fr.*, 62: 281–286.
143. Wolfflin E (1926): Beitrag zur pathologischer Anatomie der Retinitis exsudativa Fall mit Knochenbildung in noch sehfähigen Auge. *Von Graefe's Arch. Ophthalmol*, 117: 33–39.
144. Woods A C and Duke J R (1963): Coats' disease. I. Review of the literature, diagnostic criteria, clinical findings and plasma lipid studies. *Br. J. Ophthalmol*, 47: 385–412.
145. Wulff J D, Lin. J T and Kepes J J (1982): Inflammatory facioscapulohumeral muscular dystrophy and Coats' syndrome. *Ann. Neurol*, 12: 398–401.
146. Young J W S and Harris G S (1976): Coats' disease: a study of cholesterol transport in the eye. *Can. J. Ophthalmol*, 11: 61–68.
147. Zinsser F (1929): Beitrag zur Kenntnis der exsudativen Netzhauterkrankungen (fünf Fälle von Retinitis exsudativa, ein Fall von Angiomatosis retinae). *Arch. f. Ophthalmol*, 121: 686–714.

9 Idiopathic juxtafoveolar retinal telangiectasis

In 1973 Ehlers and Jensen described what they called central retinal angiopathy in three members of a family. They first examined a 40 year old woman with bilateral visual loss and later found similar fundus lesions in her 66 year old mother and a 38 year old brother, although their visual acuity was normal. Hutton et al. [16] observed in four patients – two of them were sisters – telangiectasis, localized to the temporal perifoveal area of both eyes.

A similar ophthalmoscopic aspect had already been described earlier [15] and such cases were included in series of patients with Leber-Coats' disease [1, 11, 21]. Although these cases, at least in some instances, probably represent a subgroup of Leber's disease with later onset of visual symptoms and milder prognosis, there are indications that they may also be an expression of an acquired disease. For this reason, idiopathic juxtafoveolar retinal telangiectasis is discussed separately from Leber-Coats' disease.

I. Incidence

Although parafoveal telangiectasis has only recently be considered as a separate entity, the number of cases reported in the literature suggests that is not an exceptional disease. Some large series have been published (Gass and Okayawa: 27 cases; Casswell et al.: 46 cases; Millay et al.: 28 cases) as well as smaller series or individual cases [5, 6, 9, 14–16, 18, 19]. Up to now, there are at least 118 cases reported in the literature.

As in Leber-Coats' disease there is a definite male predominance. Of the 118 cases, 82 were men (70%) and 36 women.

The disease often affects both eyes. Fifty eight of the 118 cases were bilateral (49%). In unilateral cases there is no obvious preference for right or left eye.

The youngest patient in whom juxtafoveolar retinal telangiectasis was diagnosed was a 6 year old girl with bilateral disease [13] and the eldest, a 84 year old woman, also with both eyes affected [16]. The mean age at discovery of the fundus lesions in Gass and Oyakawa's series was 39 years for unilateral cases, 56 years for bilateral parafoveolar cases and 41 years for bilateral perifoveolar cases [13]. The mean age was 51.3 years in the series of Casswell et al. [4] and of 60.2 years in the series of Millay et al. [17].

II. Heredity

Ehlers and Jensen [9] first described the familial occurrence of parafoveal retinal telangiectasis in a brother and sister and their mother. Other familial cases have since been published: Hutton et al. [16]; two sisters; Putteman et al. [19]: a father and his son in one family and two brothers in another family.

Chew et al. [5] described bilateral parafoveal telangiectasis in a 65 year old diabetic man. His brother, who was not diabetic by history, was also affected with similar retinal vascular lesions, which resulted in a clinical picture resembling pseudovitelliform dystrophy. All familial cases were bilateral, except possibly one case of Putteman et al. [19].

No other familial cases were reported but as the symptoms may be extremely discrete, a negative family history is not sufficient to rule out a possible hereditary factor.

III. Clinical aspects

1. Presenting symptoms

The most common complaints are blurred vision, metamorphopsia or a positive scotoma [13]. In some cases the macular lesion was found during a routine ophthalmological examination or at the occasion of a family screening [14, 16, 19]. In bilateral cases involvement of the second eye was sometimes discovered after the first visit [4].

The visual acuity is usually only mildly affected. Combining the three largest series of such cases [4, 13, 17] 68% of the affected eyes have 20/40 vision or better (26.5% with 20/20 vision), 27% have a vision between 20/50 and 20/200 and only 5% have a vision of less than 20/200. In bilateral cases both eyes are usually not similarly affected.

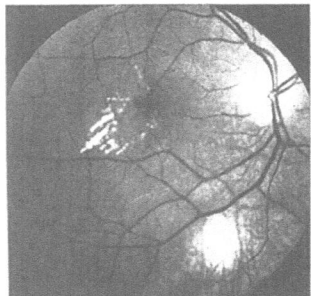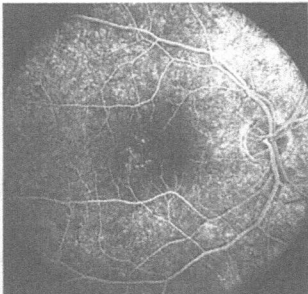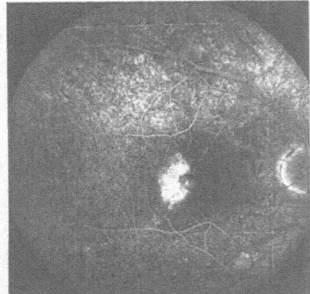

Figure 9–1.   Parafoveal retinal telangiectasis in the right eye of a 32 year old man. The lesions are limited to the temporal part of the fovea and leak profusely. This results in a foveal cystic lesion.

2. *Ophthalmoscopic appearance*

In typical cases the vascular changes predominantly affect the temporal aspect of the macula. The lesions may be extremely subtle and only clearly to be seen with slitlamp biomicroscopy or better with fluorescein angiography. Fluorescein angiography reveals the presence of dilated capillaries with microaneurysms. They are either limited to the temporal site of the fovea (Fig. 9–1) or surround it completely (Fig. 9–4). In unilateral cases the area with telangiectatic capillaries is usually larger and extends to about 2 disc diameters, whereas in bilateral cases it is often limited to the temporal part and less than one disc diameter in size. The vascular anomalies are almost equally distributed in the area above and below the horizontal raphe. This differentiates juxtafoveolar telangiectasis from capillary changes as a result of a previous retinal branch vein occlusion.

Especially in bilateral cases [13] but also in unilateral cases [17] right angled venules may be seen draining the telangiectatic capillaries in the deep retinal plexus.

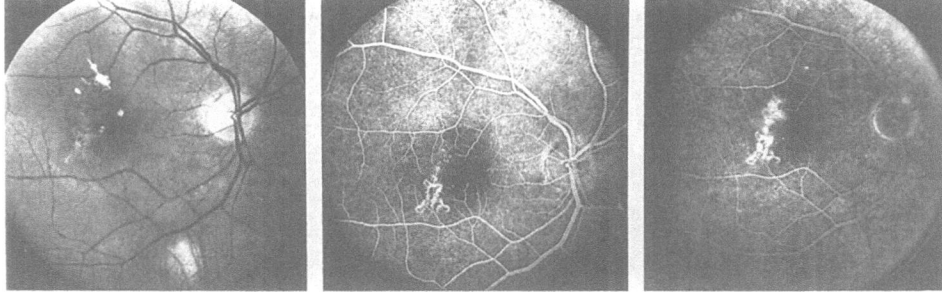

Figure 9–2. Same eye as Fig. 9–1 four months after focal laser treatment. Partial regression of the lipoid exudates and disappearance of the foveolar cyst. Presence in the superotemporal quadrant of still leaking capillaries.

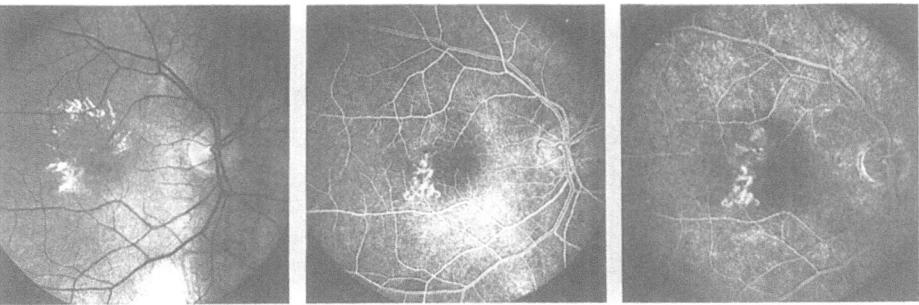

Figure 9–3. Same eye as Fig. 9–1 three years after treatment. Lipoid exudates surround the still leaking capillaries already visible in Fig. 9–5.

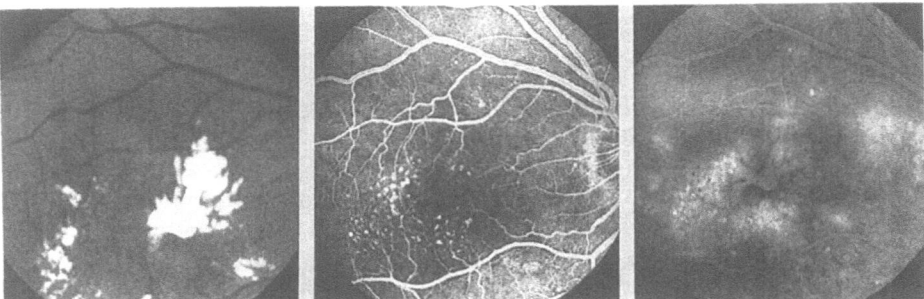

Figure 9–4.   Extensive perifoveolar telangiectasis in a 65 year old man. Visual acuity was reduced to finger counting, but improved to 2/10 after lasercoagulation in the temporal part of the macula.

The amount of leakage is variable. Macular edema may even be absent in cases with minimal vascular changes, usually the second eye in asymmetrical bilateral disease [4]. In some cases a foveolar cyst may be formed (Fig. 9–1) which may even progress to a macular hole [18]. The vascular lesions are frequently associated with lipid deposits in their vicinity, sometimes located in a stellar or in a circinate fashion (Fig. 9–5) [4, 13, 15]. In advanced cases these deposits may form a macular plaque (Fig. 9–4).

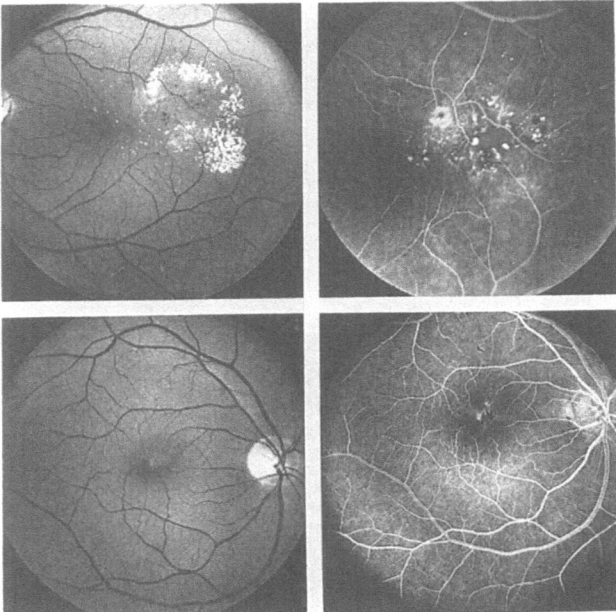

Figure 9–5.   Left and right eye of a 63 year old man. In the left eye paramacular telangiectasis is seen, whereas the right eye presents perifoveolar pigmentary changes suggestive of adult onset vitelliform degeneration.

Gass and Oyakawa [13] divided their cases in 4 groups:
- group 1: unilateral parafoveolar telangiectasis
- group 2: bilateral parafoveolar telangiectasis
- group 3: bilateral perifoveolar telangiectasis
- group 4: consisting of a 47 year old man with bilateral perifoveolar lesions and capillary occlusion. This patient also had optic disc pallor and hyperactive tendon reflexes.

In the 1987 edition of his stereoscopic atlas of macular diseases Gass [12] however considered group 2 and 3 together.

Parafoveal retinal telangiectasis may be associated with peripheral telangiectasis [4]. In such cases the peripheral lesions are mild and not complicated by massive lipoid exudation or retinal detachment.

Telangiectatic lesions with right angled venules are at risk of developing subretinal changes, subretinal pigmenthyperplasia or even choroidal neovascularization [13]. Focal hyperpigmentation has been found in a number of cases [4, 5, 13, 16]. We had the opportunity to examine a 63 year old man who in the left eye presented paramacular telangiectasis and in the right eye foveal pigmentary changes, suggestive of pseudovitelliform macular degeneration (Fig. 9–5).

Except in cases with peripheral telangiectasis, the fundus appears otherwise normal. The vitreous is clear. There are no signs of inflammation and no clinical indications of a diffuse retinal vascular disorder.

3. Prognosis

The progression of these lesions is slow. A progressive increase of the exudation may be observed. However, spontaneous reabsorption of the exudates is also possible [4, 13]. The vision may remain unchanged or only slightly deteriorate over a period of several years [4, 13, 17] except of course, when the development of subretinal neovascular membrane results in rapid visual loss.

IV. Differential diagnosis

1. Diabetic maculopathy

Chew et al. [5] observed in five patients with mild non-proliferative diabetic retinopathy the presence of parafoveal telangiectasis, similar to cases which were previously described. The affected area was less than one disc diameter in size and limited to the temporal site of the fovea. None of these patients presented diffuse leakage from the capillaries elsewhere in the fundus. In some of these eyes localized subretinal pigment epithelial hyperplasia was also seen. Millay et al. [17] did glucose tolerance tests in their patients with juxtafoveolar telangiectasis. Six of nine patients with bilateral telangiectasis (one patient was not examined) had evidence of abnormal glucose metabolism as well as six of the seventeen unilateral cases.

Although at least in a number of cases, and especially those with bilateral disease, diabetes must play a role in the development of these vascular lesions, perifoveal telangiectasis appears different from the classical diabetic maculopathy, which is associated with other manifestations of diabetic retinopathy. It differs also from isolated diabetic macular edema as described by Schatz and Patz [20] and by Bonnet et al. [2].

2. *Retinal vein occlusion*

Localized macular edema may be a consequence of retinal branch vein occlusion. In such cases however the dilatation does not affect symmetrically the capillaries in the area below and above the horizontal raphe. Also mostly collaterals are seen. Some of these cases are however difficult to differentiate (Fig. 9–6).

Cystoid macular edema is a well known complication of central retinal vein occlusion. However, the clinical history is usually quite different, with an episode of sudden visual loss and often opticociliary vessels are seen on the optic disc, indicating the previous vascular accident.

3. *Pseudovitelliform macular degeneration*

The pigmentary scar which is not uncommonly seen in juxtafoveolar telangiectasis looks similar to the lesions described by Fishman et al. [10] as pseudovitelliform macular degeneration. As a number of their patients showed perifoveal leakage from the retinal capillaries, it may well be that the cases Fishman described, were in fact genuine examples of juxtafoveolar telangiectasis. The typical adult onset vitelliform macular degeneration represents probably the endresult of a previous retinal pigment epithelial detachment [7] and is unrelated to retinal vascular disease.

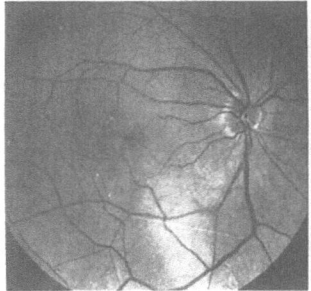 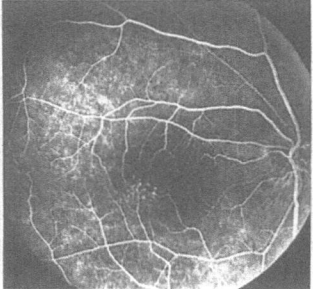 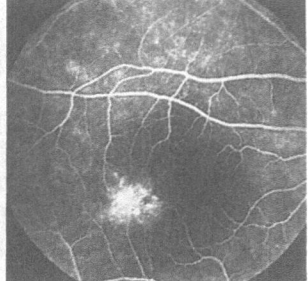

Figure 9–6. A 46 year old man with localized parafoveolar capillary dilatation. Idiopathic retinal telangiectasis or consequence of retinal branch vein occlusion?

4. Dominant cystoid macular edema

Deutman et al. [8] described dominantly inherited cystoid macular edema in two families. In these cases the vascular anomalies affected a larger area of the posterior pole. These cases also presented a subnormal EOG which indicated widespread involvement of the retinal pigment epithelium, which in older patients could also be demonstrated fluoroangiographically.

5. Other differential diagnoses

Other differential diagnoses include carotid artery occlusion [3], radiation retinopathy [13, 16], macular edema in retinitis pigmentosa (see chapter 10), other inflammatory causes of macular edema and other causes of choroidal neovascularization.

V. Histopathology

Green et al. [14] examined with light and electron microscopy the eye of a 53 year old woman. She was examined clinically before elective orbital exenteration for a squamous cell carcinoma of the left maxillary anthrum with probable orbital extension. During this examination bilateral parafoveal telangiectasis was diagnosed. On histopathology there was no evidence of telangiectasis. The walls of the retinal capillaries appeared thickened, resulting in the narrowing of the lumen. The authors showed evidence of a multilaminated basal membrane, degeneration of endothelial cells and especially a loss of pericytes. These changes were not limited to the parafoveal area but were seen to a lesser degree throughout the retina. The retinal pigment epithelium appeared normal in light and in electron microscopy.

VI. Pathogenesis

It is probable that unilateral cases, especially those associated with peripheral telangiectasis, are congenital in origin and represent a mild form of Leber-Coats' disease. Most other cases are likely to be acquired.

A possible causal relationship with diabetes whether clinical or latent is suggested by the findings of Chew et al. [5] and Millay et al. [17]. Also the pathological changes observed by Green et al. [14] may occur in diabetic retinopathy. [5, 17].

Gass [12] suggested the possible role of chronic venous obstruction occurring over a period of many years. He also considered the subretinal changes (localized pigment epithelial hyperplasia and subretinal neovascularization) as a consequence of chronic macular edema. On the other hand, Casswell et al. [4] hypothesized that the retinal capillary leakage could be related to a localized disease of the retinal pigment epithelium. This is difficult to accept as it does not explain the observation that the temporal parafoveal region is most commonly affected. Also the retinal pigment epithelium appeared morphologically normal in the case of Green et al. [14] and in clinical cases the pigment epithelial lesions, if present, are relatively limited. Up to now, no EOG studies have been performed in these cases to study the functional status of the retinal pigment epithelium.

VII. Treatment

We have seen that the vision may remain stable for a prolonged period of time in patients with juxtafoveolar retinal telangiectasis. Treatment is thus only considered if increase of exudation or edema results in progressive visual loss. Photocoagulations close to the fovea may result in permanent and very annoying loss of paracentral visual field or cause central retina distorsion and metamorphopsia [13]. To avoid these complications it is advised to use small low intensity burns placed in a grid fashion. A successful treatment results in regression of lipid exudates and edema (Fig. 9–2) and sometimes visual improvement [6]. However, if there are still leaking vessels, new exudates may appear which possibly may require a second treatment (Fig. 9–3).

References

1. Bonnet M (1980): Le syndrome de Coats. *J Fr Ophtalmol* 3: 57–66.
2. Bonnet M, Bensoussan B, Grange J D, Pingault C, and Francoz M (1982): Capillaropathie oedémateuse aigue du diabétique insulino-dépendant. *J Fr Ophtalmol* 5: 303–316.
3. Campo R V and Reeser F H (1983): Retinal telangiectasis secondary to bilateral carotid artery occlusion. *Arch. Ophthalmol*, 101: 1211–1213.
4. Casswell A G, Chaine L, Rush P and Bird A C (1986): Paramacular telangiectasis. *Trans. Ophthalmol. Soc. U.K.*, 105: 683–692.
5. Chew E Y, Murphy R P and Newsome D A (1986): Parafoveal telangiectiasis and diabetic retinopathy. *Arch. Ophthalmol*, 104: 71–75.
6. Chopdar A (1978): Retinal telangiectasis in adults: fluorescein angiographic findings and treatment by Argon laser. *Br. J. Ophthalmol*, 62: 243–250.
7. De Laey J J (1989): Adult onset vitelliform macular lesion and pattern dystrophy of the retinal pigment epithelium, in: M. Zingirian and F Cardillo-Piccolino (ed.), *Retinal pigment epithelium*. Kugler and Ghedini Publications: Amsterdam, pp. 87–99.
8. Deutman A F, Pinckers A J L G and Aan de Kerk A L (1976): Dominantly inherited cystoid macular edema. *Am. J. Ophthalmol*, 82: 540–548.
9. Ehlers N and Jensen V A (1973): Hereditary central retinal angiopathy. *Acta Ophthalmol*, 51: 171–178.
10. Fishman G A, Trimble S, Rabb M T and Fishman M (1977): Pseudovitelliform macular degeneration. *Arch. Ophthalmol*, 95: 73–76.
11. Gass J D M (1968): A fluorescein angiographic study of macular dysfunction to retinal vascular disease. V Retinal telangiectasis. *Arch. Ophthalmol*, 80: 592–605.

12. Gass J D M (1987): Stereoscopic atlas of macular diseases. Diagnosis and treatment. Third edition, the C V Mosby C°, 390–394.

13. Gass J D M and Oyakawa R T (1982): Idiopathic juxtafoveolar retinal telangiectasis. *Arch. Ophthalmol*, 100: 769–780.

14. Green W R, Quigley H A, De la Cruz Z and Cohen B (1980): Parafoveal retinal telangiectasis. Light and electron microscopy study. *Trans. Ophthalmol. Soc. U.K.*, 100: 162–170.

15. Gruber M (1951): Beobachtungen über einem Fall von Miliaraneurysmaretinitis 'Leber'. *Ophthalmologica*, 121: 91–94.

16. Hutton W L, Snijder W B, Fuller D and Vaiser A (1978): Focal parafoveal retinal telangiectasis. *Arch. Ophthalmol*, 96: 1362–1367.

17. Millay R H, Klein M L, Handelman I L and Watzke R C (1986): Abnormal glucose metabolism and parafoveal telangiectasis. *Am. J. Ophthalmol*, 102: 363–370.

18. Patel B, Duvall J and Tullo A B (1988): Parafoveal telangiectasis and macular hole. *Br. J. Ophthalmol*, 72: 550–551.

19. Putteman A, Toussaint D, Graff E and Verougstraete C (1984): Téléangiectasies rétiniennes juxtafovéolaires idiopathiques familiales. *Bull. Soc. Belge Ophtalmol*, 209: 81–90.

20. Schatz H and Patz A (1976): Cystoid maculopathy in diabetics. *Arch. Ophthalmol*, 94: 761–769.

21. Spitznas M, Joussen F, Wessing A and Meyer-Schwickerath G (1975): Coats' disease. An epidemiologic and fluorescein angiographic study. *Von Graefe's Arch. Clin. Exp. Ophthalmol*, 195: 241–250.

10 Coats' syndrome and retinitis pigmentosa

In 1956 Zamorani [47] described as first the association of Coats-like lesions and retinitis pigmentosa. His patient was a sixteen year old girl who had always complained of night blindness. She presented a total cataract in her left eye. Her right eye had a vision of 1/10 and a tubular visual field. The fundus was typical of retinitis pigmentosa but in the temporal periphery retinal neovascularization, aneurysms and exudates were also noted.

The association of retinitis pigmentosa and lesions resembling Coats' disease has been observed by a number of authors [1, 4, 10, 17, 21, 23, 26, 30, 33, 37–41, 45–47]. We have personally seen six such cases (Table 1).

I. Incidence

The association of Coats' syndrome and retinitis pigmentosa is relatively rare. In a series of 329 retinitis pigmentosa patients Kajiwara [26] found only two cases with such a combination. Newsome [34] did not see a single case in his study of 78 retinitis pigmentosa patients and Krill [28] only mentions the possibility of such an association. We observed six such cases (Table 1).

Coats' syndrome has been seen in association with various hereditary forms of retinitis pigmentosa: autosomal recessive [30, 37, 38, our cases 2 and 3], autosomal dominant [40, our fifth case] or sporadic cases. To the best of our knowledge no cases have yet been seen in association with sex-linked retinitis pigmentosa. Schuman et al. [39] observed it in a patient with familial renal-retinal dystrophy.

Grizzard et al [22] noted perivenous fluorescein accumulation in identical twins with cone-rod dystrophy and Gass [21] observed the development of a Coats' syndrome in a patient with localized pseudo-retinitis pigmentosa caused by trauma.

In families with retinitis pigmentosa not all affected members necessarily develop Coats' syndrome [37], although this combination has been seen in two or more members of a same family, up to now always in the same generation [30, 38, 40, our cases 2 and 3].

Of the 25 cases we could find in the literature (including our 6 cases), 16 were women and 9 men. The age when the vascular lesion was diagnosed, varies between 12 years [30] and 50 years (our fourth patient). Usually the diagnosis is made during the second or third decade.

Table 1. Retinitis pigmentosa and Coats' lesions

Author	N°	Age	Sex	Eye	Site of peripheral lesion	Vision at presentation OD	OS	Aspect of macula	
Zamorani [47]		16	F	OD	temp. periph.	0.1	NLP	nm	OS: total cataract, no further informations
Morgan and Crawford [33]	1	34	F	OU	infero-temp.	20/40	FC	nm	OD: treated with photo-coagulation, no recurrence one year later OS: untreated; progression to exudative retinal detachment
	2	16	F	OU	inferior	20/200	FC	CME (OD)	OD: progression despite repeated photo-coagulation OS: intravitreous hemorrhage
Schmidt and Faulborn [38]	1	42	M	OU	inferior	0.1	HM	nm	Progressed to chronic uveitis and secondary glaucoma
	2	26	F	OU	inferior	0.5	0.5	nm	
Lanier et. al [30]	1	17	F	OU	inferior	LP	LP	PE changes	These three patients are brother and sisters; members of a family with autosomal recessive R.P.
	2	12	M	OU	inferior	FC	FC	PE changes	
	3	18	F	OU	inferior	20/200	20/60	PE changes	
Ayesh et al. [1]		15	F	OU	inferior	5/60	6/18	PE changes	
Fogle et al. [17]		38	M	OU	OD superior and inferior	20/30	LP	CME	OS: enucleated for secondary glaucoma
Spalton et al. [41]		31	M	OS	nm	6/18	6/60	CME	OD: pars plana exudates
Heckenlively [23]		32	F	OD	inferior	5/200	5/200	PE atrophy	Patient with thalassemia minor

		Age	Sex	Eye	Location	VA	VA	Macula	Comments
Yuguchi and Majima [46]		13	F	OU	inferior	0.3	0.15	CME	First treated with photocoagulation. As the lesions progressed, cryocoagulation was performed. This resulted in resorption of exudates.
Spallone et al. [40]	1	18	F	OU	inferior	4/20	2/20	CME	Family of dominant R.P.; sister of case 1
	2	23	M	OU	inferior	FC	2/20	CME	
Schuman et al. [39]		20	M	OD	nm	nm	nm	OS preret. fibrosis	Familial renal-retinal dystrophy. OD developed neovascular glaucoma and was enucleated.
Gass [21]		18	F	OD	inferior	nm	nm	CME	The exudates cleared spontaneously over a period of 3 years.
Personal cases	1	21	F	OU	inferior	0.1	0.1	CME followed by PE atrophy	OD: progressed to retinal detachment and total cataract. OS: had repeated vitreous hemorrhages. No recurrences since cryotherapy.
	2	30	F	OU	inferior	0.1	0.1	PE changes	Lesions first treated with Xenon, later with laser. Appeared cicatricial 2 years after second treatment.
	3	24	F	OU	inferior	0.05	FC	Diffuse exudates	Sister of patient 2. Extensive exudates which include the macula. Treated with Xenon. Later developed iritis with secondary glaucoma first in the right eye, later in the left eye.

Table 1 (Continued).

Author	N°	Age	Sex	Eye	Site of peripheral lesion	Vision at presentation OD	OS	Aspect of macula	
Personal cases	4	50	M	OS	inferior	NLP	0.4	CME	OD: lost by neovascular glaucoma and total retinal detachment OS: treated with the laser The exudates regressed, but the neovascularization is still present 4 years after treatment.
	5	47	M	OU	inferior	0.3	FC	PE atrophy	Family of dominant RP. A younger brother is blind by retinal detachment, supposedly due to bilateral Coats' disease.
	6	36	F	OS	inferior	LP	0.2	CME	OD: lost by retinal detachment and secondary glaucoma OS: treated with cryotherapy

nm = not mentioned   FC = finger counting
HM = hand movements   LP = light perception

Most cases are bilateral. Sometimes one eye is already lost before the association of Coats' syndrome and retinitis pigmentosa is recognized [47, our cases 4 and 6). Only a few genuine unilateral cases have been described [21, 23, 39, 41].

II. Clinical characteristics

In most cases retinitis pigmentosa was diagnosed long before the retinal vascular lesions appeared, or at least there was a family history of retinitis pigmentosa or a long history of night blindness. Exudative changes seem thus to be a late complication of the dystrophic process [17, 33].

Visual acuity is usually very poor even in the least affected eye. This is the consequence of marked macular changes: macular edema, exudates, macular pigment epithelial atrophy or preretinal fibrosis. Cystoid macular edema may be present before the appearance of peripheral retinal vascular lesions [21]. Cystoid macular edema is common (Figs. 10–1, 10–6) and diffuse edema of the posterior pole is also possible (Fig. 10–4). Macular edema may regress spontaneously resulting in pigment epithelial atrophy (Figs. 10–1, 10–2).

As a result of retinitis pigmentosa the visual fields are markedly constricted, the dark adaptation curve is elevated and the ERG is extinguished.

In a number of eyes the retinal vascular lesion was discovered because the patient noticed sudden vision loss due to vitreous hemorrhage or because one eye developed neovascular glaucoma [17, 30, 33, 39, 47, our cases 4 and 6].

A characteristic finding is the sometimes very impressive inflammatory reaction in the vitreous. The aspect of retinal pigment dystrophy is variable. Sometimes it is very marked (Figs. 10–3, 10–8), in other cases more

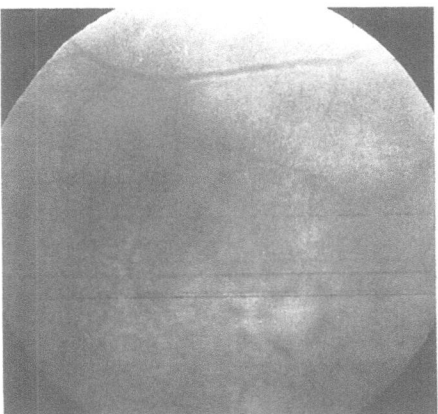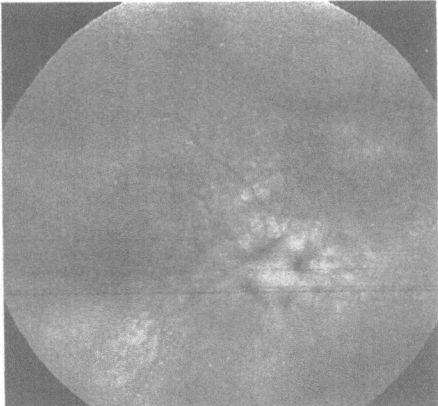

Figure 10–1.　　Case 1. Aspect in April 1971. Marked cystoid macular edema.

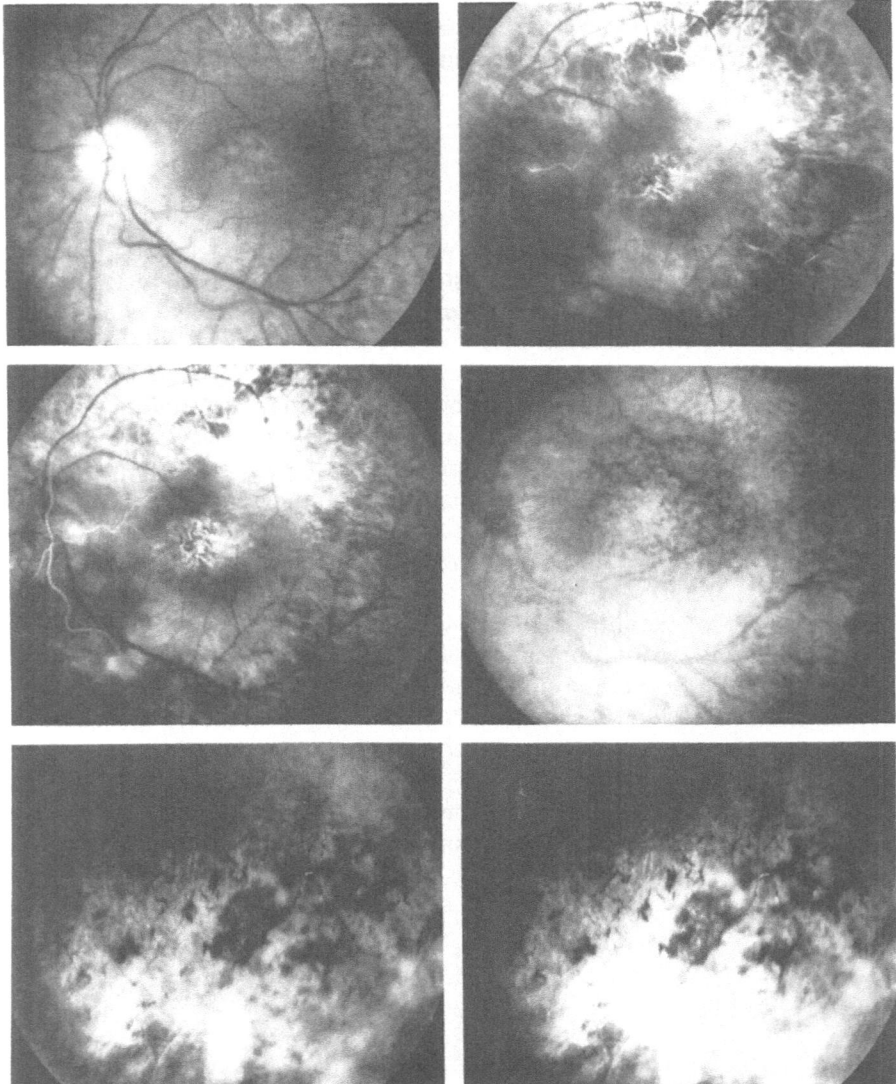

Figure 10–2.   Case 1. Aspect in June 1984. The right eye was meanwhile lost by retinal detachment. In the left eye an atrophic macular lesion is seen as well as areas of retinal vascular leakage in the inferior periphery.

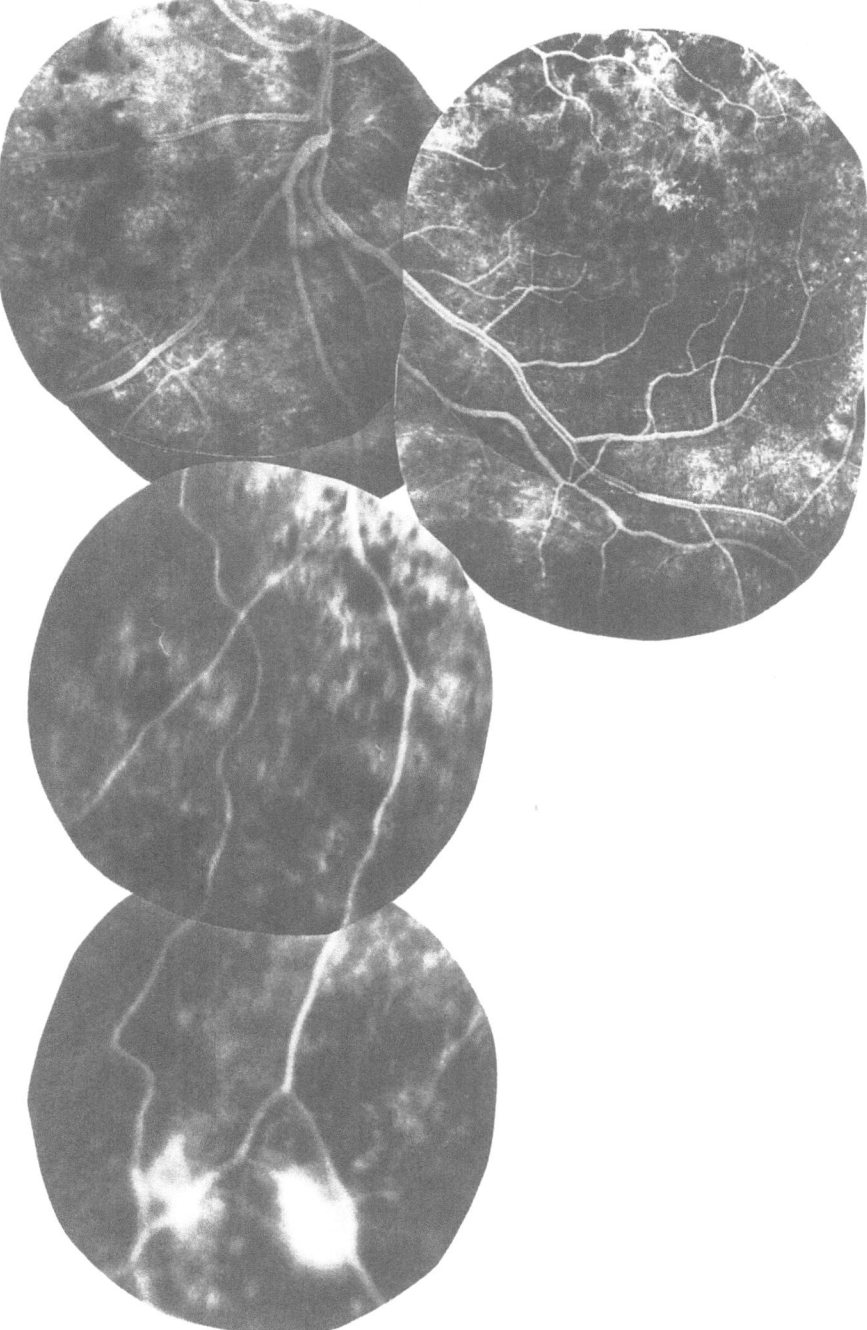

Figure 10-3. Case 2. Photomontage of the fluoroangiography of the left eye. Diffuse pigmentary changes also affecting the macular region. Area of retinal newvessels in the inferior periphery.

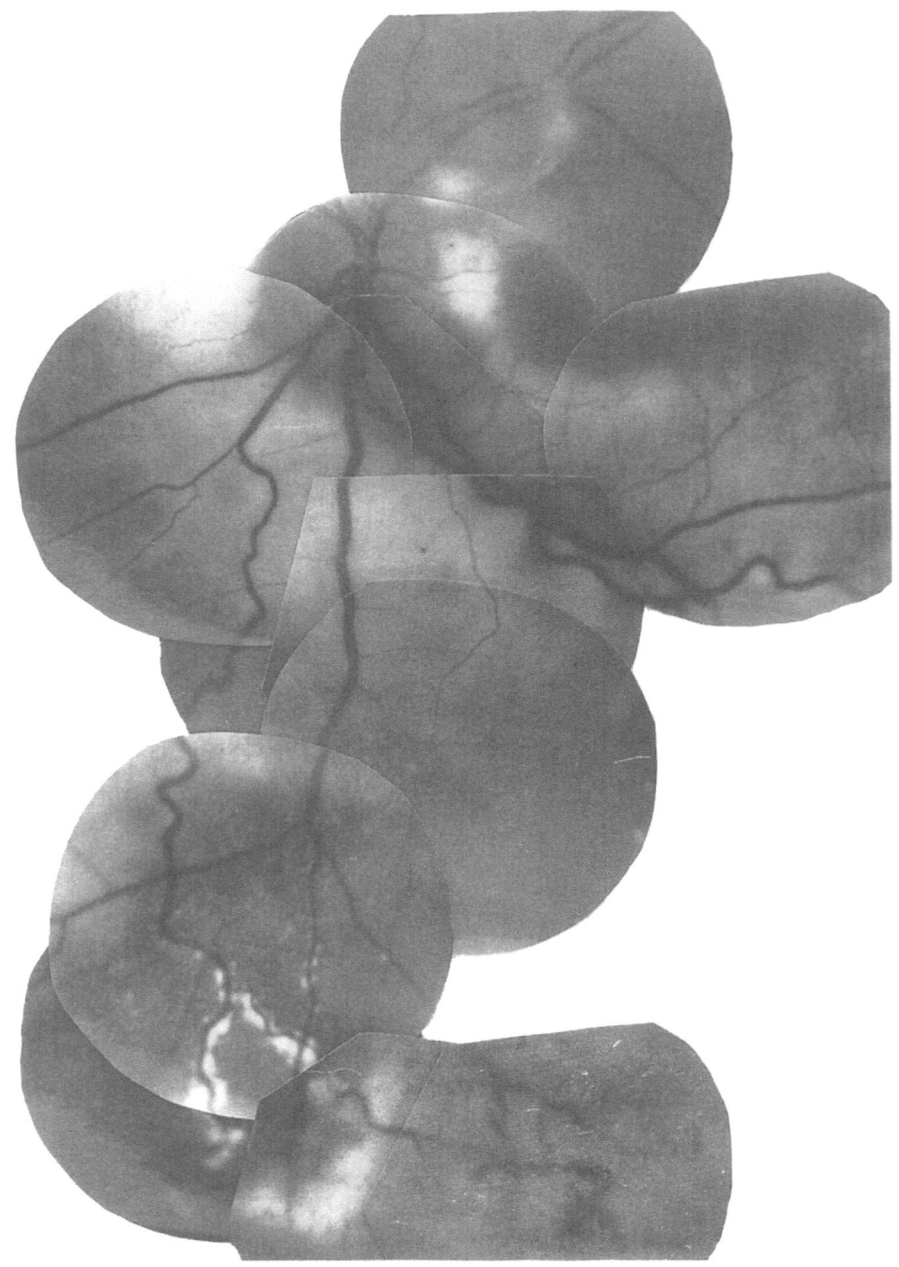

Figure 10–4.   Case 3 (younger sister of case 2). Massive exudation extending up to the posterior pole. Preretinal fibrosis above the macula. Telangiectatic lesions in the inferior periphery.

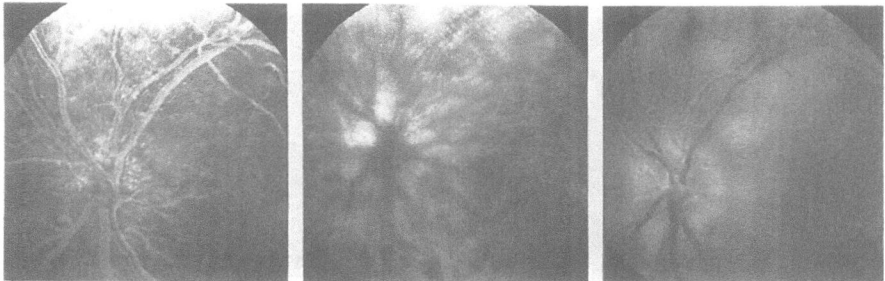

Figure 10–5. Case 3. Fluoroangiography of the posterior pole. Diffuse fluorescein leakage and massive retinal edema.

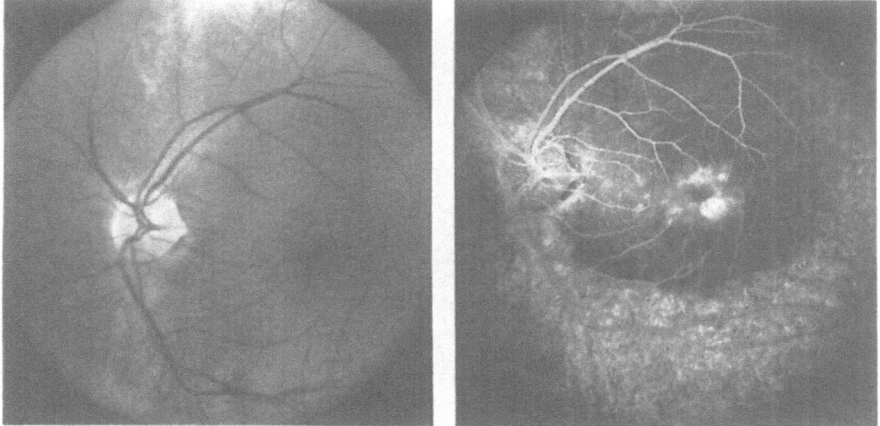

Figure 10–6. Case 4. Cystoid macular edema and attenuated retinal vessels.

discrete (Fig. 10–6) or masked by the exudative response (Figs. 10–4, 10–5). In retinitis pigmentosa the retinal vessels are usually extremely narrow. In some of our cases they appeared on the contrary markedly dilated, at least at some point of the disease process (Figs. 10–1 and 10–4). Papiledema and drusen of the optic discs are sometimes noted [30] (Figs. 10–5, 10–8).

The Coats-like lesion is most frequently situated in the inferior periphery. Multiple foci of telangiectasis may be present [30]. The lesion may initially consist of a cluster of new vessels, surrounded by some hemorrhages and lipid exudates (Figs. 10–3, 10–7). In more progressed cases subretinal exudation is present and the lesion acquires a pseudotumoral aspect covered by dilated vessels, telangiectasis and neovascularization (Fig. 10–9).

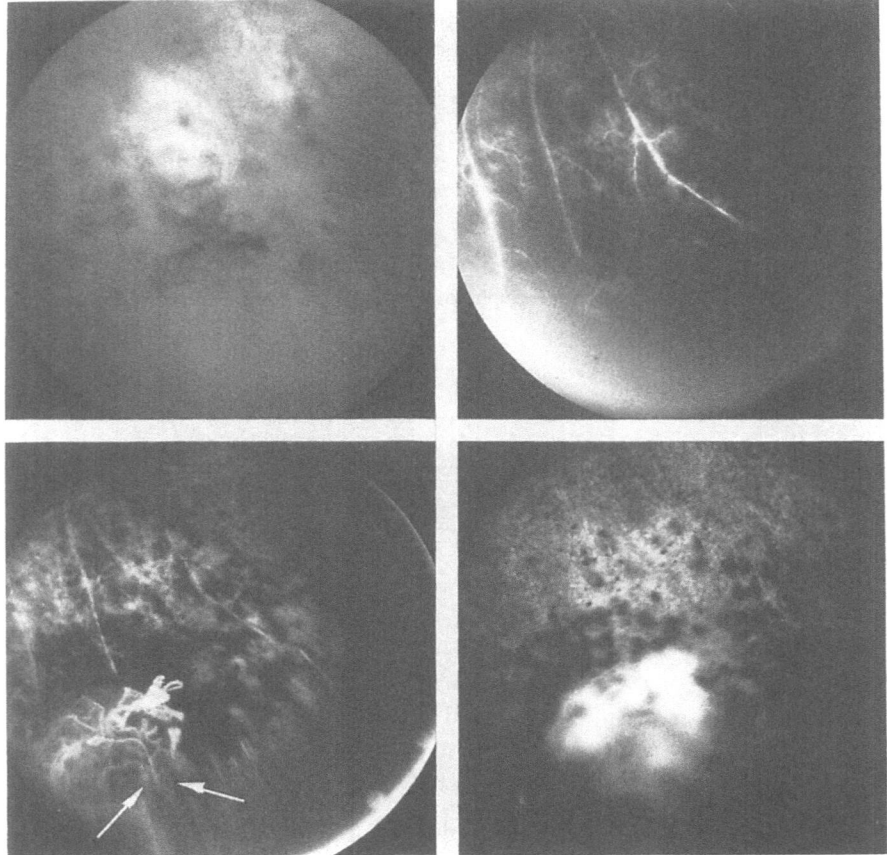

Figure 10–7.   Case 4. Neovascular lesion in the inferior periphery. Possible retino-choroidal anastomoses (see arrows). The lesion has already been surrounded by laser photocoagulation. This resulted in regression of the lipoid exudates.

The retinal exudation may be extremely marked and progress up to the posterior pole (Fig. 10–4), obscuring the ophthalmoscopic features of retinitis pigmentosa as in our third case. However, the family history, the aspect of the lesions in the sister, the complaints of night blindness since childhood and the extinct ERG response are sufficient reasons to accept the diagnosis of retinitis pigmentosa in this case. Our fifth patient is a member of a dominant retinitis pigmentosa family. The disease is present in members of three successive generations. His younger brother was examined elsewhere at the age of 23 years and bilateral Coats' disease was diagnosed. He eventually lost vision in both eyes by exudative detachment. Unfortunately no informations concerning his ocular condition before that age are avail-

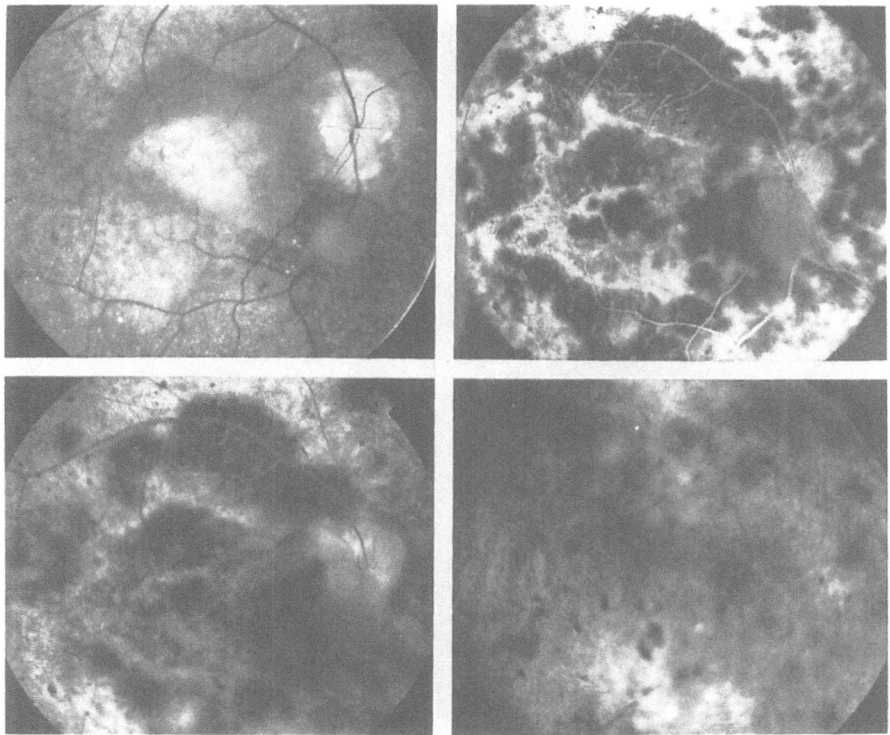

Figure 10–8.   Case 4. Extensive pigmentary changes. Drusen of the optic disc. Narrow retinal vessels. Atrophic macular lesion and fluorescein leakage in the inferior periphery (d).

able, except that his vision had always been poor. It is not unreasonable to suggest that he too presented bilateral Coats' syndrome in relationship to retinitis pigmentosa.

Fluorescein angiography demonstates the frequent presence of leakage in the posterior pole and underlines the vascular lesions in the inferior periphery. Communications of the preretinal fibrovascular tissue with the choroid through breaks of Bruch's membrane have been demonstrated histologically [17]. In one of our patients fluorescein angiography suggests a possible retinochoroidal anastomose (Fig. 10–7).

Spontaneous disappearance of the exudates has been documented [21]. However a number of cases tend to progress to exudative detachment and intractable neovascular glaucoma. Other complications are chronic uveitis [37, case 3] or recurrent vitreous hemorrhage (case 1). Even if the exudative reaction can be arrested, the dystrophic fundus lesions further progress, so that the visual prognosis is very bleak.

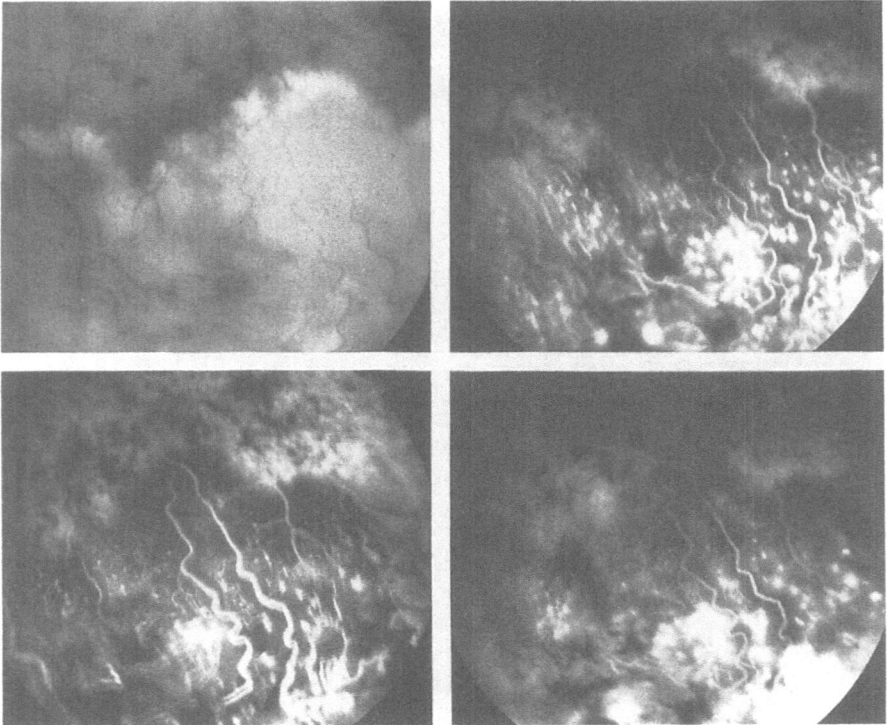

Figure 10–9. Pseudotumoral lesion in the inferior periphery with marked dilatation of the retinal vessels, telangiectasis and massive exudation.

III. Differential diagnosis

A number of other hereditary fundus disorders may be associated with retinal vascular involvement. This is particularly the case with Goldman-Favre syndrome [16], Wagner's disease [44], dominant exudative vitreoretinopathy [7, 44] and X-linked juvenile retinoschisis [2, 44]. In none of these cases do the retinal vascular anomalies progress to a pseudotumoral lesion. Also the vascular lesions are not predominantly found in the inferior periphery and are not associated with inflammatory signs.

Neovascular fundus abnormalities may also be present in eyes with peripheral uveitis [11]. These anomalies sometimes form angioma-like lesions located on the snowbank in the inferior ora serrata region and appear very similar to acquired retinal angiomatosis (see chapter 11). But patients with peripheral uveitis do not present the early signs and symptoms of retinitis pigmentosa and only in very progressed cases is the ERG possibly extinct. Also no familial incidence is known.

These cases also differ from congenital retinal telangiectasis or Leber-Coats' disease as described in chapter 8. Not only because of the possible familial incidence, the fact that women are relatively more commonly affected, the older age of the patients and the frequent bilateral involvement but also the ophthalmoscopic lesions appear different. Whereas in Leber-Coats' disease telangiectases are most frequently located in the (supero) temporal periphery, in cases associated with retinitis pigmentosa they are predominantly found in the inferior periphery. The capillary bed in the affected area, although sometimes very dilated, does not present that coarse aspect so typical for congenital telangiectasis. Light bulbs are less frequently found whereas retinal neovascularization and pseudotumoral aspects are relatively more common than in Leber-Coats' disease. Still because of the extreme exudative response it is quite understandable that the vascular lesions seen in some cases of retinitis pigmentosa have been considered as the combination of two separate diseases in a same patient.

IV. Histopathology

Coats' lesions in retinitis pigmentosa share a number of similar histological characteristics with Coats' disease [45] such as the disintegrated retina with exudative detachment, the retinal vascular changes and the presence of cholesterol slits in the gliotic retina and in the subretinal space. Lipid laden macrophages and scattered inflammatory cells are seen [17, 39]. The retinal vessels appear sclerotic. On electron microscopy they show attenuated endothelial cells with an irregular basement membrane [17, 39]. Fogle et al [17] noticed the presence of vascular communications through breaks in Bruch's membrane between the choroid, a subretinal disciform lesion and the preretinal fibrovascular membrane. Schuman et al. [39] did not observe changes at the level of Bruch's membrane. In Fogle's case the macular area was relatively well preserved although there was a mild degree of cystoid degeneration. Other histological findings such as the atrophy of the nerve fiber, ganglion cell, inner and outer nuclear layers and the marked changes of the retinal pigment epithelium are similar to what has been described in histological specimens of eyes with retinitis pigmentosa [20].

V. Pathogenesis

Three theories have been proposed to explain the association of retinitis pigmentosa with Coats' syndrome:
1. both diseases are genetically determined [30] which may explain why they can occur simultaneously in a same family.
2. the association of Coats' lesions and retinitis pigmentosa is purely co-incidental [17, 33].

3. Coats' syndrome is a complication of retinitis pigmentosa [1, 14, 21, 37, 38, 45].

This third theory best explains the late appearance of Coats' syndrome in these cases. A comparison can be made with cystoid macular edema. Cystoid macular edema has frequently been described in retinitis pigmentosa [5, 13, 18, 19, 21, 24, 31, 32] as well as more diffuse vascular leakage [14, 15]. According to Fetkenhour et al. [12] up to 70% of retinitis pigmentosa patients present some degree of cystoid macular edema.

This complication may be found in all genetic forms of retinitis pigmentosa and usually affects both eyes [34, 36]. Fishman et al. [15] observed that in such cases fluorescein leakage is not limited to the retinal vessels but may also affect the iris vasculature. Fluorophotometry in patients with retinitis pigmentosa and cystoid macular edema shows increased fluorescein concentration into the anterior chamber [36]. This is an indication that the vascular involvement is not limited to the retinal vessels. It must be also be stressed that inflammatory signs in retinitis pigmentosa are frequently observed in the vitreous. In an unilateral case of Coats' syndrome with retinitis pigmentosa, the fellow eye presented pars plana exudates [41].

The origin of cystoid macular edema in retinitis pigmentosa is still debated. There are reasons to believe that the rupture of the blood-retinal barrier mainly occurs at the level of the retinal pigment epithelium [9, 34, 43]. Yet, the retinal vessels probably also participate in the process. These reactions may be the consequence of an inflammatory response. A cellular immunity response to degenerating outer segments of the photoreceptors has been suggested [6, 8, 25, 27, 29, 35]. Other authors could not confirm this hypothesis [3, 42] even if they do not exclude the possibility that a toxic metabolite of degenerating retina might cause a breakdown of the blood-retinal barrier at the level of the vascular endothelium.

Coats' syndrome in retinitis pigmentosa probably represents an unusual severe inflammatory reaction to degenerating retinal tissue. This may explain the late onset of the vascular lesions, the association with inflammatory signs in the vitreous, the possible occurrence of uveitis and the similarity of the vascular lesions with the angioma-like lesions seen in peripheral uveitis [11]. This reaction is thus not related to a genetic type of retinitis pigmentosa but may occur in various forms of diffuse progressive degenerative processes affecting the outer retina whether this is hereditary determined or possibly even acquired. The immunological reactions in this specific group of patients have however not been studied specifically.

VI. Treatment

Although some eyes may stabilize or even show spontaneous reabsorption of the exudates [21], untreated eyes tend to progress to exudative detachment and neovascular glaucoma or present repeated vitreous hemorrhages [33, 37, 38, case 1].

The purpose of the treatment should be to destroy the vascular anomalies. These cases are however difficult to treat [4, 10]. Direct photocoagulation of the affected area either with the Xenon arc or with the Argon laser has been attempted with varying results. In some eyes this did not prevent further progression [33, 46, case 3]. Also such a treatment introduces the risk of bright-light exposure in eyes with severe retinal dystrophy. Probably a more efficient and also safer approach is repeated ab externo cryotherapy, if necessary after release of subretinal fluid in cases of associated exudative detachment.

References

1. Ayesh I, Sanders M D and Friedmann A I (1976): Retinitis pigmentosa and Coats' disease. *Br J Ophthalmol*, 60: 775–777.
2. Bec P, Ravault M, Arne J L and Trepsat C (1980): La périphérie du fond d'oeil. Ed Masson, Paris, 221–226.
3. Benezra D, Gery I, Chan C C, Nussenblatt R B, Palestine A G, Kaiser-Kupfer M, Maftzir O and Peer J (1984): Cellular and humoral immune parameters among patients with retinitis pigmentosa and other retinal disorders. *Ophthalm Paed Genet*, 4: 193–197.
4. Bonnet M (1980): Le syndrome de Coats. *J Fr Ophtalmol*, 3: 57–66.
5. Bonnet M and Pingault C (1973): Oedéme maculaire cystoïde et rétinopathie pigmentaire. *Bull Soc Ophtalmol Fr*, 73: 715–718.
6. Brinkman C J O, Pinckers A J L G and Broekhuyse R M (1980): Immune reactivity to different retinal antigens in patients suffering from retinitis pigmentosa. *Invest Ophthalmol Vis Sci*, 19: 743–750.
7. Canny C L B and Oliver G L (1976): Fluorescein angiographic findings in familial exudative vitreoretinopathy. *Arch Ophthalmol*, 94: 1114–1120.
8. Corwin J M and Weiter J J (1981): Immunology of chorioretinal disorders. *Survey Ophthalmol*, 25: 287–305.
9. Cox S M, Hay E and Bird A C (1988): Treatment of chronic macular edema with acetazolamide. *Arch Ophthalmol*, 106: 1190–1198.
10. Egerer I, Tasman W and Tomer T L (1974): Coats disease. *Arch Ophthalmol*, 92: 102–112.
11. Felder K S and Brockhurst R J (1982): Neovascular fundus abnormalities in peripheral uveitis. *Arch Ophthalmol*, 100: 750–754.
12. Fetkenhour C L, Choromokos E, Weinstein J and Shoch D (1977): Cystoid macular oedema in retinitis pigmentosa. *Trans Am Acad Ophthalmol Otolaryngol*, 83: 515–521.
13. Ffytche T J (1972): Cystoid maculopathy in retinitis pigmentosa. *Trans Ophthalmol Soc U.K.*, 92: 265–283.
14. Fiore C, Santoni G and Babel J (1984): Microangiopathie et dystrophie rétinienne. *J Fr Ophtalmol*, 7: 305–311.
15. Fishman G A, Fishman M and Maggiano J (1977): Macular lesions associated with retinitis pigmentosa. *Arch Ophthalmol*, 95: 798–803.
16. Fishman G A, Jampol L M and Goldberg M F (1976): Diagnostic features of the Favre-Goldmann syndrome. *Br J Ophthalmol*, 60: 345–353.
17. Fogle J A, Welch R B and Green W R (1978): Retinitis pigmentosa and exudative vasculopathy. *Arch Ophthalmol*, 96: 696–702.

18. Francois J, De Laey J J and Verbraeken H (1972): L'oedème kystoïde de la macula. *Bull Soc Belge Ophtalmol*, 161: 708–721.
19. Francois P, Turut P and Desnouck B (1976): Les altérations maculaires de la rétinopathie pigmentaire. *Arch Ophtalmol*, 36: 5–20.
20. Gartner S and Henkind P (1982): Pathology of retinitis pigmentosa. *Ophthalmology*, 89: 1425–1432.
21. Gass J D M (1987): *Stereoscopic atlas of macular diseases*. 3rd ed. The C V Mosby Co, St. Louis, pp. 274–278.
22. Grizzard W S, Deutman A F and Pinckers A J L G (1978): Retinal dystrophies associated with peripheral retinal vasculopathy. *Br J Ophthalmol*, 62: 188–194.
23. Heckenlively J (1981): Retinitis pigmentosa, unilateral Coats' disease and thalassemia minor. A case report. *Metab Ped Ophthalmol*, 5: 67–72.
24. Hyvarinen L, Maumenee A E, Kelly J and Cantollino S (1971): Fluorescein angiographic findings in retinitis pigmentosa. *Am J Ophthalmol*, 71: 17–26.
25. Jain I S, Singh K P and Dhir S P (1981): Serum ceruloplasmin and immuno-globulins in retinitis pigmentosa: *Ann Ophthalmol*, 13: 733–734.
26. Kajiwara Y (1980): Ocular complications of retinitis pigmentosa. Association with Coats' syndrome. *Jap J Clin Ophthalmol*, 34: 947–955.
27. Keltner J L, Roth A M and Shihman C R (1983): Photoreceptor degeneration. Possible auto-immune disorder. *Arch Ophthalmol*, 101: 564–569.
28. Krill A E (1977): *Hereditary retinal and choroidal diseases*. Harper and Row Publishers, Hagerstown (Md.) p. 538.
29. Kumar M, Gupta R M and Nema H V (1983): Role of auto-immunity in retinitis pigmentosa. *Ann Ophthalmol*, 15: 838–840.
30. Lanier J D, McCrary III J A and Justice J (1976): Autosomal recessive retinitis pigmentosa and Coats' disease. A presumed familial incidence. *Arch Ophthalmol*, 94: 1737–1742.
31. Merin S (1970): Macular cysts as an early sign of tapeto-retinal degeneration. *J Ped Ophthalmol*, 7: 225–228.
32. Metge P, Chovet M, Ebagosti A and Tassy A (1974): Oedème maculaire cystoide dans la rétinopathie pigmentaire. *Bull Soc Ophtalmol Fr*, 74: 119–123.
33. Morgan W E III and Crawford J B (1968): Retinitis pigmentosa and Coats' disease. *Arch Ophthalmol*, 79: 146–149.
34. Newsome D A (1986): Retinal fluorescein leakage in retinitis pigmentosa. *Am J Ophthalmol*, 101: 354–360.
35. Rahi A H S (1973): Auto-immunity of the retina. II. Raised serum IgM levels in retinitis pigmentosa. *Br J Ophthalmol*, 57: 904–909.
36. Schauwvlieghe P and De Laey J J (1985): Fluorophotometry in retinitis pigmentosa. *Bull Soc Belge Ophtalmol*, 215: 87–4.
37. Schmidt D and Faulborn J (1970): Retinopathia pigmentosa mit Coats-Syndrom. *Klin Mbl Augenheilk*, 157: 643–652.
38. Schmidt D and Faulborn J (1972): Familiäres Vorkommen von Coats-Syndrom kombiniert mit Retinopathia pigmentosa . *Klin Mbl Augenheilk*, 160: 158–163.
39. Schuman J S, Lieberman K V, Friedman A H, Berger M and Schoeneman M J (1985): Senior-Loken syndrome (familial renal-retinal dystrophy) and Coats' disease. *Am J Ophthalmol*, 100: 822–827.
40. Spallone A, Carlevaro G and Ridling P (1985): Autosomal dominant retinitis pigmentosa and Coats-like disease. *Int Ophthalmol*, 8: 147–151.
41. Spalton D J, Bird A C and Gleary P E (1978): Retinitis pigmentosa and retinal oedema. *Br J Ophthalmol*, 62: 174–182.
42. Spalton D J, Rahi A H S and Bird A C (1978): Immunological studies in retinitis pigmentosa, associated with retinal vascular leakage. *Br J Ophthalmol*, 62: 183–187.
43. Tso M O M (1981): Pathology and pathogenesis of cystoid macular edema. *Ophthalmologica*, 183: 46–54.

44. Van Nouhuys C E (1982): Dominant exudative vitreoretinopathy and other vascular developmental disorders of the peripheral retina. Dr. W. Junk Publishers.

45. Witschel H (1974): Retinopathia pigmentosa und 'Morbus Coats'. *Klin Mbl Augenheilk*, 164: 405–411.

46. Yuguchi M and Majima A (1984): A case of retinitis pigmentosa associated with Coats' syndrome. *Ophthalm Paed Genet*, 4: 177–182.

47. Zamorani G (1956): Una rare associazione di retinite di Coats con retinite pigmentosa. *G It Oftalmol*, 2: 429–433.

11 Presumed acquired retinal angiomatosis (Adult Coats' disease)

In chapter 8 it was concluded that the term Coats' disease should be reserved to cases of exudative retinopathy due to the presence of congenital telangiectasis. Leber-Coats' disease mainly occurs in younger individuals. However, an ophthalmoscopic aspect characterized by retinal vascular anomalies and progressive exudation may also be found in adults [6, 17].

Henkind and Morgan [10] used the term 'adult Coats' disease' for these cases, while Shields et al. [14] proposed the name of 'presumed acquired retinal angiomas'. However, in our opinion it would be better to speak of 'angiomatosis' instead of 'angiomas'.

I. Incidence

The number of cases of presumed acquired retinal angiomatosis published in the literature is still small [1, 2, 5, 6, 9–12, 14, 17].

Yet, Shields et al. [14] reviewed 12 cases seen between March 1975 and January 1982 in the oncology service of Will's Eye Hospital in Philadelphia and Laqua and Wessing [12] described 10 cases which they examined between 1980 and 1982. In 1985 we published four cases [4] and have since seen five new cases. These 9 cases are summarized in Table 1.

Table 1.

Case	Sex	Age	Eye	Vision at presentation	Macula	Site of the lesion	Feeder vessels	Lipoid exudates	Hemorrhages
1	M	55	R	0.7	mac. edema	infero-temp.	+	+ +	+
2	F	74	R	0.4	preret. fibr.	inferior	+ +	−	+
3	F	63	L	0.2	exudates	inferior	+	+ +	+
4	F	55	R	0.1	preret. fibr.	inferior	+ +	−	+
5	F	63	R	0.3	mac. edema	inferior	+	+ +	+
6	M	43	L	0.3	mac. edema	inferior	+	+	+ +
7	M	53	L	0.8	mac. exud.	inferior	+	+ + +	−
8	F	70	R	0.8	nl.	inferior	−	+	+
9	F	71	L	0.2	mac. edema	inferior	−	+ +	+

Spitznas et al. [16] in an epidemiological study of Coats' disease noted a high incidence of the disease before the age of 20 years and after the age of

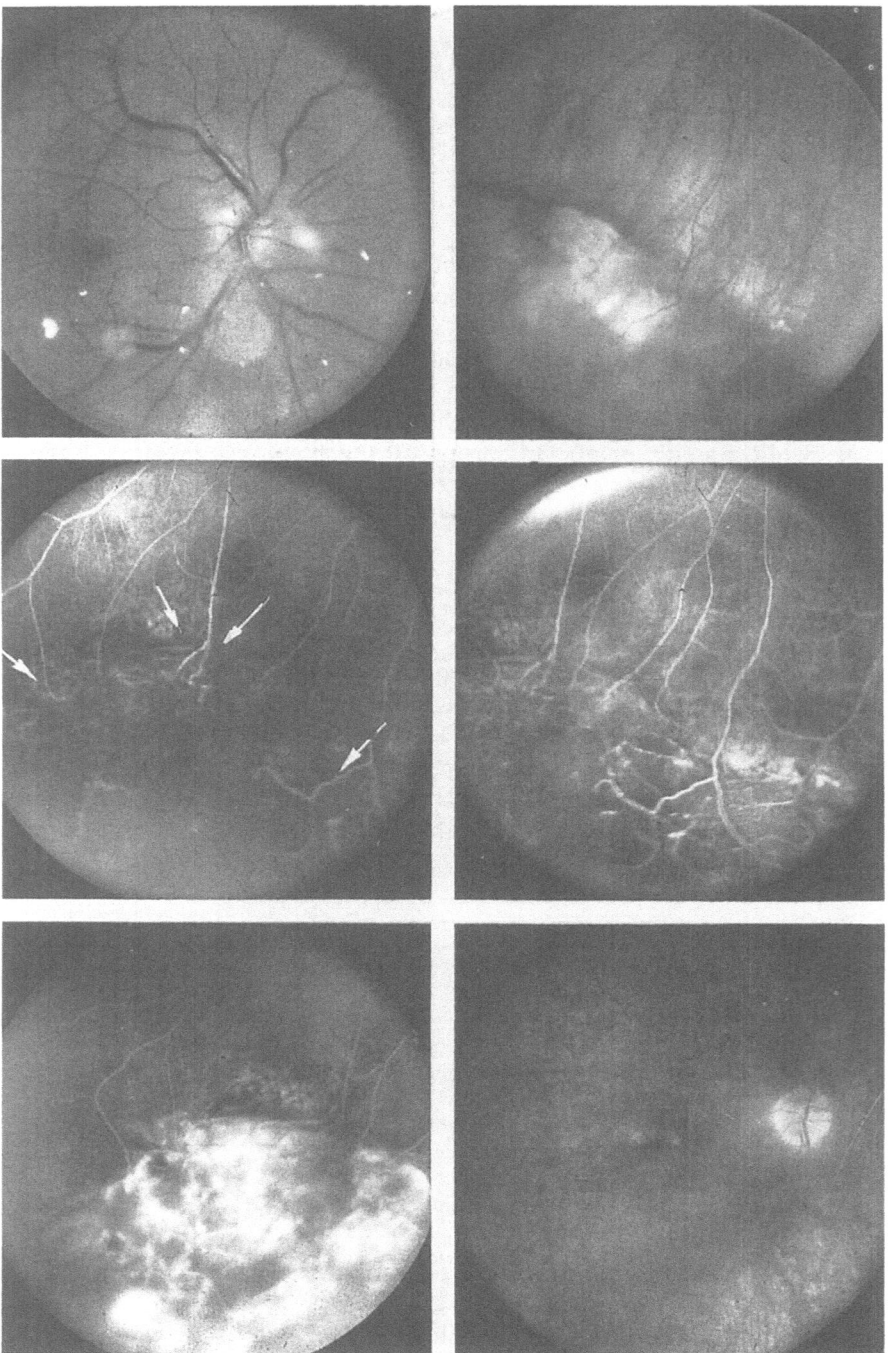

Figure 11–1. Case 1. Mild macular edema and vascular lesion in the inferior periphery. Presence of multiple retinal feeding and draining vessels (c, arrows).

40 years. Most probably in this second group a number of acquired retinal angiomatosis are included. In our series the ages at presentation vary between 43 and 71 years. The youngest patient in Shields' series was 34 years old and the eldest 85 years.

Six of our 9 patients were women. An increased incidence in women was also noticed by Shields et al. [14] but not by Laqua and Wessing [12].

The disease usually affects only one eye, although bilateral cases have been described [17].

The family history is unremarkable. In none of these cases were signs or symptoms observed of von Hippel-Lindau's disease.

II. Clinical aspects

The patient usually complains of floaters or of blurred vision mainly due to associated macular edema. The patient may even be asymptomatic at the moment the lesions are discovered [12]. A number of cases were referred for a suspected malignancy [12, 14, our first case]. Some patients may have a history of uveitis [17].

In all our cases the anterior segment appeared normal except for occasional senile cataract. The posterior vitreous was detached and preretinal fibrosis or prepapillary gliosis was noticed in the posterior pole in some eyes (Figs. 11–2, 11–4, 11–6).

Vitreous cells and asteroid hyalosis are sometimes seen. Macular edema was confirmed by fluorescein angiography in 6 of our 9 cases. The retinal vascular lesion, which is the hallmark of this disease, is most commonly situated in the inferior of infero-temporal periphery. It is surrounded by lipoid exudates and may present the aspect of a highly vascularized tumoral mass (Figs. 11–1, 11–2 and 11–4). The vasculature of the lesion appears to derive from the retinal vasculature (Figs. 11–1 and 11–4), although a possible relationship with choroidal vessels cannot be ruled out in other cases (Fig. 11–2). Feeder and draining vessels were observed in most of our cases but they did not have the extremely dilated calibre which is typical of von Hippel's disease. Multiple feeders were noticed in a few instances (Fig. 11–1). Although the capillaries are dilated, the coarse aspect typical of Coats' disease is seldom seen. Capillary occlusion peripheral to the vascular lesion can sometimes be observed and may possibly cause retinal neovascularization (Fig. 11–4).

An exudative detachment is commonly seen [14] and may be quite impressive (Fig. 11–3). Progression of the exudates in the macular region, exudative detachment, recurrent hemorrhages or even total retinal detachment and neovascular glaucoma are possible complications of this lesion.

Laqua and Wessing [12] divided their cases into three stages:
– Stage 1: small peripheral lesion (1 or 2 disc diameter in width) with fine microvascular abnormalities in relation to peripheral vessels. The sur-

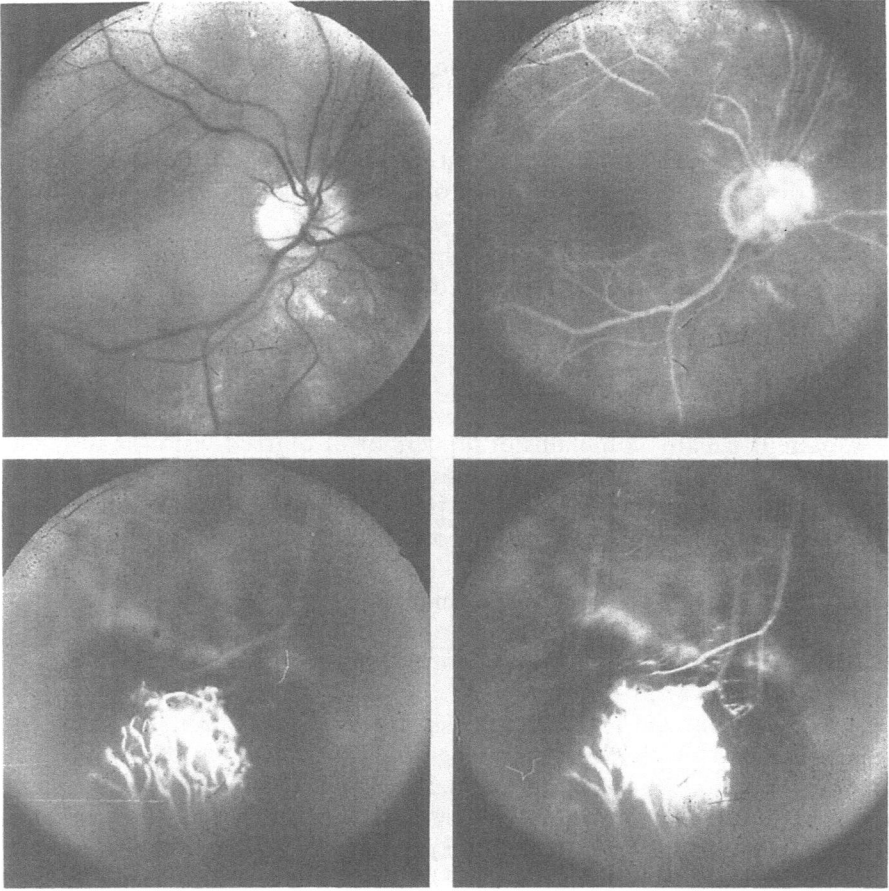

Figure 11–2.   Case 2. Posterior vitreous detachment and markedly vascularized tumor in the inferior periphery.

rounding retina is slightly edematous and few lipoid exudates may be seen.
- Stage 2: the lesion is more prominent than in stage 1 and is often multilobulated. These telangiectases are associated with organized scar tissue which is avascular.
- Stage 3: prominent peripheral lesion with heavy exudates and retinal detachment.

The lesions described by Shields et al. [14] correspond to stage 3 of Laqua and Wessing.

The lesions are not always demonstrable with echography. In the cases where analysis is possible, A-scan echography shows high internal reflectivity and B-scan the absence of choroidal excavation (Fig. 11–5).

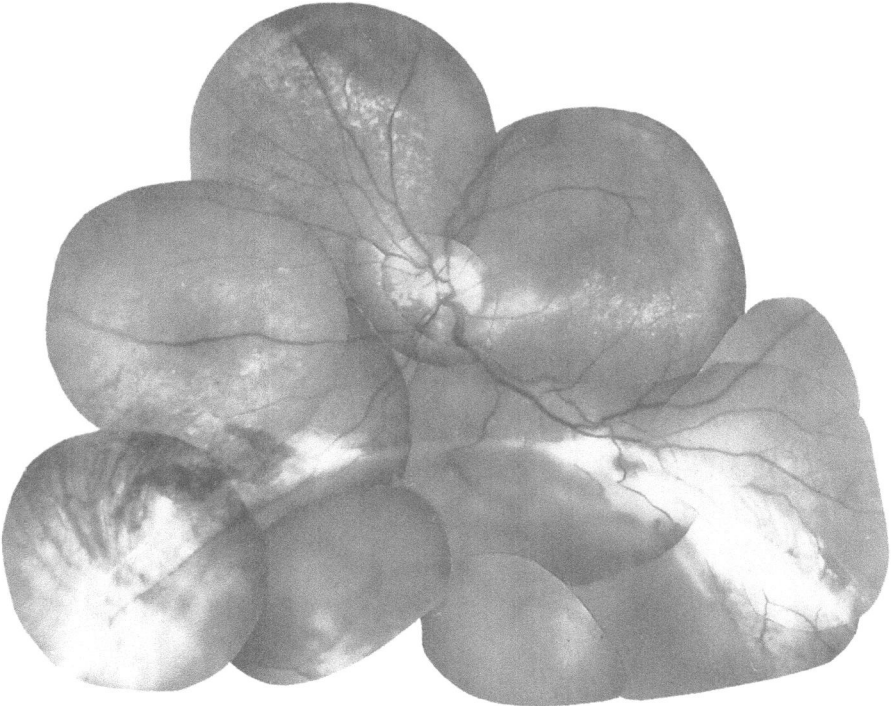

Figure 11–3.   Case 3. Photomontage of the lesions in the left eye. (Courtesy of Dr. A. Leys, Leuven)

III. Differential diagnosis

The condition described here must be differentiated from:
1. congenital retinal telangiectasis or Leber-Coats' disease (see chapter 8);
2. von Hippel's disease (see chapter 2);
3. vascular complications of peripheral uveitis;
4. malignant melanoma of the choroid;
5. vascular changes in long standing retinal detachment.

1. Congenital retinal telangiectasis

We mentioned already that acquired retinal angiomas have been called 'adult Coats' disease' [10, 17]. However, typical congenital telangiectasis is rare in patients older than 30 years and predominantly affects male patients. It is however hazardous to differentiate both conditions mainly on the basis of the age of the patient. Both conditions have a number of common characteristics: they are unilateral, are associated with retinal and subretinal

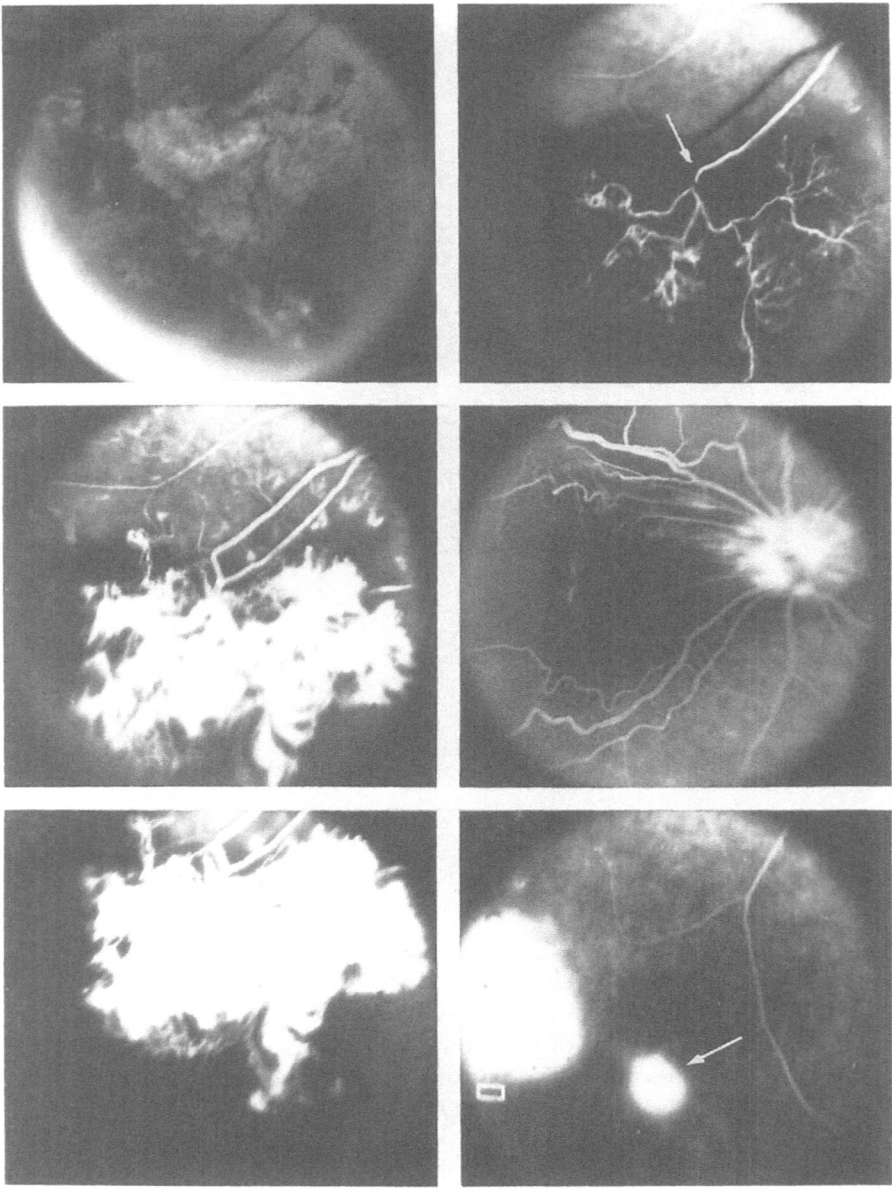

Figure 11-4.   Case 4. Ophthalmoscopic and fluoroangiographic aspect of the lesion in the infero-temporal periphery. The vessels of the tumor are fed by the infero-temporal retinal artery (a). Peripheral ischemic area. Marked distorsion of the retinal vessels in the posterior pole (d). Secondary retinal neovascularization outside the tumor (f, arrows). (Courtesy of Dr. A. Leys, Leuven)

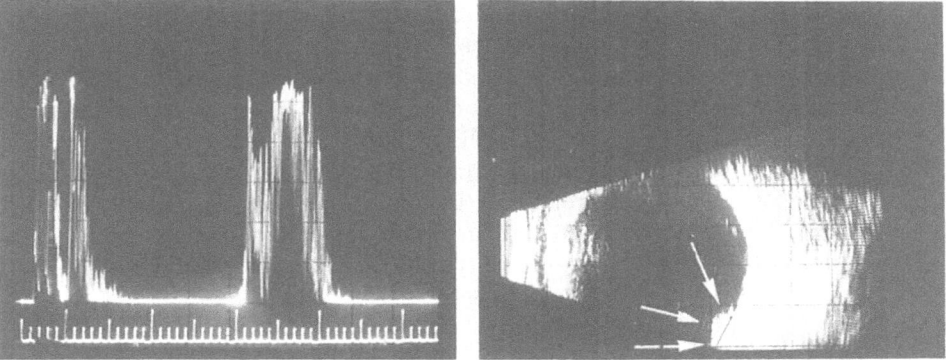

Figure 11–5. Case 5. A- and B-scan echography prior to treatment. High internal reflectivity of the lesion; absence of choroidal excavation.

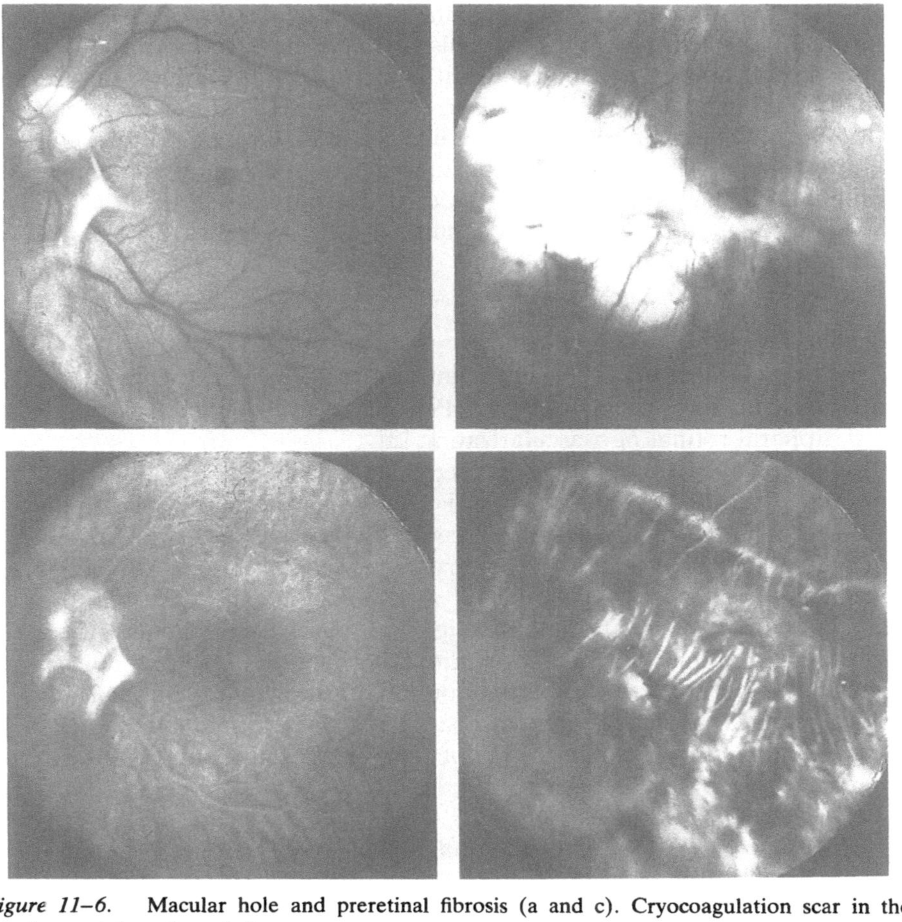

Figure 11–6. Macular hole and preretinal fibrosis (a and c). Cryocoagulation scar in the inferior periphery (b and d).

exudation and may result in retinal detachment and neovascular glaucoma. The telangiectasis in Coats' disease is usually situated in the (supero) temporal periphery, whereas it is mainly found inferiorly in acquired retinal angiomas. Juvenile Coats' disease is characterized by a very coarse aspect of the affected capillaries and typical 'light bulbs' are seen on retinal arteries, capillaries or veins. In acquired retinal angiomatosis the lesions are more localized. Light bulbs are relatively uncommon but feeder vessels are often seen. Such feeder vessels are not a feature of congenital retinal telangiectasis, neither the tumoral aspect so typical for acquired retinal angiomatosis.

2. Von Hippel's disease

Von Hippel's angiomatosis is quite different from the lesions described here. Although feeder vessels are commonly found, they are not markedly dilated. The lesion is also solitary, whereas in von Hippel's disease one or multiple cysts are found. Also the site and the aspect of the lesions are different. Mature angiomas in von Hippel's disease appear as homogenuous masses with smooth borders, usually red but sometimes white in color. Both eyes are affected in 50% of the cases. Von Hippel-Lindau's disease is dominantly inherited and the ocular lesions may be associated with one or more visceral manifestations of the disease. In presumed acquired retinal angiomatosis no familial cases have yet been described, the lesion only affects one eye and the patient has no signs of concommittant disease. Also the histopathological aspect is quite different.

3. Peripheral uveitis

Woods and Duke [17] reported a clinical history or signs of uveitis in their patients with adult Coats' disease. Peripheral uveitis may be complicated by peripheral retinal neovascularization [3].

Felder and Brockhurst [7] observed angioma-like lesions in six of eleven patients with adult Coats' disease. Peripheral uveitis may be complicated These lesions were situated on a classic snowbank, usually in the inferior periphery and could lead to secondary detachment and exudates. However, peripheral uveitis is usually seen at a younger age, is often bilateral and associated with some inflammatory signs in the anterior segment of the eye. In acquired retinal angiomatosis the fellow eye is usually normal and snowbanks are not seen. The common finding in acquired retinal angiomatosis of cells in the vitreous and of cystoid macular edema may be indications of an inflammatory reaction; it is not possible to tell if the inflammation is the cause or the result of the peripheral lesions.

4. Malignant melanoma of the choroid

A number of patients were referred with the clinical diagnosis of malignant melanoma [12, 14, our first case] and the third patient of Henkind and

Morgan [10] was enucleated for that reason. The differential diagnosis is usually easy. Lipoid exudates and preretinal fibrosis are uncommon in choroidal melanomas. Also the fluoroangiographic aspect is quite different. Even when a marked congestion of the own vasculature of a malignant melanoma is caused when the tumor has perforated Bruch's membrane, the surrounding portion of the tumor still shows pigmentary changes which lead to the correct diagnosis [4]. Also retinal feeder vessels are not found in malignant melanomas of the choroid. Echography and diaphanoscopy are of course helpful. In exceptional cases nevertheless, the differentiation may be difficult and Shields et al. [15] described a case of choroidal melanoma simulating a retinal angioma.

5. Vascular changes in longstanding rhegmatogenous retinal detachment

Longstanding rhegmatogenous retinal detachment may be associated with alterations of the retinal capillary bed. In these cases telangiectasis and even angioma-like lesions may be found in the equatorial and pre-equatorial region of the detached retina [8, 13]. It is worth mentioning that cases 2 and 4 of Henkind and Morgan [10] had a history of longstanding retinal detachment before the eye was enucleated. In case 2 the nature of the detachment is not specified, but in case 4 there was a suggestion of a horseshoe tear in the involved eye. In the other cases in the literature and in our own series longstanding rhegmatogenous retinal detachment is unlikely to be the cause of the peripheral vascular lesion.

IV. Histopathology

The histopathology of eyes with presumed acquired retinal angiomatosis was described by a few authors [1, 10, 17]. They all insist on the similarities with Coats' disease.

Henkind and Morgan [10] as well as Apple et al. [1] observed telangiectatic vessels with hyalinized walls, pigment proliferations, subretinal albuminous exudates, lipid loaden macrophages, ghost cells and cholesterol clefts. The affected retina is degenerated. The endothelial cells of the abnormal vessels are either absent of markedly disturbed [1]. The choroid may be atrophic but shows no signs of inflammation.

V. Pathogenesis

The pathogenesis of presumed acquired retinal angiomatosis is still not clear. These angioma-like lesions are quite similar to the peripheral vascular lesions seen in some cases of retinitis pigmentosa (see chapter 10), in cases with uveitis [7] or longstanding retinal detachment [8, 13]. Association with uveitis was noticed [17] and Duke and Woods [6] also insisted on the constant finding of hypercholesterolemia in their cases. They considered the role of a previous uveal inflammation as a trigger mechanism initiating the deposition of cholesterol in the tissues. However, most cases of presumed acquired retinal angiomatosis do not present evidence of a previous inflammation or of a dystrophic retinal process.

VI. Treatment

In some cases the lesion is not very progressive. Treatment is mainly advised when subretinal fluid or retinal exudates extend to the macular area and threaten central vision [4].

The treatment of choice is cryocoagulation [4, 9] using the freeze-thaw technique [14]. Multiple sessions may be necessary. If the retina is detached, a buckling procedure must be considered. After successful treatment regression of the tumor and reabsorption of the exudation are noticed. Complications of such a treatment are rare. In one of our cases however we observed an increase of the preretinal fibrosis in the posterior pole and the appearance of a macular hole (Fig. 11–6).

References

1. Apple D J, Gieser D K and Goldberg M F (1981): Pathologische Befunde bei einem Erwachsener mit Morbus Coats. *Klin Mbl Augenheilk*, 179: 336–339.
2. Bernard J A, Vallat M, Quentel G, Durevil J, Rammaert B and Adenis J P (1979): Nonperfusion du lit capillaire rétinien périphérique avec hémorragie du vitré et néovascularisation pseudo-angiomateuse. Cause ou conséquence? *Bull Soc Ophtalmol Fr*, 79: 471–475.
3. Brockhurst R J, Schepens C L and Okamura I D (1960): Uveitis. II. Peripheral uveitis: clinical description, complications and differential diagnosis. *Am J Ophthalmol*, 49: 1257–1266.
4. De Laey J J (1976): Fluorescein angiographic aspects of choroidal melanomas. *Doc Ophthalmol Proc Series*, 7: 221–236.
5. De Laey J J, Devuyst A and Leys A (1985): Acquired retinal angiomatosis or adult Coats' disease. *Bull Soc Belge Ophtalmol*, 211: 99–108.
6. Duke J R and Woods A C (1963): Coats' disease. II. Studies on the identity of the lipids concerned and the probable role of mucopolysaccharides in its pathogenesis. *Br J Ophthalmol*, 47: 413–434.
7. Felder K S and Brockhurst R J (1982): Neovascular fundus abnormalities in peripheral uveitis. *Arch Ophthalmol*, 100: 750–754.
8. Felder K S and Brockhurst R J (1982): Retinal neovascularization complicating rhegmatogenous retinal detachment of long duration. *Am J Ophthalmol*, 93: 773–776.
9. Gass J D M (1974): Differential diagnosis of intraocular tumours: a stereoscopic presentation. The C V Mosby C°, St. Louis, pp. 260–261.
10. Henkind P and Margan G (1968): Peripheral retinal angioma with exudative retinopathy in adults (Coats' disease). *Br J Ophthalmol* , 50: 2–11.
11. Keith C G (1973): Angiomatosis retinae. *Br J Ophthalmol*, 57: 593–594.

12. Laqua H and Wessing A (1983): Peripheral retinal telangiectasis in adults, simulating a vascular tumor or melanoma. *Ophthalmology*, 90: 1284–1291.
13. Malbran E S, Dodds R A and Hulsbus R (1979): Retinal telangiectasia associated with longstanding retinal detachment as a prognostic sign. *Mod Probl Ophthalmol*, 20: 96–100.
14. Shields J A, Decker W L, Sanborn G E, Augsburger J J and Goldberg R E (1983): Presumed acquired retinal hemangiomas. *Ophthalmology*, 90: 1292–1300.
15. Shields J A, Joffe L and Guibor P (1978): Choroidal melanoma clinically simulating a retinal angioma. *Am J Ophthalmol*, 85: 67–71.
16. Spitznas M, Joussen F, Wessing A and Meyer-Schwickerath G (1975): Coats' disease. An epidemiologic and fluorescein angiography study. *Von Graefe's Arch Clin Exp Ophthalmol*, 195: 241–250.
17. Woods A C and Duke J R (1963) Coats' disease. I. Review of the literature, diagnostic criteria, clinical findings and plasma lipid studies, *Br Ophthalmol*, 47, 385–412.

12 Acquired retinal macroaneurysms

Aneurysms are common lesions in retinal vascular diseases, whether congenital or acquired. A number of these diseases as von Hippel's disease, cavernous retinal hemangioma, retinal telangiectasis and acquired retinal angiomatosis have been discussed at large in previous chapters. In other diseases such as diabetic retinopathy, hypertensive retinopathy, radiation retinopathy, Takayasu's disease, hyperviscosity syndrome, carotid insufficiency, retinal vein occlusion ..., capillary microaneurysms are characteristic findings.

Retinal arteriolar macroaneurysms are however far less frequent. The first case was reported in 1881 by Loring [35]. Raehlman in 1889 [48] described as first a pulsating arterial macroaneurysm. A number of cases described in the early literature [28, 35, 46] concern young, apparently healthy individuals and are possibly examples of congenital retinal telangiectasis rather than acquired retinal arterial macroaneurysms [47].

In 1973 Robertson [51] introduced the term arterial macroaneurysm to distinguish these dilatations of major retinal arterial branches from the classical aneurysm of the capillary or venous plexus. He described 13 patients presenting such macroaneurysms and stressed their mean common features:

1. situation on a main retinal artery, usually within the first three bifurcations of the central retinal artery;
2. frequent association with hemorrhages and exudates;
3. frequent association with longstanding arterial hypertension;
4. natural tendency to become fibrosed.

I. Incidence

Acquired retinal arteriolar macroaneurysms are not rare and since Robertson's description a number of large series have been published: Cleary et al. [12]; 20 patients; Lewis et al. [34]: 16 patients; Lavin et al. [32]; 40 patients; Palestine et al. [44]; 35 patients (update of Robertson's original series); Attali et al. [4]: 17 patients; Abdel-Khalek et al. [1]: 19 patients; Rabb et al. [47]: 60 patients. The largest series is the collaborative study of Schatz et al. [56] which comprises 132 patients. Other authors have published smaller series or individual cases [2, 3, 5, 6, 9, 10, 14, 15, 18–23, 28, 30, 31, 39–43, 45, 57, 59, 60].

Acquired arterial macroaneurysm is a disease of the elderly. The mean age of the patients at presentation varies in large series between 66 years [32] and 73 years [4].

The disease is twice to four times more frequent in women than in men [1, 18, 32, 44, 47].

Macroaneurysms are not limited to the human species alone. They have also been observed in monkeys [24].

Usually only one eye is affected. Bilaterality has been found in 1 of 30 cases by Cleary [11], in 4 of 40 cases by Lavin et al. [32], in 2 of 19 cases by Attali et al. [4], in 5 of 80 cases by Rabb et al. [47] and in 11 of 132 cases by Schatz et al. [56]. In a personal survey of 23 cases seen at the University of Ghent we had only one bilateral involvement.

Although François [18] stated that the right eye is involved in 80% of the cases, a survey of 308 cases published in the literature (including 23 personal cases) indicates that the right eye was affected in 107 patients and that in 31 patients retinal macroaneurysms were found in both eyes.

II. Clinical manifestations

1. Presenting symptoms

By itself a retinal macroaneurysm may be asymptomatic, so that a number of cases are incidental findings of a routine fundus examination. Acute visual loss may result from a hemorrhage in the macular region or less frequently into the vitreous [32] due to the rupture of a macroaneurysm. Progressive visual loss is usually the result of exudation in the macular area. Visual acuity may thus vary from 10/10 in cases of asymptomatic macro-aneurysms to light perception when the rupture of a macroaneurysm causes a massive vitreous hemorrhage.

Some patients may present major field defects due to the occlusion of the affected arteriole [34].

2. Ophthalmoscopic findings

Macroaneurysms are observed at the major branches of the central retinal artery. They are nearly always found temporal to the disc [1, 18, 34, 41, 47, 55, 57] and according to Lavin et al. [32] more commonly in the superotemporal quadrant. In our series of 23 patients (one bilateral case) one eye presented macroaneurysms on a superotemporal and an infero-temporal artery. The macroaneurysms were situated on a supero-temporal artery in 16 cases (64%), an infero-temporal artery in 7 cases (28%) a supero-nasal artery in 1 case (4%) and an infero-nasal artery in another case (4%).

Involvement of a cilioretinal artery [20, 34] or of an artery on the optic nerve head [10, 44, 47, 55] is rather exceptional. Macroaneurysms are more frequently seen within the first three orders of arterial bifurcation and remain thus usually confined to the posterior pole [18, 51].

In Lewis' series [34] seven of 17 separate arteriolar macroaneurysms occurred at an arterial bifurcation and three more at an arteriovenous crossing.

There are two main types of arterial macroaneurysms: saccular or blowout aneurysms and fusiform or cuffed aneurysms [1, 17]. Sometimes they present a loop formed by the apparent fusion of adjacent macroaneurysms [17]. Most often the aneurysm is isolated, however multiple aneurysms either on the same arteriole or on different arterioles of the same eye are not uncommon (Fig. 12–1). Macroaneurysms are frequently haloed (Fig. 12–2) and this cuff may represent a thickening of the arteriolar wall [22] or an accumulation of white blood cells [51].

Pulsating aneurysms have already been described in 1889 [48]. Robertson [51] found one pulsatile aneurysm in 13 cases. Pulsating aneurysms may be a sign of impending vessel rupture and serious bleeding [21, 51, 57]. They may also regress spontaneously [9, 51].

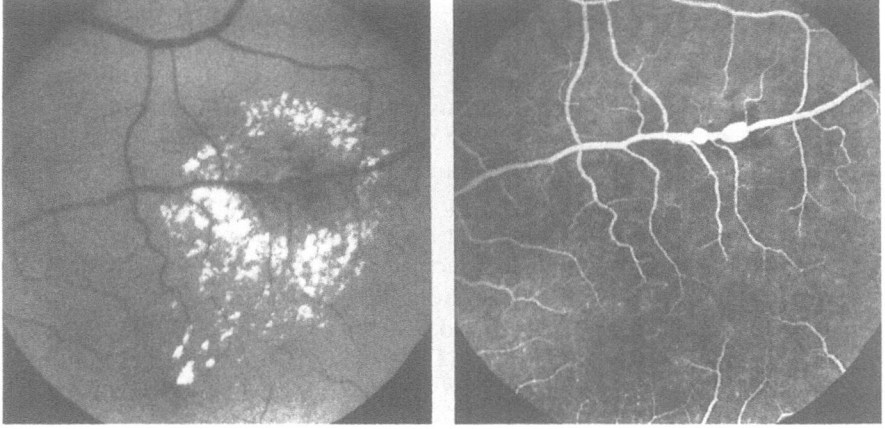

Figure 12–1. Double retinal macroaneurysm along the supero-temporal retinal arteriole of the left eye in a 73 year old lady.

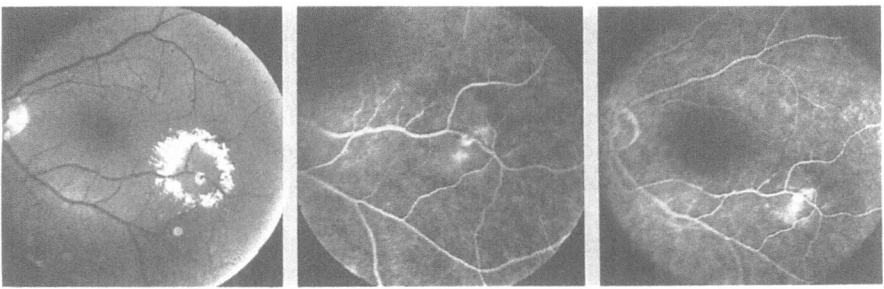

Figure 12–2. Typical haloed macroaneurysm surrounded by circinate lipoid deposits.

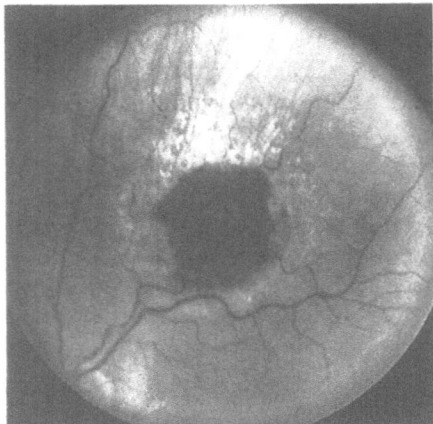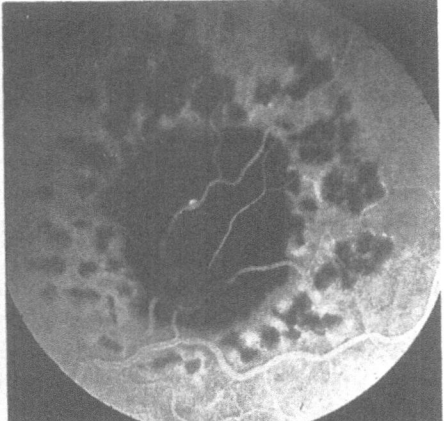

Figure 12–3.   Large retinal hemorrhage obscuring a retinal macroaneurysm, which became only visible after partial reabsorption. At first examination the hemorrhage was considered as resulting of a possible retinal tear and therefore a double ring of photocoagulations was applied around the hemorrhage.

Macroaneurysms are frequently associated with hemorrhages, retinal edema, lipoid exudates and serous or hemorrhagic detachment of the neuroretina.

The dominant feature in most macroaneurysms is hemorrhage [32], which may even initially obscure the lesion (Fig. 12–3). This is possibly one of the reasons why macroaneurysms are still so frequently misdiagnosed. Hemorrhages may be the only sign if the macroaneurysm spontaneously thromboses. Hemorrhages can be precipitated by a Valsalva manoeuvre [6]. Intra- and subretinal hemorrhages are found but also preretinal and intravitreal hemorrhages [1, 4, 18, 34, 44, 47, 51]. Subretinal and preretinal hemorrhages are not unfrequently associated [47, 57]. In our series hemorrhages were a prominent feature in 14 of 24 eyes, and in two of these a vitreous hemorrhage was present.

Saccular or blow-out aneurysms are more prone to bleed. The intensity and site of the hemorrhage possibly depends on the size of the aneurysm and where the rupture occurs. If it is at the anterior site of the macroaneurysm, the hemorrhage is likely to be situated in the preretinal or vitreous space, whereas a rupture of the posterior or postero-lateral wall leads to intra- and subretinal hemorrhages [1]. Macroaneurysms close to the optic disc are more prone to bleed than others. Retinal hemorrhages are not necessarily due to a massive rupture of the vessel wall but may be the consequence of oozing of blood from small dehiscences in the wall [3]. Repeated hemorrhages may occur [41] but are relatively rare and they may be related to the rupture of another aneurysm in the same eye [47].

An exudative response is frequently observed in macroaneurysms

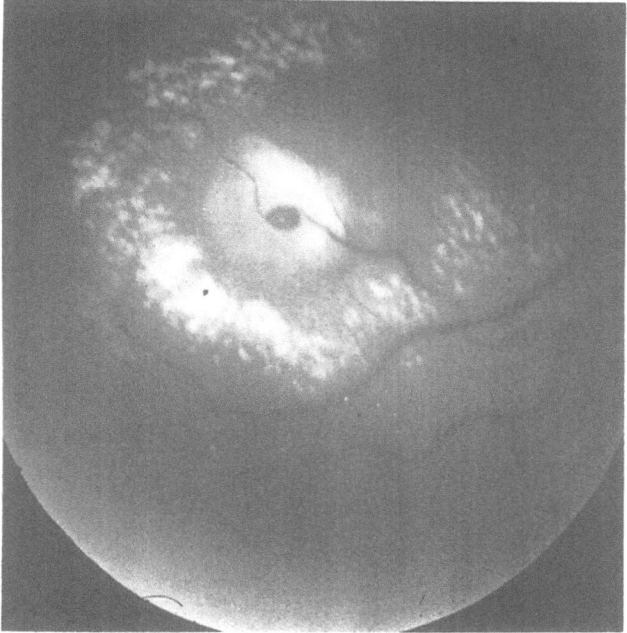

Figure 12–4.   Single aneurysm with macular edema and exudates involving the macular area.

Around the aneurysm an area of retinal edema may be seen, frequently surrounded by lipoid deposits in a circinate pattern [1, 18, 19, 32, 47, 51, 59]. Lipoid exudates may sometimes accumulate in the macular region and thus provoke visual loss even if the macroaneurysm is at an apparently save distance of the macula (Fig. 12–4). A serous detachment of the neuroretina surrounding the macroaneurysm is a possible complication [4, 44, 47]. An exudative response is more commonly observed than hemorrhages in macroaneurysms associated with retinal vein occlusion.

3. Fluorescein angiographic findings

Retinal macroaneurysms generally fill simultaneously with the filling of the affected artery [15, 18, 19, 23]. The distal part of the artery may present delayed filling (Fig. 12–5).

On occasion, ophthalmoscopically typical macroaneurysms fill incompletely or not at all. This suggests the obliteration of the lumen by a thrombotic process. Leakage of dye in varying amount frequently occurs from the macroaneurysm or from the surrounding arteriolar wall. Because of the presence of hemorrhages a detailed study of the capillary bed around the macroaneurysm is not always possible. In some instances capillary dilatation may be observed [23] (Fig. 11–5). The involved artery as well as

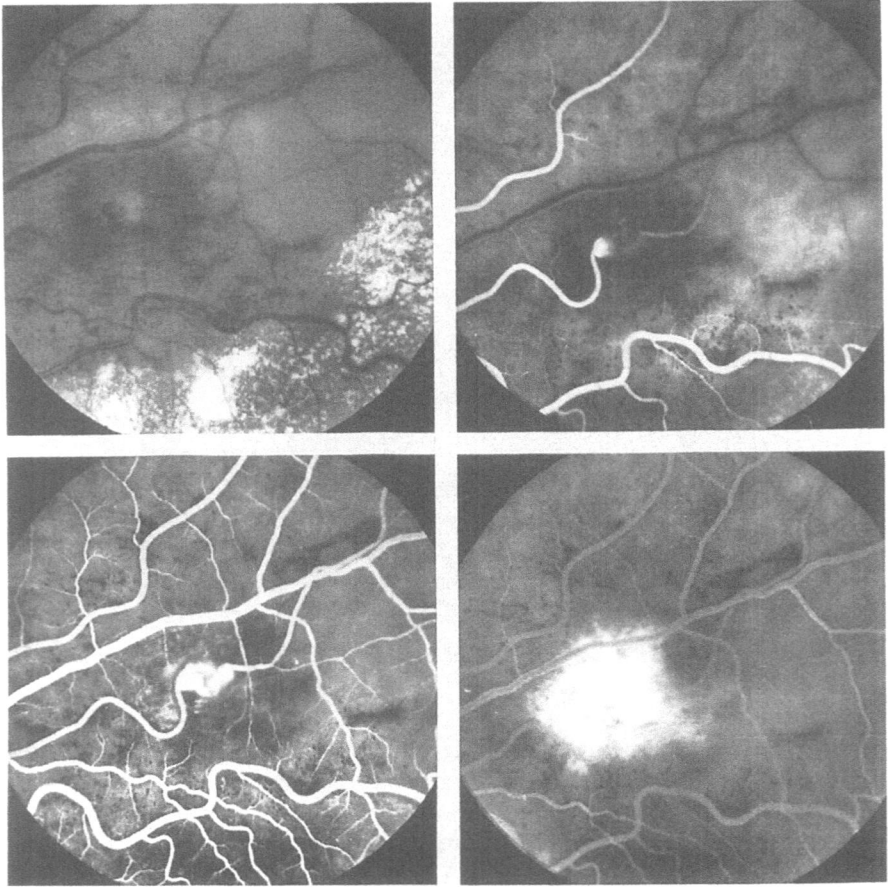

Figure 12–5.   Single macroaneurysm with massive exudative response. Note the delayed filling and the irregularity of the arterial portion distal to the aneurysm.

others in the same eye usually show marked irregularity, focal narrowing and tortuosity.

4. Classification and evolution

Several authors have attempted a classification of macroaneurysms.

Lavin et al. [32] differentiate between quiescent, exudative and hemorrhagic macroaneurysms. Quiescent macroaneurysms are associated with hemorrhages or exudates extending for less than one disc diameter and sparing the macula. In exudative macroaneurysms exudation is the major component measuring more than one disc diameter and in hemorrhagic macroaneurysms the hemorrhage extending more than one disc diameter is more extensive than the associated exudation.

Palestine et al. [44] identify three groups.

In the first group the lesions are located within the vascular arcade and cause visual loss. In the second group the lesions, also situated within the vascular arcade, are not associated with loss of central visual acuity, whereas in the third group the lesions are situated outside the vascular arcade and pose no threat to macular function.

Abdel-Khalek et al. [1] differentiate between acute and chronic aneurysmal decompensation. Acute decompensation is characterized by sudden visual loss due to presumed aneurysmal rupture; in chronic decompensation the ophthalmoscopic picture is dominated by the presence of exudates and edema.

Macroaneurysms may remain stationary for a long period of time [3], others may slowly increase in time. Intraretinal hemorrhages generally resolve spontaneouly as well as vitreous hemorrhages. In both cases visual acuity is usually restored. After a preretinal hemorrhage a fibrotic plaque may remain for a prolonged period of time [4] and subsequently disappear leaving however in some instances preretinal fibrosis. The prognosis is less favourable in subretinal hemorrhages, where changes in the retinal pigment epithelium and in the neuroretina result in permanent visual loss. Retinal pigmentary changes after subretinal hemorrhages are commonly observed [4, 32, 47].

The prognosis of hemorrhagic macroaneurysms is relatively favourable as after hemorrhage these aneurysms tend to occlude spontaneously [11, 12]

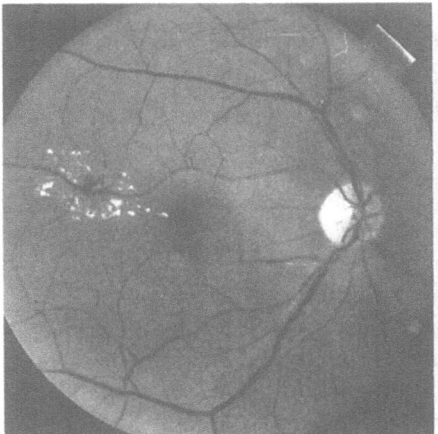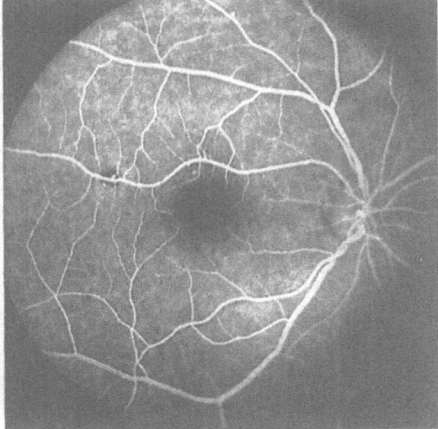

Figure 12–6. Small macroaneurysm, still recognizable in ophthalmoscopy, but which does not stain on fluorescein angiography suggesting spontaneous closure. A few microaneurysms are visible around the lesion. The affected arteriole is permeable.

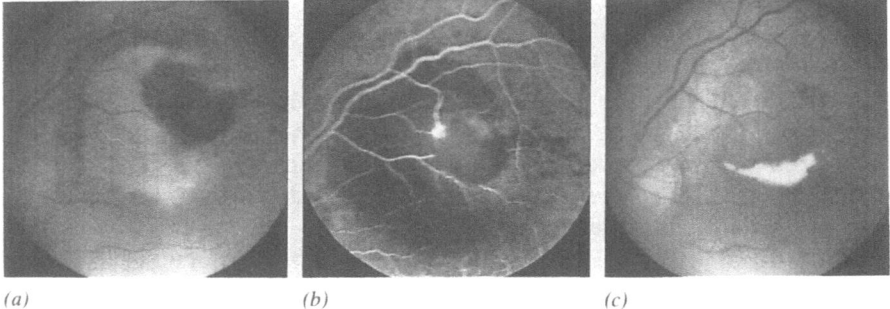

(a)   (b)   (c)

Figure 12–7.   Single aneurysm with preretinal and subretinal hemorrhages. a, b. aspect in May 1978. c. aspect in September 1978: spontaneous resolution of the hemorrhages but exudates in macular region.

(Figs. 12–6, 12–7). In few instances however a hemorrhagic lesion may progress to chronic exudation (Fig. 12–7).

In exudative cases the prognosis is less favourable and their course is much more chronic. Chronic exudation may result in macular hole formation [21] or permanent structural alterations of the macula. Exudation is the most common cause of poor visual outcome of macroaneurysms [12, 44, 55].

III. Associated diseases

1. Associated retinal diseases

Macroaneurysms are frequently associated with other signs of arteriosclerosis [51]. Irregular arterial calibre, arteriolar plaques and retinal emboli are found [31]. A common observation is the association with retinal arterial or venous occlusions in the same or in the fellow eye [1, 9, 12, 17, 26, 30–32] (Fig. 12–9).

In Lavin's series [32] hemorrhagic macroaneurysms were significantly less frequently associated with retinal vein occlusion as compared to non-hemorrhagic macroaneurysms.

Augsburger and Henry [5] observed the appearance of arterial, capillary and venous aneurysms in a young boy with chronic renal failure who developed cytomegalovirus infection after repeated renal transplantation.

Not surprisingly in an older population macular drusen, senile cataract and open angle glaucoma are more frequently seen.

Myelinated fibers were noted by Brown and Weinstock [10] and by Pringle [46]. Although such as association is probably coincidental, it is remarkable that these myelinated fibers were present in the same areas as the macroaneurysms.

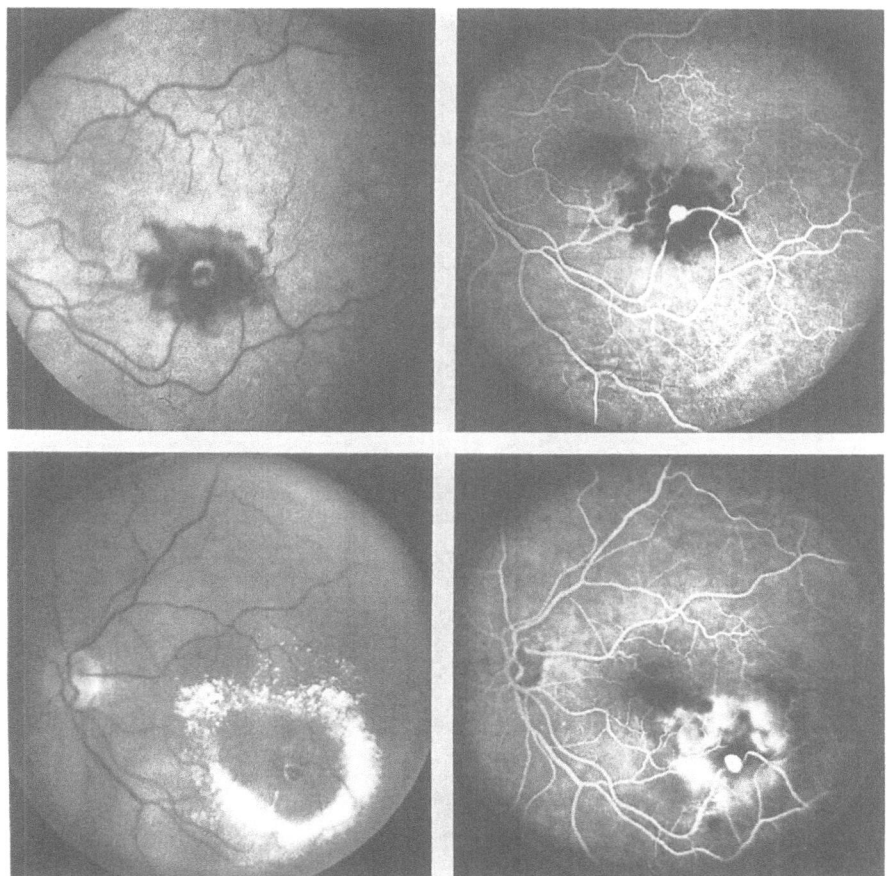

Figure 12–8. Single macroaneurysm. (Top) aspect at presentation in May 1982: the macro-aneurysm is surrounded by dense intraretinal hemorrhages. (Bottom) same eye in September 1982: spontaneous resolution of the hemorrhages but marked retinal edema and circinate retinopathy around the vascular lesion.

2. General diseases

A large number of patients present arterial hypertension and arteriosclerotic disease [3, 9, 12, 23, 44, 51, 56]. It is worthwhile to underline that aneurysmal dilatations of cerebral blood vessels have also been described in arterial hypertension [13, 52]. As retinal macroaneurysms, cerebral aneurysms are more frequent in women than in men. They appear in arteries of size comparable to retinal arterioles.

Diabetes, with or without hyperlipidemia, is less frequently associated with retinal macroaneurysms [4] and in those cases arterial hypertension is present as well [4, 34].

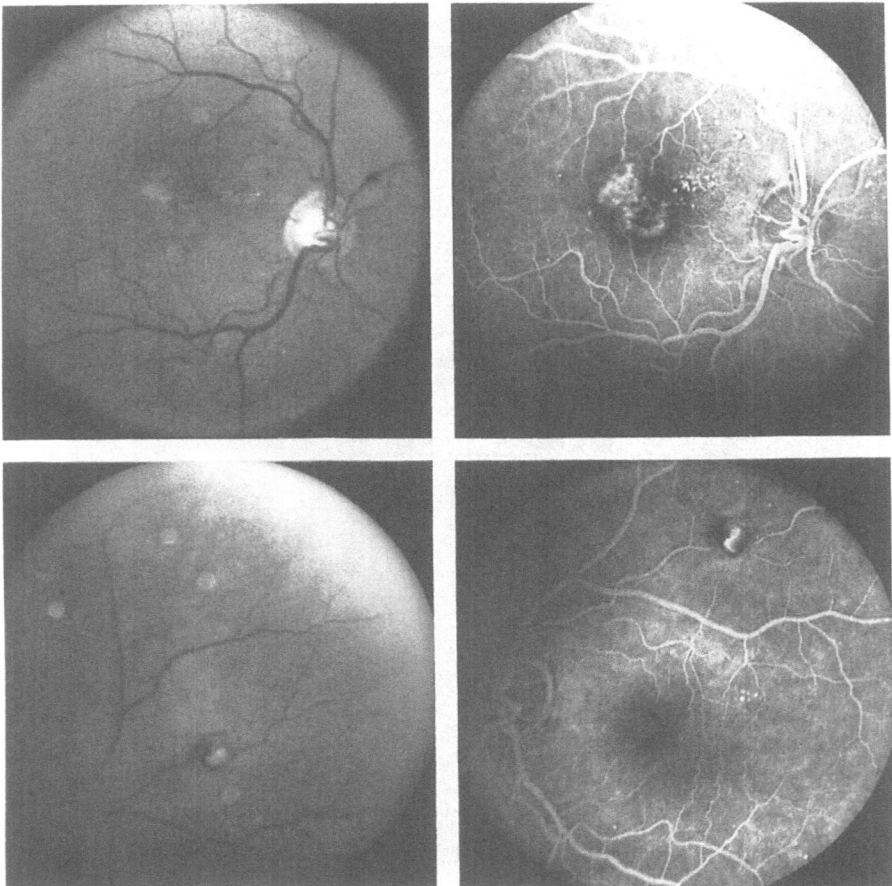

Figure 12–9.   Both eyes of the same patient. The right eye presents signs of a previous branch vein occlusion and in the left eye an asymptomatic macroaneurysm is seen on the supero-temporal artery.

Lavin et al. [32] found that patients with macroaneurysms have a significantly higher blood packed cell volume (hematocrit) than controls. Hematocrits over 45% were found in 55% of patients with macroaneurysms and in 20% of the controls.

The presence of retinal arterial macroaneurysms is a strong indication of a generalized vascular disease. It is thus not surprising that a number of these patients present life threatening vascular complications such as myocardial infarction or cerebrovascular accidents [12, 32, 34, 41]. Eleven of twenty patients of Cleary et al. [12] had a history of myocardial ischemia or a previous cerebrovascular accident. One of these patients died of a myocardial infarction and another as a result of a cerebrovascular insult.

Four of the sixteen patients of Lewis et al. [34] died between 9 months and 5 1/4 years after presentation, one of stroke, two of combined myocardial infarction and stroke and one after resection of a symptomatic abdominal aortic aneurysm. Two of the forty patients of Lavin et al. [32] died of complications of vascular disease.

IV. Histopathology

As macroaneurysms were only characterized clinically in 1973 it is not surprising that their histopathological description is also relatively recent [17, 22, 45]. The cases of McDonald and Sarin [36], described as intraretinal angioma, could be similar to isolated retinal arterial aneurysms [22].

The microscopic characteristics of macroaneurysms are illustrated in Figs. 12–10 to 12–13.

Both the artery and the surrounding retina may show varying histological pictures according to the duration of the disease and the level of the lesion which was examined. Aneurysms have been described located anterior to an

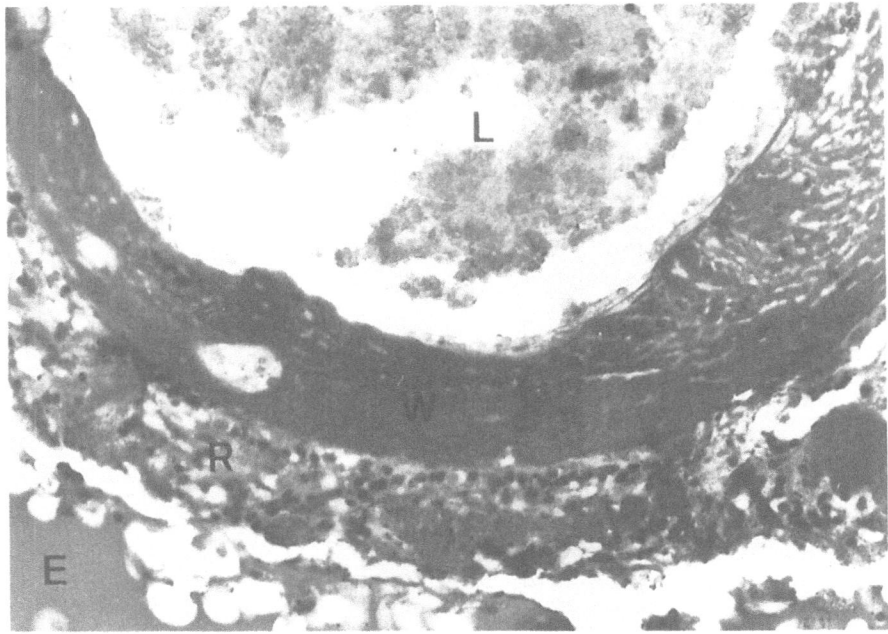

Figure 12–10. Large retinal macroaneurysm (case 5906.86). The wall is focally enlarged by a laminated fibrin clot. (L = lumen, W = enlarged wall, R = degenerated retina, E = subretinal exudate).

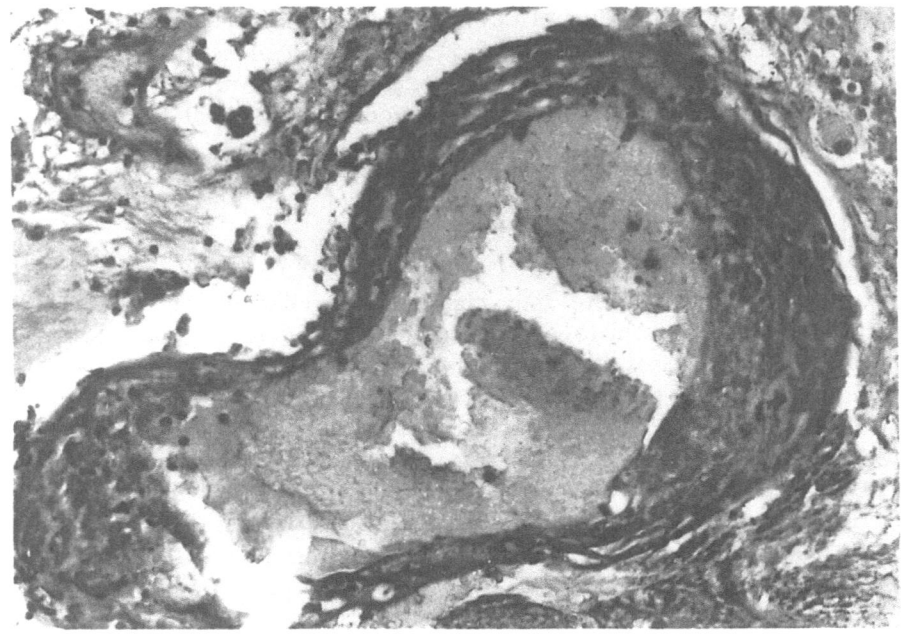

Figure 12–11.   Retinal macroaneurysm with laminated fibrin clot. Degenerated surrounding retina (case 5906.86).

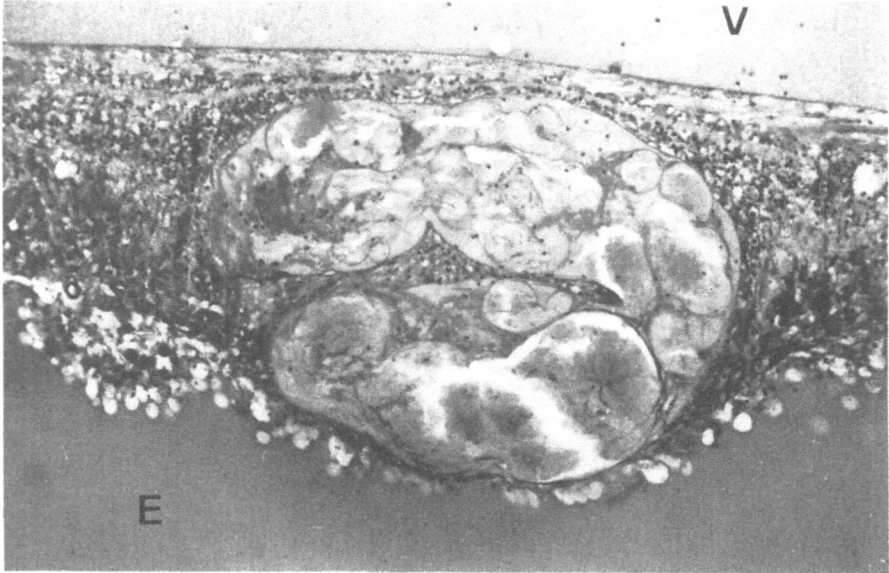

Figure 12–12.   Retinal macroaneurysm with compartmentalized structure. Surrounding degeneration. Retinal detachment by subretinal exudates (case 5906.86). (V = vitreous, E = subretinal exudate).

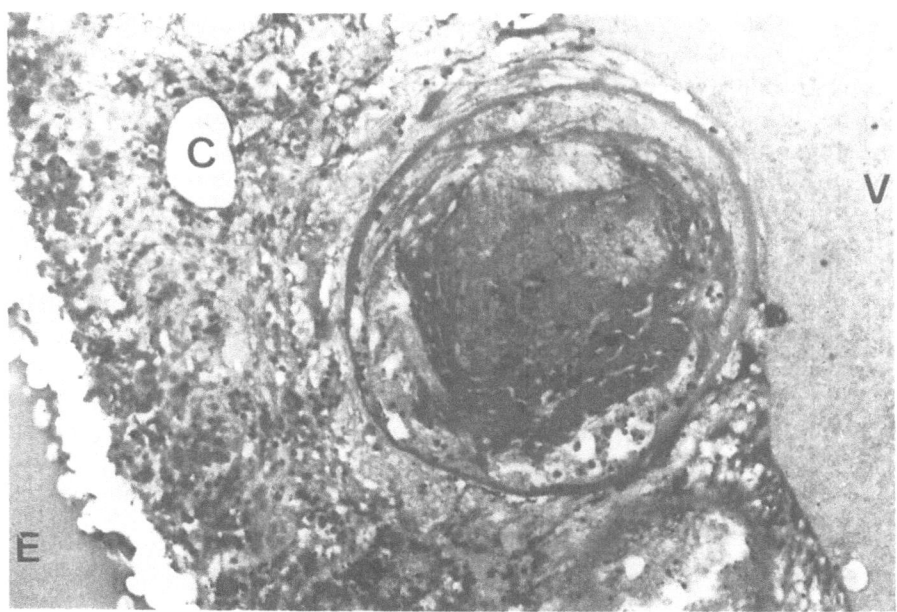

Figure 12–13. Thrombosed retinal macroaneurysm (case 5906.86). The surrounding retina is swollen and degenerated. (C = dilated capillary, E = subretinal exudate, V = vitreous).

arteriovenous crossing [17]. They may be saccular [22] or compartmentalized [17] and partially obliterated by scar tissue [22]. Some aneurysms may be as large as 600 × 350 μm [22]. The wall of the artery may be thickened [22] or focally enlarged by a laminated fibrin clot with hypertrophy of the muscularis [17]. The internal elastic lamina shows focal breaks [22] or fragmentation and reduplication [17]. The adjacent endothelium is disrupted with extravasation of red blood cells and fibrin [17]. Hemorrhage, fibrin and occasional foamy macrophages are interspersed through the thickened wall [17].

In older organized cases there may be a main eccentric lumen and several lumina within a thick collagenized wall with lipid macrophages and a few round cells [17].

Densely pigmented hemosiderin deposits, indicative of an old hemorrhage, are sometimes found around the artery, which may also be buried in a mass of intense fibroglial reaction and collagenous tissue with lipid loaden histiocytes, cholesterol clefts and hemosiderin [22].

A large spheroid nodule, composed of precipitated fibrin, was also found adjoining a widely dilated artery. It represented a laminated clot adjacent to a ruptured saccular aneurysm [45].

The corresponding vein may show chronic inflammatory infiltration [17, 22]. The significance of the lymphocytes around the vein is unknown, but this is probably a secondary phenomenon [17].

The retina may be swollen or thickened; the photoreceptors in the affected area are degenerated or focally destroyed [17, 45] but without discontinuity of the retinal pigment epithelium [45]. The outer retinal layers are sometimes compressed by the material around the artery and the vein. There may even be a complete disruption of the retinal architecture. Proteinaceous exudates are occasionally seen in the outer plexiform layer and lipoid exudates and lipid filled histiocytes may be present from the inner nuclear layer into the subretinal space. Numerous dilated capillaries have been observed in the surrounding retina [22].

Extensive retinal hemorrhages are found in all layers in some cases or mainly in the ganglion cell and nerve fibers layers in other cases. Subretinal hemorrhages may break through the retina into the vitreous. In some instances excessive bleeding has caused misinterpretation of the lesion which was taken for a malignant melanoma [17, 45].

V. Pathogenesis

Various causes such as old age, atherosclerosis, arterial hypertension or other vascular diseases, have been proposed as contributing factors in the development of solitary retinal macroaneurysms [8, 16, 45, 51, 57].

Lewis et al. [34] made the observation that a number of macroaneurysms occur at an arterial bifurcation or at a point of arteriovenous crossing and that they may be associated with arteriolar emboli. These findings suggest that macroaneurysms may result from a focal damage of the vascular wall.

Leishman [33] demonstrated that in involutional sclerosis contractile elements of the arterial wall are replaced by collagen. This is accompanied by a decrease in cellularity and a thinning of the wall, which probably offers less resistance to increased intraluminal pressure. As indicated previously most patients suffer from arterial hypertension.

We have already mentioned the frequent association with retinal venous occlusion. It is not possible however to indicate if there is a possible causal relationship between venous occlusion and macroaneurysm formation or if both are only the result of the same basic disease. Macroaneurysms are not confined to arteries but may occur on retinal veins [25, 37, 54, 58] and in the capillary bed [56]. Venous and capillary macroaneurysms are associated with retinal vein occlusion and are also the consequence of increased intraluminal pressure on a degenerated vessel wall.

Fatty exudates occur clinically around the aneurysm and form large circinate rings. The pathophysiology of this non-specific finding is unknown. It may be that disturbance in flow through the involved artery may lead to decreased perfusion and hypoxia of the adjacent capillary bed with subsequent leakage of fluid. Preferential resorption of proteinaceous materials by surrounding healthy capillaries may then secondarily lead to deposition of lipid material and to the formation of a ring [22].

VI. Differential diagnosis

1. Retinal telangiectasis

The characteristics of retinal telangiectasis, whether congenital or acquired, have been described at large in previous chapters. Some cases of macroaneurysms described in young patients [18, 28, 35, 46] probably represent a variant of congenital telangiectasis rather than acquired retinal macroaneurysms.

2. Retinal angiomatosis

Retinal angiomatosis and angiomatosis of the optic disc are discussed in chapters 2 and 3. In small angiomas the differentiation is not always evident [36], especially as the characteristic feeder vessels are missing. However, these tumors are not situated along the retinal arterioles and are mostly found in the peripheral fundus. Quite often, angiomas in various stages of evolution are found in the same fundus. Except in acquired angiomatosis (see chapters 10 and 11), retinal angiomas are found in a younger age group than acquired retinal macroaneurysms.

3. Retinal cavernous hemangiomas

This disease is discussed in chapter 4. The lesions are multiple and unassociated with exudative reaction. They may however be the cause of massive hemorrhage.

4. Congenital vascular anomalies of the optic disc

Awan [4] observed an unusual dilatation of the inferior papillary artery resembling a small aneurysm of that artery. That appearance was the result of a sudden backward turn of one of the branches at the origin.

Joffe et al. [9] termed varix of the optic disc an unusual vascular dilatation of the central retinal vein at the optic disc. The patient was asymptomatic.

5. Disciform macular degeneration

Retinal and subretinal hemorrhages from a ruptured macroaneurysm in the posterior pole may mimic a senile disciform macular degeneration especially if the other eye presents senile macular drusen. Fluorescein angiography may be extremely helpful in identifying the source of bleeding unless the hemorrhage is too important. Usually the follow-up will allow the differentiation.

6. Malignant melanoma

Hemorrhages from isolated arterial aneurysms may simulate a malignant melanoma of the choroid [15] or a tumor of the disc [10]. Careful observation, echography and fluorescein angiography must permit an accurate diagnosis.

7. Vitreous hemorrhages from other causes

Although retinal macroaneurysms are a relatively unfrequent cause of vitreous hemorrhage, this possibility must be kept in mind.

VII. Treatment

The question whether a macroaneurysm needs treatment depends on its site [44] and the risk of macular involvement and massive hemorrhage. The risk of bleeding appears to be significantly greater in pulsating aneurysms [57]. It must however be kept in mind that spontaneous occlusion of the aneurysm with recovery of vision is possible [41, 51, 59]. The prognosis is usually better if the macroaneurysm is complicated by hemorrhages as compared to the cases with chronic exudation [12, 56, 59]. The hemorrhage is frequently followed by a spontaneous obliteration of the aneurysm, whereas exudative macroaneurysms usually have a protracted course. Cases with serous retinal detachment carry a poor prognosis [56, 59].

As aneurysms complicated by hemorrhages tend to have a benign evolution, it seems reasonable in those cases to observe the natural evolution. Photocoagulation is however to be considered in cases were the chronic exudation jeopardizes macular function. The purpose of the treatment is to induce fibrosis in and around the aneurysm.

Photocoagulation can be applied either with the Xenon lamp [18, 28, 34] or with the Argon laser [1–4, 14, 18, 39, 40, 43–44, 59]. More recently, dye yellow laser treatment was also advised [38].

The treatment can be applied directly to the aneurysm. However, there is a risk of provoking an arterial occlusion resulting in a permanent scotoma (Fig. 12–14).

Indirect treatment with low intensity coagulations of the retina in the immediate vicinity of the aneurysm is probably a safer procedure. Occlusion of the aneurysm can be obtained with preservation of the patency of the affected vessel. The procedure has sometimes to be repeated.

A successful treatment results in the reabsorption of edema and exudates.

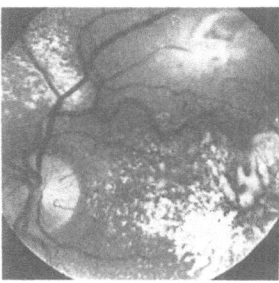 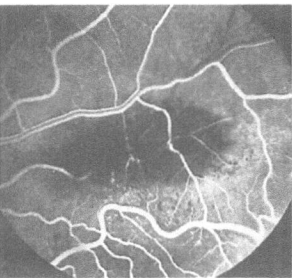 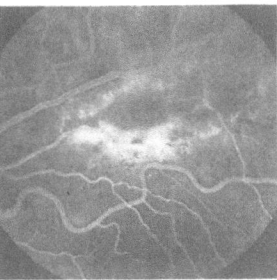

Figure 12–14. Same eye as Fig. 12–5 after direct Xenon arc photocoagulation. Complete occlusion of the arteriole distal to the macroaneurysm.

In longstanding edema however this will not necessarily improve visual acuity. Therefore patients should be treated rapidly if the macula is at risk.

Complications of treatment are not common. We already mentioned the possibility of causing arteriolar occlusion [3]. This complication is perhaps more frequent in direct heavy photocoagulation and possibly also with the use of dye yellow laser [53]. It must be stressed that because of the marked edema in the surrounding retina the selection of desirable energy is not always easy.

Other complications such as cellophane retinopathy [34] may be the consequence of too heavy coagulation and were observed after Xenon treatment.

References

1. Abdel-Khalek M N, and Richardson J (1988): Retinal macroaneurysm: natural history and guidelines for treatment. *Br J Ophthalmol*, 70: 2–11.
2. Amalric P, Dauban F, Courtois M, and Broqua J P (1979): Signes cliniques et angiographiques des macroanévrysmes artériels rétiniens. *Bull Soc Ophtalmol Fr*, 79: 109–111.
3. Asdourian G K, Goldberg M F, Jampol L, and Rabb M (1977): Retinal macroaneurysms. *Arch Ophthalmol*, 95: 624–628.
4. Attali P, Sterkers M, and Coscas G (1984): Les macroanévrysmes artériels rétiniens. *J Fr Ophtalmol*, 7: 697–710.
5. Augsburger J J, and Henry R Y (1978): Retinal aneurysms in adult cytomegalovirus retinitis. *Am J Ophthalmol*, 86: 794–797.
6. Avins L R, and Krummenacher T K (1983): Valsalva maculopathy due to a retinal macroaneurysm. *Ann Ophthalmol*, 15: 421–423.
7. Awan K J (1977): Arterial vascular anomalies of the retina. *Arch Ophthalmol*, 95: 1197–1202.
8. Ballantyne A J (1937): The evolution of retinal vascular disease. *Trans Ophthalmol Soc UK*, 57: 301–341.
9. Bleckmann H (1983): Pulsierendes Makroaneurysma einer retinalen Arterie. *Klin Mbl Augenheilk*, 182: 91–93.
10. Brown G C, and Weinstock F (1985): Arterial macroaneurysm on the optic disc presenting as a mass lesion. *Ann Ophthalmol*, 17: 519–520.

11. Cleary P E (1977): Retinal macroaneurysms: a specific cause of retinal haemorrhage, pp. 159–160, in J. François (ed.), *Fifth Congress of the European Society of Ophthalmology, Hamburg 1976*. F. Enke Verlag: Stuttgart.

12. Cleary P E, Kohner E M, Hamilton A M, and Bird A C (1975): Retinal macroaneurysms. *Br J Ophthalmol*, 59: 335–361.

13. Cole F M, and Yates P D (1967): The occurrence and significance of intracerebral microaneurysms. *J Pathol Bacteriol*, 93: 393–411.

14. Constantinides G, and Hochart G (1981): Macroanévrysme artériel rétinien. *Bull Soc Ophtalmol Fr*, 81: 579–581.

15. Dewachter A, and De Laey J J (1982): Acquired retinal macroaneurysms. *Bull Soc Belge Ophtalmol*, 201: 105–111.

16. Fernandez F M (1920): Multiple aneurisms of the retinal arteries. *Am J Ophthalmol*, 3: 641–643.

17. Fichte C, Streeten B W, and Friedman A H (1978): A histopathologic study of retinal macroaneurysms. *Am J Ophthalmol*, 85: 509–518.

18. Francois J (1979): Acquired macroaneurysms of the retinal arteries. *Int Ophthalmol*, 1: 153–161.

19. Gass J D M (1987): Stereoscopic atlas of macular diseases. Diagnosis and treatment. Third Edition, the C V Mosby C°, St Louis, 362–369.

20. Giuffre G, Montalto F F, and Amodei G (1987): Development of an isolated retinal macroaneurysm of the cilioretinal artery. *Br J Ophthalmol*, 71: 445–448.

21. Godel V, Blumenthal L, and Regenbogen L (1977): Arterial macroaneurysm of the retina. *Ophthalmologica*, 175: 125–129.

22. Gold D H, La Piana F G, and Zimmerman L E (1976): Isolated retinal arterial aneurysms. *Am J Ophthalmol*, 82: 848–857.

23. Gold D H, and Walsh J B (1976): Fluresccein angiographic patterns of retinal arterial aneurysms. *Doc Ophthalmol Proc Series*, 9: 541–548.

24. Henkind P (1976): in discussion Gold D H, and Walsh J B Fluorescein angiographic patterns of retinal arterial aneurysms. *Doc Ophthalmol Proc Series*, 9: 547–548.

25. Henkind P, and Walsh J B (1980): Retinal vascular anomalies. Pathogenesis, appearance and history. *Trans Ophthalmol Soc UK*, 100: 425–433.

26. Holland P M (1984): Evolution of a retinal arterial macroaneurysm. *Ann Ophthalmol*, 16: 1167–1170.

27. Hudomel J, and Imre G (1973): Photocoagulation treatment of solitary aneurysm near the macula lutea. Report of a case. *Acta Ophthalmol (Kbh)*, 51: 633–638.

28. Jennings J E (1918): Aneurysms of the retinal arteries. *Am J Ophthalmol*, 1: 12–13.

29. Joffe L, Annesley W H, Shields J A, and Federman J L (1978): Varix of the optic disc. *Am J Ophthalmol*, 86: 520.

30. Kayazawa F (1980): Bilateral retinal arterial macroaneurysms. *Ann Ophthalmol*, 12: 1218–1222.

31. Khalil M, and Lorenzetti D W C (1979): Acquired retinal macroaneurysms. *Can J Ophthalmol*, 14: 163–168.

32. Lavin M J, Marsh R J, Peart S, and Rehman A (1987): Retinal arterial macroaneurysms : a retrospective study of 40 patients. *Br J Ophthalmol*, 71: 817–825.

33. Leishman R (1957): The eye in general vascular disease. Hypertension and arteriosclerosis. *Br J Ophthalmol*, 41: 641–701.

34. Lewis R A, Norton E W D, and Gass J D M (1976): Acquired arterial macroaneurysms of the retina. *Br J Ophthalmol*, 60: 21–30.

35. Loring F B (1881): Peculiar anatomical development of one of the central arteries of the retina. *Trans Am Ophthalmol Soc*, 3: 40–42.

36. McDonald P R, and Sarin L K (1970): The treatment of intraretinal angiomas. *Trans Am Ophthalmol Soc*, 68: 129.

37. Magargal L E, Augsburger J J, Hyman D, and Townsend R (1980): Venous macroaneurysm following branch retinal vein obstruction. *Ann Ophthalmol*, 12: 685–688.

38. Mainster W A, and Whitacre M M (1988): Dye yellow photocoagulation of retinal arterial macroaneurysms. *Am J Ophthalmol*, 105: 97–98.
39. Makabe R (1981): Netzhautblutung bei Makroaneurysma der Netzhautarterien. *Klin Mbl Augenheilk*, 178: 471–472.
40. Makabe R (1984): Argon laser coagulation of retinal arterial macroaneurysms *Doc Ophthalmol Proc Series*, 36: 115–121.
41. Nadel A J, and Gupta K K (1976): Macroaneurysms of the retinal arteries. *Arch Ophthalmol*, 94: 1092–1096.
42. Norton E W D (1974): Arteriolar aneurysms in the adult. An acquired defect. in K Shimizu ED., Fluorescein Angiography, Igaku Shoin, Tokyo, 131–133.
43. Orsoni-Dupont C (1984): Traitement au laser à l'Argon d'un cas de dégénérescence maculaire hémorragique et exsudative par macroanévrysme rétinien. *Bull Soc Ophtalmol Fr*, 84: 85–86.
44. Palestine A G, Robertson D M, and Goldstein B G (1982): Macroaneurysms of the retinal arteries. *Am J Ophthalmol*, 93: 164–171.
45. Perry H D, Zimmerman L E, and Benson W E (1977): Hemorrhage from isolated aneurysm of a retinal artery: report of two cases simulating malignant melanoma. *Arch Ophthalmol*, 95: 281–283.
46. Pringle J A (1917): A case of multiple aneurysms of the retinal arteries. *Br J Ophthalmol*, 1: 87–92.
47. Rabb M F, Gagliamo D A, and Teske M P (1988): Retinal arterial macroaneurysms. *Survey Ophthalmol*, 33: 73–96.
48. Raehlman E (1889): Ueber ein pulsierendes Dehnungsaneurysma der Arteria Centralis Retinae. *Klin Mbl Augenheilk* 27: 203–214
49. Raehlman E (1902): Ueber die ophthalmoscopische Diagnose sklerotischer Erkrankungen der Netzhautgefässe. *Ztschr Augenheilk*, 7: 425–451.
50. Reimar M (1899): Ueber Retinitis haemorrhagica infolge von Endarteritis proliferans mit mikroskopischer Untersuchung eines Falles. *Arch Augenheilk*, 38: 209–256.
51. Robertson D M (1973): Macroaneurysms of the retinal arteries. *Tr. Am Acad Ophtalmol Otolaryngol*, 77: 55–67.
52. Russell R W R (1963): Observations on intracerebral aneurysms. *Brain*, 86: 425–442.
53. Russell S R, and Folk J C (1987): Branch retinal artery occlusion after dye yellow photocoagulation of an arterial macroaneurysm. *Am J Ophthalmol*, 104: 186–187.
54. Sanborn G E, and Magargal L E (1984): Venous macroaneurysm associated with branch retinal vein obstruction. *Ann Ophthalmol*, 16: 464–468.
55. Schatz H, Yannuzzi L A, Gitter K A, and Irvine A R (1980): Retinal arterial macroaneurysms. A large collaborative study: clinical findings and natural history. Presented at the American Academy of Ophthalmology Annual Meeting, Chicago.
56. Schulman J, Jampol L M, and Goldberg M F (1981): Large capillary aneurysms secondary to retinal venous obstruction. *Br J Ophthalmol*, 65: 36–41.
57. Shults W T, and Swan K C (1974): Pulsatile aneurysms of the retinal arterial tree. *Am J Ophthalmol*, 77: 304–309.
58. Spencer W H (1985): Ophthalmic pathology. An atlas and textbook. Third Edition, ed. W B Saunders C°, vol. 2, 707–710.
59. Van Nouhuys E, and Deutman A F (1980): Argon laser treatment of retinal macroaneurysms. *Int Ophthalmol*, 2: 45–53.
60. Witmer R (1978): Retinitis circinata. Leitsymptom aneurysmatischer Erkrankungen der Netzhautgefässe. in J François Ed., 5. *Kongress der Europäischen Gesellschaft für Ophthalmologie*, Hamburg, 1976, Ed. F Enle, Stuttgart, 124–127.

Monographs in Ophthalmology

1. P.C. Maudgal and L. Missotten (eds.): *Superficial Keratitis.* 1981
   ISBN 90-6193-801-5
2. P.F.J. Hoyng: *Pharmacological Denervation and Glaucoma.* A Clinical Trial Report with Guanethidine and Adrenaline in One Eyedrop. 1981
   ISBN 90-6193-802-3
3. N.W.H.M. Dekkers: *The Cornea in Measles.* 1981   ISBN 90-6193-803-1
4. P. Leonard and J. Rommel: *Lens Implantation.* 30 Years of Progress. 1982
   ISBN 90-6193-804-X
5. C.E. van Nouhuys: *Dominant Exudative Vitreoretinopathy and Other Vascular Developmental Disorders of the Peripheral Retina.* 1982 ISBN 90-6193-805-8
6. L. Evens (ed.): *Convergent Strabismus.* 1982   ISBN 90-6193-806-6
7. A. Neetens, A. Lowenthal and J.J. Martin (eds.): *The Visual System in Myelin Disorders.* 1984   ISBN 90-6193-807-4
8. H.J.M. Völker-Dieben: *The Effect of Immunological and Non-Immunological Factors on Corneal Graft Survival.* A Single Centre Study. 1984
   ISBN 90-6193-808-2
9. J.A. Oosterhuis (ed.): *Ophthalmic Tumours.* 1985   ISBN 90-6193-528-8
10. O. van Nieuwenhuizen: *Cerebral Visual Disturbance in Infantile Encephalopathy.* 1987   ISBN 0-89838-860-0
11. E.A.C.M. Sanders, R.J.W. de Keizer and D.S. Zee (eds.): *Eye Movement Disorders.* 1987   ISBN 0-89838-874-0
12. R. Živojnović: *Silicone Oil in Vitreoretinal Surgery.* 1987
    ISBN 0-89838-879-1
13. A. Brini, P. Dhermy and J. Sahel: *Oncology of the Eye and Adnexa.* Atlas of Clinical Pathology / *Oncologie de l'Œil et des Annexes.* Atlas Anatomo-Clinique / *Onkologische Diagnostik in der Ophthalmologie.* Vergleichender Klinisch-Pathologischer Atlas. 1990   ISBN 0-7923-0409-8
14. J.J. De Laey and M. Hanssens: *Vascular Tumors and Malformations of the Ocular Fundus.* 1990   ISBN 0-7923-0750-X

KLUWER ACADEMIC PUBLISHERS – DORDRECHT / BOSTON / LONDON